MW00469008

From the publishers of the *Tarascon Pocket Pharmacopoeia*®

Edited by

Amit Chandra, MD, MSc

Attending Physician
New York Hospital Queens
Department of Emergency Medicine
Flushing, NY

Matthew Dacso, MD, MSc

Adjunct Assistant Professor of Medicine
University of Pennsylvania School of Medicine
Botswana-UPenn Partnership
Gaborone, Botswana

JONES AND BARTLETT PUBLISHERS
Sudbury, Massachusetts
BOSTON   TORONTO   LONDON   SINGAPORE

World Headquarters
Jones and Bartlett
Publishers
40 Tall Pine Drive
Sudbury, MA 01776
978-443-5000
info@jbpub.com
www.jbpub.com

Jones and Bartlett
Publishers Canada
6339 Ormindale Way
Mississauga, Ontario L5V 1J2
Canada

Jones and Bartlett
Publishers International
Barb House, Barb Mews
London W6 7PA
United Kingdom

Jones and Bartlett's books and products are available through most bookstores and online booksellers. To contact Jones and Bartlett Publishers directly, call 800-832-0034, fax 978-443-8000, or visit our website, www.jbpub.com.

Substantial discounts on bulk quantities of Jones and Bartlett's publications are available to corporations, professional associations, and other qualified organizations. For details and specific discount information, contact the special sales department at Jones and Bartlett via the above contact information or send an email to specialsales@jbpub.com.

Production Credits
Senior Acquisition Editor: Nancy Anastasia
Duffy
Production Assistant: Sara Cameron
Production Director: Amy Rose
Production Editor: Daniel Stone
VP Manufacturing and Inventory
Control: Therese Connell

Composition: Newgen Imaging Systems Pvt
Ltd, India
Cover Design: Kristin E. Parker
Cover Credit: © Michael Halbert

Library of Congress Cataloging-in-Publication Data

Chandra, Amit.
  Tarascon Global Health Pocketbook / Amit Chandra, Matthew Dacso.
    p. ; cm.
  Other title: Pocket guide to global health
  Includes bibliographical references and index.
  ISBN 978-0-7637-7889-7 (alk. paper)
  1. World health—Handbooks, manuals, etc. I. Dacso, Matthew. II. Title.
III. Title: Pocket guide to global health.
  [DNLM: 1. World Health—Handbooks. 2. Disease—Handbooks.
  3. Public Health—Handbooks. WA 39 C456t 2011]
  RA441.C45 2011
  362.1—dc22

2010012069

6048

Printed in the United States of America
14 13 12 11 10   10 9 8 7 6 5 4 3 2 1

Dedication

To our families: Subash, Sarla, Priya, Mridu, Cliff, Sheri, Mara, and Rebecca

Acknowledgments

The authors would like to acknowledge the contributions made by the following individuals: Mrs. Sheryl Dacso, Dr. Kaushal Shah, Ms. Rashi Khilnani, Ms. Shirin Pakfar, Dr. Jennifer Stratton, Dr. Heidi Ladner, Ms. Anna Breznan, Dr. Sandy Saintonge, Dr. Nassim Assefi, Dr. Dalibor Blazek, Dr. Charles Carpenter, Ms. Hiba Abu Swaid, Ms. Maha Jaafar, Ms. Cassie Jones, and Dr. Mary Kestler.

The authors are interested in receiving your feedback regarding the publication of this book. You can reach them at: pocketglobalhealth@gmail.com. They welcome recommendations, critiques, and/or requests for any possible future editions.

Tarascon Global Health Pocketbook

Table of Contents

List of Contributors

Jonathan Bertram, MD
Department of Family Medicine
University of Western Ontario
Schulich School of Medicine
London, Ontario, Canada

Priya Blazkova-Chandra, MHSA
Brno, Czech Republic

Gar Ming Chan, MD
Consultant, New York Poison Control Center
Assistant Professor of Emergency Medicine
New York University School of Medicine
New York, NY

Amit Chandra, MD, MSc
Attending Physician
New York Hospital Queens
Department of Emergency Medicine
Flushing, NY

Matthew Dacso, MD, MSc
Adjunct Assistant Professor of Medicine
Botswana-UPenn Partnership
Gaborone, Botswana

Clifford C. Dacso, MD, MPH, MBA
Chairman of General Internal Medicine
The Methodist Hospital
Professor of Clinical Medicine
Weill Cornell Medical College
Houston, TX

Fadi El-Jardali, MPH, PhD
Assistant Professor
Faculty of Health Science
American University of Beirut
Beirut, Lebanon

Cheri Finalle, MD
Chief Resident
Emergency Medicine
New York Hospital Queens
Flushing, NY

Rodney Finalle, MD
Attending Physician
The Children's Hospital of Philadelphia
Philadelphia, PA

Jacqueline Firth, MD, MPH
Department of Medicine/Pediatrics
Warren Alpert School of Medicine at Brown University
Providence, RI

Stephen Gluckman, MD
Professor of Medicine
University of Pennsylvania School of Medicine
Philadelphia, PA

Amit K. Gupta, MD
Medical Toxicology Fellow
North Shore University Hospital
Manhasset, NY

Sanjey Gupta, MD
Clinical Assistant Professor of Emergency Medicine
Weill Cornell Medical College
New York, NY

Daniel Irving, MD
Chief Resident, Emergency Medicine
New York Hospital Queens
Flushing, NY

Diana Jamal, MPH
Senior Research Assistant
Faculty of Health Science,
American University of Beirut
Beirut, Lebanon

Nasreen Jessani, MSPH
International Development Research Center—Canada (based in Kenya)
Nairobi, Kenya

Andrew Kestler, MD
Head of Emergency Medicine
University of Botswana School of Medicine
Gaborone, Botswana

Umakant Kori, MD
Chief Resident, Department of Family Medicine
The Cleveland Clinic/Fairview Hospital
Cleveland, OH

Mitchell Levy, MD
Professor of Medicine
Brown Medical School
Providence, RI

Premal Patel, MD, MSc
Internal Medicine Specialist
Baylor International Pediatric AIDS Corps
Gaborone, Botswana

Dmitriy Pereyaslov, MD, MPH
Technical Officer Virologist
WHO Regional Office for Europe (Copenhagen)
Copenhagen, Denmark

Craig Spencer, MD
New York Hospital Queens
Flushing, NY

Catherine Todd, MD, MPH
Department of OB/GYN
Columbia University
New York, NY

Nand Wadhwani
The Rehydration
Hong Kong, China

Joseph Walline, MD
Instructor
Department of Surgery (Division of Emergency Medicine)
Saint Louis University School of Medicine
Saint Louis, MO

Samuel Yingst, DVM, PhD
US Army Medical Research Institute for Infectious Diseases
Fort Detrick, MD

Nicola Zetola, MD, MPH
Assistant Professor
Division of Infectious Diseases
University of Pennsylvania (based at Princess Marina Hospital)
Gaborone, Botswana

Abbreviations

ABG	Arterial Blood Gas
ACLS	Advanced Cardiac Life Support
AFB	Acid Fast Bacilli
AIDS	Acute Immunodeficiency Syndrome
AMS	Acute Mountain Sickness
APP	Acute Pesticide Poisoning
ART	Antiretroviral Therapy
ARV	Antiretroviral
ATT	Antituberculosis Treatment
BCG	Bacille Calmette-Guerin Vaccine
BMI	Body Mass Index
BRV	Bovine-Human Reassortant Vaccine
CAM	Complementary and Alternative Medicine
CBC	Complete Blood Count
CBF	Cerebral Blood Flow
CDC	United States Centers for Disease Control and Prevention
CHF	Congestive Heart Failure
CIDA	Canadian International Development Agency
CNS	Central Nervous System
COPD	Chronic Obstructive Pulmonary Disease
CPK	Creatine Phosphokinase
CPR	Cardiopulmonary Resuscitation
CSF	Cerebral Spinal Fluid
DHF	Dengue Hemorrhagic Fever
DOTS	Directly Observed Treatment Short-Course
DPT	Diphtheria/Pertussis/Tetanus
EKG	Electrocardiogram
ELISA	Enzyme-Linked Immunosorbent Assay
EPI	Expanded Program on Immunization
FAO	Food and Agriculture Organization
GAVI	The Global Alliance for Vaccines and Immunizations
GHI	Global Hunger Index
HAART	Highly Active Antiretroviral Treatment

HACE	High Altitude Cerebral Edema
HAH	High Altitude Headache
HAPE	High Altitude Pulmonary Edema
HBV	Hepatitis B Virus
Hib	Hemophilus Influenza Virus Type B
HIV	Human Immunodeficiency Virus
ICP	Intracranial Pressure
IDP	Internally Displaced Person
IPT	Isoniazid Preventative Therapy
IRIS	Immune Reconstitution Inflammatory Syndrome
KS	Kaposi's Sarcoma
LDC	Less Developed Country
LTBI	Latent Tuberculosis Infection
MDG	Millenium Development Goal
MDR TB	Multidrug Resistant Tuberculosis
MMR	Measles Mumps Rubella
MR	Measles Rubella
MSM	Men having Sex with Men
MTCT	Mother to Child Transmission
NGO	Nongovernmental Organization
NSAID	Nonsteroidal Anti-Inflammatory Drug
OI	Opportunisistic Infection
OPV	Oral Polio Vaccine
ORS	Oral Rehydration Salts
ORT	Oral Rehydration Therapy
PAHO	Pan American Health Organization
PATH	Program for Appropriate Technology in Health
PCR	Polymerase Chain Reaction
PEP	Post-Exposure Prophylaxis
PEPFAR	United States President's Emergency Plan for AIDS Relief
PPD	Purified Protein Derivative
PTB	Pulmonary Tuberculosis
SARS	Severe Acute Respiratory Syndrome
TB	Tuberculosis
TCM	Traditional Chinese Medicine
UN	The United Nations

UNDP	The United Nations Development Program
UNICEF	The United Nations Childrens Fund
USAID	United States Agency for International Development
WFP	World Food Program
WHO	The World Health Organization
XDR TB	Extensively Drug Resistant Tuberculosis

I ■ INTRODUCTION

Matthew Dacso, MD, MSc

Amit Chandra, MD, MSc

The world of medicine as we know it is changing rapidly. Across the globe, population demographics, affected by unprecedented emigration and immigration, are in a state of constant flux. With these shifts has come a transformation in the dynamics of public health. Whether the motivation is for education, research, or advocacy, healthcare professionals seek experience in this new international setting. Recent data suggests that over 25% of medical trainees participate in some type of international activity, as compared with only 6% in 1984.[1] This number can be expected to increase as borders become blurred, nations become increasingly interdependent, and a new discipline of research and practice—global health—emerges.

WHAT IS GLOBAL HEALTH?

In the early 1900s, the United States was at a unique point in history. Along with Teddy Roosevelt's concept of a Square Deal for every American came the promise of expansion of manufacturing and trade across national borders. The country was in the midst of an industrial revolution producing such innovations as the airplane and the automobile.

At this time, Latin America promised a wealth of raw materials and a potential market for manufactured goods. Transborder issues however, pertaining to quarantine and inspection, became difficult obstacles to freedom of trade. With the goal of standardizing these procedures, the first formal international public health alliance was founded in 1902 with the creation of the International Sanitary Bureau of the American Republics.

The end of World War II brought a new set of challenges, leaving most of Western Europe in ruins. The United States, to aid its Allied powers, created the Marshall Plan—a model for the reconstruction of Western Europe that relied on a spirit of international cooperation and transnational support. Out of this effort the United Nations (UN) was born.

In 1948, several European organizations met in Geneva, Switzerland alongside the Sanitary Bureau of the American Republics and together conceived the World Health Organization (WHO), a body to be operated under the auspices of the UN that would focus on the health of nations. It is against this backdrop that the concept of *global health* has emerged. It has evolved into an idea and philosophy that the health of individuals and populations is a concern to us all.

Globalization is a term that refers to the process of international interconnectivity. Over the past two decades, there has been an exponential increase in the capacity to form relationships across borders. The creation of the Internet and the increasing ease of transnational travel have amplified this phenomenon on a scale unprecedented in human history.

The globalization of health is not a new phenomenon. The colonization of the Americas brought with it epidemics of smallpox, measles, and diphtheria. Global health as an area of research and discourse, however, is a relatively novel idea.

Much of the discussion surrounding global health has traditionally focused on communicable diseases such as tuberculosis, malaria, and HIV/AIDS. Over the past several years however, newer data have led to an increased international focus on the prevalence and incidence of so-called *chronic diseases*—heart disease, kidney disease, stroke, cancer, and most recently, obesity.

There are no standard guidelines or definitions for what we now call global health. It is a term that means different things to different people. It is a discipline that finds itself at the intersection of a messy amalgam of social sciences (e.g., anthropology, political science, economics, public health) and medicine. How we study global health is one thing—how we practice it is another.

If you bought this book, then you are likely traveling to another country to do medical work. You may be going to a hospital or a clinic. You may be located in a big city or in a small village. You may be treating individual patients or working on a public health initiative. Similar to "doing development," "doing global health" implies doing some*thing* to some*one*. It is imperative to keep in mind a respect for community and individual autonomy in your travels. Consider the historical, cultural, and economic context that surrounds your work, and think about how your work will continue when you leave. It is our hope that with the ideas raised in this book, you will not be able to hear or see the words *global health* without a questioning ear and eye.

INTERNATIONAL MEDICAL VOLUNTEERS

The increase in international activity by physicians, nurses, and other medical professionals has not been accompanied by a significant change in their didactic curricula to include formal training in health economics, international development, or public health. Nevertheless, international medical volunteerism has continued to develop on a variety of fronts.

Many students of the health professions begin their training with an interest in global health and many of them have prior experience traveling abroad. For some, their exposure to global health issues inspired them to pursue a career in health care. Their international experiences can be planned by organizations specialized in providing housing, language training, and clinical exposure in exchange for widely ranging fees. Some academic medical institutions participate in ongoing programs overseas, and students are invited to participate. Others choose to contact specific practicing physicians or training programs in an attempt to coordinate their own experiences.

After medical school, resident physicians often have less time to participate in global health electives. Nevertheless, some residency programs encourage international travel. Academic hospitals with their own international partnerships and clinical activities usually draw upon their pool of residents to staff these programs.

For residency-trained physicians, certified nurses, and public health specialists, a variety of short- and long-term volunteer opportunities exist. Religious and secular organizations often plan short-term ventures involving their participants in an overseas project that might include staffing an existing clinic, establishing a temporary clinic, or joining local counterparts to provide disaster relief. Other opportunities are available to staff the long-term program commitments of large international relief organizations like *Médecines sans Frontières* (Doctors Without Borders), *Médecines du Monde* (Doctors of the World), the International Rescue Committee (IRC), and the International Committee of the Red Cross (ICRC).

A select few medical professionals turn their experiences with international medical volunteerism into careers in global health and development. Their employers include governmental aid agencies (e.g., United States Agency for International Development [USAID] and the Canadian International Development Agency [CIDA]), the UN, the World Bank, and a myriad of nongovernmental organizations (NGOs). Their positions may involve clinical responsibilities, program coordination, research, or organizational management.

WHAT IS DEVELOPMENT?

At the core of their mission statements, international medical participants and agencies aim to improve the health of their target populations. Their activities may be in response to a recent natural disaster or an ongoing conflict, or they may target public health indicators to reduce the regional burden of disease. In either case, they are agents of development. *Development* is a concept that has, until recent years, been bound to economic measures such as the gross domestic product (GDP) and income. Since 1990, it has been expanded to include a larger spectrum of human existence with the creation of the human development index. Inspired by the work of Nobel Prize winning economist Amartya Sen, this index formally matches economic indicators with advancements in education and health. When discussing development activities under this new regime, themes of sustainability, participation, and evaluation are placed on equal footing with income growth.

All global health activities must be evaluated regularly to ensure that they are effectively and efficiently achieving their stated goals. Well-designed projects often create parallel evaluation programs to provide ongoing feedback and quality improvement. Beyond measuring the immediate impact of a clinic or vaccination program, a program must be assessed for its sustainability, i.e., how will a development project's beneficial outcomes continue when the external resources and agents leave?

The theories of Paulo Freire, a 20th century Brazilian philosopher, have been used to link sustainability with the ideas of participation and empowerment. International agencies should involve local physicians, village leaders, and community activists in the planning and execution of local development projects. They can be empowered with training, resources, and organizational support to determine their own specific goals. Out of their "critical consciousness," local NGOs and communal activities will continue long beyond the tenure of international partners.

TRADITIONAL MEDICINE

Failure to address traditional medical practices would mean ignorance of a vital form of primary health care. In many parts of the world, traditional, or complementary and alternative medicine (CAM), serves as a supplement to (and often a replacement of) "western" medicine. The WHO estimates that up to 80% of the population of Africa relies on traditional medicine for its health needs.[2] Across East Asia, Central and Latin America, South Asia, and the Middle East traditional forms of healing are often the first-line options for treatment.

There are many reasons that individuals turn to traditional medicine for their healthcare needs:

Availability: Many traditional forms of medicine are grown, produced, and performed locally. Prescribed pharmaceuticals are not available free of charge in most countries in the world, so antibiotics, antiretrovirals, and medications for diabetes, hypertension, and heart disease are often more expensive than local alternatives.

Familiarity: In many communities, healing is a mind/body/spirit process that incorporates local rites, mores, and customs. Spiritual leaders and traditional healers are revered and trusted members of the community. Traditional medicine also has time on its side—most local healers practice techniques that pre-date western biomedical science.

Distrust: In some communities, the western biomedical model of practice is seen as more effective or more prestigious. Others however, regard it with suspicion and see it as intrusive, foreign, and unwelcome.

Traditional medicine is a valuable part of the international healthcare system. Many forms of traditional medicine such as analgesics, massage, and heat therapy can provide excellent adjuncts to care. Some traditional therapies however, can have severe side effects and are not well understood. The pharmacologic mechanisms of naturopathic remedies are poorly defined and their efficacy is not well studied.

When working or living abroad, healthcare practitioners should familiarize themselves with local forms of traditional medicine in a nonjudgmental and inquisitive manner—they may learn how to integrate local healing techniques into their practice.

PRACTICING MEDICINE IN RESOURCE-LIMITED SETTINGS

If you are reading this book in English then it is likely that you came from the United States, Western Europe, or Canada. In these countries, physicians utilize a variety of diagnostic tests, each with its own sensitivity and specificity, to rule in or rule out disease. When seeing patients in resource-limited settings, lab facilities, CT scans, MRIs, and invasive or noninvasive diagnostic technologies (endoscopy, echocardiography, etc.) are often unavailable. If they are available, patients may have to pay for each test ordered. In these instances, it is important to utilize a combination of clinical suspicion, history, and physical exam maneuvers to optimize the diagnosis and management of illness in a manner that is fair to the patient. We recommend using Bayesian reasoning as a clinical decision tool. Simply put, Bayes' Theorem is a mathematical algorithm that explains how clinical suspicion, a proxy for pretest probability, changes based on evidence and circumstance.

Table 1-1 Example: Patient A has a cough and fever

New information	Lives in France	Lives in Kenya
Probability of TB	Low	High
Probability of viral URI	High	Low

In this example, the pretest probability of the patient having TB changed based on the information provided—the calculation of that probability relies on knowledge of regional prevalence data.

Another useful concept in resource-limited settings is that of *satisficing*. Satisficing refers to the idea that an adequate solution to a problem is sometimes preferable to an optimal one. It posits that human beings are not designed to maximize outcomes, rather that there is a paradox of choice in which psychological satisfaction is inversely related to the number of choices in a decision process.[3] In medicine, the concept of satisficing can be used to simplify diagnostic and therapeutic decisions to ensure adequate quality care is delivered to the greatest number of people. Ultimately, the use of Bayes' Theory and satisficing in concert can enhance clinical suspicion and guide empirical treatment decisions.

HOW TO USE THIS BOOK

This book was designed as a global health curriculum. It begins by reviewing major themes in international health including water safety, respiratory infections, and HIV/AIDS. The second section is comprised of region specific chapters, each describing country-specific endemic diseases, historical context, and available resources. All of our authors have extensive experience with their respective topics. We recommend reading the disease chapters in their entirety, then the regional overview pertaining to your prospective location, and finally the relevant country profile. Prior to traveling, review recent political events in the news pertaining to that country, any travel warnings (see the U.S. State Department Travel Web site), and current recommendations for travel vaccinations (see the CDC Traveler's Health Web site).

We hope our readers will ask themselves the following questions, and that this book will be a tool to find the answers.

- What are my roles and responsibilities?
- What do I hope to learn from this experience?
- What is the long-term impact of this program?
- How will our work be evaluated?
- What are other organizations doing in the region?
- Will I be involved in capacity building?
- Is this project sustainable?
- Is there an exchange of knowledge with local participants?

REFERENCES

1. Panosian C, Coates TJ. The New Medical "Missionaries"—Grooming the Next Generation of Global Health Workers. *N Engl J Med.* 2006;354(17): 1771–1773.
2. World Health Organization. *WHO Traditional Medicine Strategy 2002–2005.* Geneva, Switzerland: World Health Organization; 2002.
3. Schwartz B. *The Paradox of Choice—Why More is Less.* NY: Harper Perennial; 2004.

II ■ WATERBORNE ILLNESS: DIARRHEA, DEHYDRATION, AND WORMS

Amit Chandra, MD, MSc
Nand Wadhwani

INTRODUCTION

The World Health Organization (WHO) estimates that over 500 million children suffer from an episode of diarrhea every year. Every year, 2 million of these children die from the disease. Despite advancements in sanitation, hygiene, and treatment, it remains a leading cause of childhood mortality, particularly in developing countries. While some might consider diarrhea to be an inconvenient irritation, it can rapidly progress to life threatening dehydration.

Intestinal worms (helminth species) are spread through similar mechanisms and may or may not precipitate diarrhea. It is estimated that over 700 million people worldwide suffer from worm infections.

ETIOLOGY

Diarrhea is predominantly an infectious illness, though it can also occur as a medication side effect, a symptom of hormonal imbalance, intestinal malignancy, or inflammatory process. Infectious causes of diarrhea include viruses, bacteria, and parasites. The intestines are naturally populated with a variety of bacteria. Diarrhea can occur if a pathologic strain from the environment colonizes the system, or if one of these naturally occurring strains dominate (as seen with *Clostridium difficile* overgrowth after antibiotic use).

Infectious organisms are transmitted via the oral route by way of contaminated food or water. Infected individuals then spread these agents to other members of their households unless they adhere to strict principles of hygiene. If their sanitation system is inadequate, their fecal matter can spread the infectious agents back to their community's water supply.

Infectious diarrhea can be classified as either secretory, inflammatory, or dysentery. Secretory diarrhea occurs when either the secretion of liquid is induced or the reabsorption of fluids is inhibited. These processes occur as a result of infectious toxins acting on cells lining the intestinal wall. Inflammatory diarrhea occurs when infectious agents cause damage to the intestinal wall, resulting in a local reaction that impairs the absorption of fluid from the stool. Dysentery occurs when infectious agents invade the intestinal cell walls, causing severe diarrhea with mucous and blood.

7

Table 2-1 Common Viruses, Bacteria, and Parasites[1]

Pathogen	Comments	Fever	Abd Pain	Bloody Stool	N/V	Fecal WBC
Toxins (staph, B. cereus, C. perfringens)	Incubation < 6 to 24 hr.	–	+	–	++	–
Salmonella	Community acquired, food-borne	++	++	+	+	++
Campylobacter	Community acquired, undercooked poultry	++	++	+	+	++
Shigella	Community acquired, person-to-person	++	++	+	++	++
Shiga toxin-producing E. Coli (e.g., O157:H7)	Food-borne outbreaks, under-cooked beef; bloody stool w/o fever	–	++	++	–	–
C. difficile	Nosocomial, post-antibiotics; marked leukocytosis in 50%	+	+	+	–	++
Vibrio	Seafood	+/–	+/–	+/–	+/–	+/–
Yersinia	Community acquired, food-borne	++	++	+	+	+
E. histolytica	Tropical	+	+	++	+/–	+/–
Cryptosporidium	Waterborne outbreaks, travel, immune compromise; symptoms > 10 days	+/–	+/–	–	+	–
Cyclospora	Travel, food-borne; profound fatigue	+/–	+/–	–	+	–
Giardia	Waterborne, day care, IgA deficiency; symptoms > 10 days	–	++	–	+	–
Norovirus	Winter outbreaks; nursing homes, schools, cruise ships, shellfish	+/–	++	–	++	+/–

++ Common   + Occurs   +/– Variable   – Atypical or not characteristic

Worm infections are also spread through ingestion of contaminated food and water, although some species can also penetrate the skin to enter the bloodstream before colonizing the intestines. Pinworms (*Enterobius vermicularis*), cause severe anal itching. Hookworms (*Ancylostoma duodenale* and *Necator americanus*) feed off human blood and can cause occult gastrointestinal bleeding and anemia. Roundworms (*Ascaris lumbricoides*) are much larger than other infectious worms and can cause intestinal obstruction or migrate to other regions of the body and cause local effects. Trichinosis

(*Trichinella spiralis*) and tapeworms (*Taenia solium*) are transmitted via undercooked pork and beef, and colonize the GI tract. The guinea worm (*Dracunculus medinensis*) is transmitted through contaminated water, and can migrate from the GI tract to the skin where it slowly emerges from a painful blister. Schistosomiasis (*Schistosoma*) is found in freshwater reservoirs and enters human blood circulation through the skin, causing anemia, and intestinal and bladder pathology.

SIGNS AND SYMPTOMS

Diarrhea is often accompanied by nausea, vomiting, abdominal pain, and fever. Mucous or blood may be present in the diarrhea. Chronic diarrhea may lead to malnutrition caused by an inability to absorb nutrients. Severe diarrhea, especially when associated with nausea and vomiting, can lead to dehydration. Signs of dehydration include lethargy, fatigue, skin tenting, tachycardia (greater than 110 beats per minute in a 5 year old), decreased urine output, and hypotension leading to death.

Worm infections can present with anal itching, diarrhea, weakness from anemia, and a variety of skin and ocular complaints.

DIAGNOSIS

In general, laboratory serum and stool analysis is not required for routine cases of gastroenteritis and traveler's diarrhea. In patients presenting with

Table 2-2 Evaluating the Degree of Dehydration

Characteristic	Mild (< 5%)	Moderate (6–9%)	Severe (> 10%)
Heart rate	Normal	Mild increase	Marked increase
Mucous membranes	Normal	Dry	Very dry
Mental status	Alert	Irritable or listless	Lethargic or obtunded
Urine output	Normal	Diminished	Markedly decreased
Skin turgor	Normal	Decreased	Markedly decreased
Fontanelle	Normal	Slightly sunken	Sunken
Eyes	Normal	Sunken orbits	Deeply sunken orbits
Skin	Pink and warm	Capillary refill > 2 seconds	Cool and mottled

a fever, bloody stool, or dehydration, blood should be sent to the laboratory for a complete blood count and metabolic profile. A stool sample can be sent for a culture and screen and analysis for ova and parasites. A positive microscopic analysis for leukocytes or a positive assay for lactoferrin (a leukocyte marker) indicate a bacterial etiology. *C. difficile* toxin assay should be sent if the diarrhea is nosocomial or associated with recent antibiotic use. The stool should be tested for shiga toxin if bloody stools or hemolytic uremic syndrome is present (associated with E. coli O157:H7). If vibrio is suspected (e.g., following shellfish consumption), a special culture medium is required.

Table 2-3 Clinical Features of Diarrhea[2]

Viral Gastroenteritis	Nausea, vomiting, diarrhea, abdominal cramping, <6 stools per day, <7 days of symptoms
Bacterial Diarrhea	Recent Travel, fever, bloody diarrhea, >6 stools per day, >7 days of symptoms, severe pain, tenesmus, hemolytic uremic syndrome, +fecal leukocytes or fecal lactoferrin
Salmonella	Recent contact with amphibians, reptiles, and ducklings, or recent contaminated poultry product ingestion
Giardia	Contaminated streams and well water
Vibrio	Recent shellfish ingestion
C. difficile	Recent hospitalization or antibiotic use

Worm infections can be diagnosed via stool analysis, peripheral blood smear, or biopsy of affected organs. Eosinophilia may be present on a CBC differential.

TREATMENT

The most important initial treatment for diarrhea is rehydration. Oral rehydration solution (ORS) was invented in the 1960s and widely used after the 1971 Bangladesh war. ORS is comprised of a mix of sodium, sugar, and other electrolytes. When added to water, ORS improves the intestinal absorption of the fluid. ORS is commercially available and distributed by the WHO and UNICEF. Oral rehydration should continue until the diarrhea resolves. Caregivers and patients should be counseled that ORS does not cure diarrhea, but it does treat and prevent dehydration. If ORS is perceived as a cure, patients often discontinue it after a few days even when the diarrhea continues. Children unable to maintain hydration due to severe nausea and vomiting should be hospitalized for intravenous fluids.

Table 2-4 Rehydration Therapy

Mild	50 ml/kg ORS over 4 hours
Moderate	100 ml/kg ORS over 4 hours
Severe	20 ml/kg IV fluid bolus (normal saline), repeat until symptoms resolve, then continue IV fluids at 1.5 or 2 × maintenance (D5 ½ normal saline) until tolerating oral hydration

Anti-diarrhea medications are not recommended in children. Loperamide, which acts on opioid receptors of the large intestine, and bismuth subsalicylate can be utilized for simple cases of traveler's diarrhea in adults. A normal, age appropriate oral diet should be started as soon as it is tolerated and infants who are breastfeeding should continue to do so. The so-called BRAT diet (bananas, rice, applesauce, and toast) can provide additional supplementation, but it should not replace the foods a person normally consumes. Despite the benefits of the "continue feeding" model, it is difficult to achieve. Caregivers and patients often reduce or restrict dietary intake in an effort to slow down the diarrhea. Sometimes they replace an oral diet with an oral rehydration regimen, although they are most effective when administered together.

Malnutrition and micronutrient deficiency exacerbate the effects of diarrhea and increase the risk of death from the illness. Over recent years, the WHO and UNICEF have recommended zinc and vitamin A supplementation as an adjunct to ORS therapy. Zinc is an important micronutrient for the immune system and it becomes depleted during an episode of diarrhea. Chronic zinc deficiency can also be a predisposing factor in children with recurrent or severe symptoms (see Chapter 3). Studies have shown that a 10–14 day course of zinc can shorten the duration of the illness and may prevent the recurrence of diarrhea for several months.[3] Vitamin A supplementation has similarly shown reduced mortality associated with diarrhea (see Chapter 3).

Antibiotic therapy is recommended in certain cases of diarrhea, e.g., Shigella infections, traveler's diarrhea, and some cases of *Clostridium difficile* diarrhea.[4] The decision to start antibiotics should be guided by laboratory stool and serum analysis, although empirical treatment may be required for immunocompromised patients and those with severe systemic symptoms. In general, patients with bloody diarrhea, fever, and the presence of fecal leukocytes benefit from treatment with fluoroquinolones or trimethoprim-sulfamethoxazole. If a shiga toxin producing strain of E. coli is suspected (e.g., O157:H7), antibiotics should not be administered since they increase the incidence of hemolytic uremic syndrome.

Treatment for worm infections usually involves antihelminth agents. Pinworms are well treated with albendazole, mebendazole, piperazine, and pyrantel pamoate. Hookworms also respond to albendazole and mebendazole.

Table 2-5 Antibiotics of Choice for Common Pathogens[4]

Shigella	Flouroquinolones or trimethoprim-sulfamethoxazole
Salmonella	ABX can prolong the duration of sx, in severe case can treat with flouroquinolones, trimethoprim-sulfamethoxazole, or ceftriaxone
E. coli (enterotoxigenic, enteropathogenic, or enteroinvasive)	Flouroquinolones or trimethoprim-sulfamethoxazole
E. coli (shiga toxin producing)	Avoid ABX
Yersinia	In severe cases can treat with doxycycline + aminoglycoside, flouroquinolones, or trimethoprim-sulfamethoxazole
Vibrio cholerae	Doxycycline, tetracycline, flouroquinolones
C. Difficile	Metronidazole
Giardia	Metronidazole
Entamoeba histolytica (amebiasis)	Metronidazole + either iodoquinol or paromomycin

Note: azithromycin or erythromycin may be required for flouroquinolone resistant strains

Guinea worms must be removed from the skin slowly. Any guinea worm remnants left behind may cause severe local infections. Schistosomiasis is treated with praziquantel.

ORAL REHYDRATION THERAPY

The search for a therapy to replenish lost nutrients began centuries ago. Experiments were conducted with the ingredients of traditional treatments and these combinations were refined to optimize absorption. Research intensified around the 1950s when a formal combination of electrolytes and sugar was packaged as Oral Rehydration Salts (ORS).

The benefits of ORS were demonstrated at a cholera treatment facility in Pakistan in the late 1960s by Dr. ASM Mizanur Rahaman, Dr. Richard Cash, and Dr. David Nalin. Nurses treating different groups of patients found that the amount of fluid needed to rehydrate patients was reduced by 80% with ORS. This proved that ORS helps the body absorb fluids more efficiently. The clinical trials were then moved to Dhaka (then part of East Pakistan), due to its long history of endemic cholera.

In May 1971, the Liberation War between East and West Pakistan, which led to the creation of Bangladesh, displaced approximately 10 million people. They were housed in refugee camps in West Bengal, India. When the monsoon season arrived in June, a cholera epidemic spread throughout the camps. Before aid arrived at the camps almost one-third of the inhabitants died from cholera and other forms of diarrhea.

Given the large numbers of people with cholera it was impossible to supply enough intravenous fluid to treat dehydration. Researchers and aid workers previously involved with the ORS clinical trials decided to use ORS as the primary treatment approach for this epidemic. Dr. Dilip Mahalanabis set up two rehydration teams in Bongaon, India, near the Bangladesh-India border. From June 24 to August 30 they treated approximately 4000 people with cholera with ORS. By the peak of the epidemic more than 200 new patients were admitted for treatment each day. The overwhelmed staff could not keep up, and family members helped by feeding ORS to ailing relatives and friends.

Mahalanabis and his colleagues proved that ORS could be administered by people who had no previous healthcare training, and that the therapy was effective in large-scale emergencies.

HOW TO MAKE ORAL REHYDRATION SALTS

Ingredients:
- 1 level teaspoon of salt
- 8 level teaspoons of sugar
- 1 liter of clean drinking water or boiled water that has been cooled

Preparation Method: Stir the mixture until the salt and sugar dissolve.

PREVENTION

Diarrhea and death by dehydration can be prevented by implementing the following: latrines to prevent contamination of the local water supply, breast-feeding, universal immunization, keeping food and water clean, and thorough hand washing.

Safe drinking water is essential to good health. But in resource-poor settings, water often comes from unsafe sources and carries deadly pathogens. Of the nearly 2 million deaths from diarrhea each year, many are due to an unsafe water supply.

Breast milk is the ideal food for infants and is all they need for optimal growth and health during the first 6 months of life. Breastfeeding provides nourishment, helps develop the immune system, improves response to vaccines, and prevents many infections, including diarrhea-causing agents.

Because most acute diarrhea is related to intestinal infection that is transmitted by contaminated food or water, illness can be avoided with careful food and fluid intake and proper hygiene practices. Hand-washing campaigns alone can reduce the incidence of diarrhea by more than 40%. When the available water supply is questionable, water should be boiled and ice cubes from unsafe water should be avoided. Raw, unpeeled fruits and salads may have been washed in regular water, so they should be avoided as well. The safest food is hot and well cooked.

Research has recently focused on vaccines and protective bacteria as new prevention strategies. Immunization programs to prevent rotavirus, the leading cause of severe gastroenteritis, are increasing worldwide. There is some evidence that probiotics (such as lactobacilli and bifidobacteria) found in live yogurts, may reduce the chances of experiencing an episode of infectious diarrhea.

Worm infections are similarly prevented with proper food and water hygiene. Worm reservoirs can also be targeted to eradicate hosts necessary for their reproduction (e.g., snail control to prevent schistosomiasis)

VACCINES

The most common cause of severe diarrhea—accounting for 2 million hospitalizations and more than 500,000 deaths each year—is rotavirus. Rotavirus is highly contagious and resilient, and traditional diarrhea disease prevention measures are not enough to limit its impact.

Children in the world's poorest countries account for more than 90% of rotavirus deaths. In developing countries treatment can be hard to access and safe water is scarce, so diarrhea can be deadly.

Preventing diarrhea through immunization is a relatively new intervention, but is becoming an essential and lifesaving part of global diarrhea control strategies. Commercial vaccines are safe and effective, but they are not widely available or affordable for developing countries. In order to address this issue, organizations are working to distribute them and to accelerate the development of new formulations. New initiatives are currently underway to develop vaccines against bacteria that cause diarrhea, such as Shigella and *Escherichia coli.*

Two vaccines against rotavirus are currently in use in several countries in North and South America, Europe, and Australia. The Rotavirus Vaccine Trials Partnership between PATH, the GAVI Alliance, the WHO, and the CDC is conducting clinical trials in Africa and Asia to assess the safety and efficacy of both vaccines. Because the performance of oral vaccines like these can vary in different regions and populations, the WHO has requested these trials prior to recommending global use.

Seven developing country manufacturers and one U.S. company have licensed a candidate rotavirus vaccine, known as the bovine-human reassortant vaccine (BRV). PATH is directly supporting the development of the BRV by manufacturers in India and China, providing financial support and scientific assistance to conduct Phase 1 and 2 clinical trials.

CONCLUSION

In the 1980s and 1990s, UNICEF and the WHO led a global effort to reduce diarrhea deaths by promoting preventive measures—such as exclusive breastfeeding and improved access to clean water—and the use of ORS to counter dehydration. Despite their success, diarrhea continues to be a leading cause of death in developing countries.

Governments, the UN, and NGOs are working to refocus efforts on prevention and treatment with vaccines and new formulations of ORS that can improve on the gains made over previous decades.

Established interventions such as ORS, breastfeeding, and hygiene, plus new tools like vaccines and zinc treatment, bring new opportunities for diarrhea control. Improving water supply and sanitation, promoting safe hygiene practices, and giving urgent relief during outbreaks will also continue to reduce the impact of waterborne illnesses like infectious diarrhea and helminth infections.

FURTHER READING

Rehydration Project: http://www.rehydrate.org
The Centers for Disease Control and Prevention: http://www.cdc.gov/travel/diseases.htm#diarrhea
The World Health Organization: http://www.who.int/topics/diarrhoea/en/
Clinical Management of Acute Diarrhea: A Joint Statement by the WHO and UNICEF: http://www.who.int/child_adolescent_health/documents/who_fch_cah_04_7/en/index.html

REFERENCES

1. Adapted from Thielman, Nathan M and Guerrant, Richard L. Acute Infectious Diarrhea. The New England Journal of Medicine. 350: 38–47. 2004.
2. Esherick JS. *Tarascon Primary Care Pocketbook.* 3rd ed. Sudbury, MA: Jones and Bartlett Publishers; 2010:55–56.
3. Zinc Investigators Collaborative Group. Therapeutic Effects of Oral Zinc in Acute and Persistent Diarrhea in Children in Developing Countries: Pooled Analysis of Randomized Controlled Trials. *Am J Clin Nutr.* 2000;72:1516–1522.
4. Thielman NM, Guerrant RL. Acute Infectious Diarrhea. *N Engl J Med.* 2004;350:38–47.

III ■ MALNUTRITION

Amit Chandra, MD, MSc
Cheri Finalle, MD
Rodney Finalle, MD

INTRODUCTION

Malnutrition, the condition caused by inadequate intake of food and micronutrients, significantly impacts health around the world. Beyond mortality from starvation, it exacerbates the incidence and severity of infectious diseases, undermines education and economic programs, and perpetuates the cycle of underdevelopment.

Inadequate food supplies lead to hunger and starvation, as organ systems suffer from the lack of macronutrients: carbohydrates, protein, fat, and oils. When the variety and quality of available foods is insufficient to supply essential vitamins and minerals, micronutrient deficiency develops. Micronutrient deficiency weakens the immune system, inhibits intellectual development, and causes a variety of diseases like anemia and blindness. A lack of education and poor food choices are also major contributors to malnutrition.

Malnutrition and starvation are important aspects of global health for their severe and widespread effects. Malnutrition is an issue for all developing countries and high-risk groups in middle-income countries. An estimated 963 million people worldwide suffer from malnutrition, particularly in South Asia and sub-Saharan Africa.[1] Malnutrition is thought to be the major underlying cause of preventable child mortality around the globe. While often not cited as the cause of death, it contributes to illness severity and the body's ability to fight illness and recover from otherwise preventable diseases.

Despite advancements in agricultural science, micronutrient supplementation programs, and global food aid programs, malnutrition continues to be perpetuated and intensified by drought, famine, ineffective food distribution, patient and family education, military conflicts, and refugee crises.

MONITORING FOR MALNUTRITION

Anthropometry is the term used to describe the various methods used to measure the nutritional status of individuals. A common tool used for adults is the Body Mass Index (BMI), which equals the weight in Kg divided by the height in meters squared. A BMI of < 18.5 is considered underweight. In children, growth charts (mapping weight or height to age), and weight for height charts (mapping weight to height), are more commonly used. A low weight for a given height indicates acute malnutrition, and a stunted height

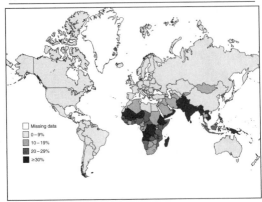

Figure 3-1 Underweight Children Under 5 in Developing Countries[2]

or low height for a given age indicates a more chronic malnutrition. Some organizations use mid-upper arm circumference, measured at the level of the mid-humerus, to determine nutritional status. An arm circumference > 16 cm is considered normal, and < 12 cm indicates severe malnourishment. This tool is most helpful during severe humanitarian crises for rapid screening of acute malnutrition.

To compare regional nutritional status, one can use the Global Hunger Index (GHI), created in 2006 by the International Food Policy Research Institute. The GHI ranks 88 countries based on an index using measures of undernourishment, the number of underweight children, and child mortality.

STARVATION: MARASMUS

According to the "rule of threes," human beings can survive three minutes without air, three days without water, and three weeks without food. Severe starvation manifests with weakness, an emaciated appearance, poor skin turgor, dehydration, infection, and ultimately death. This process of protein and energy malnutrition is known as *marasmus*.

PROTEIN MALNUTRITION: KWASHIORKOR

In contrast to marasmus, *kwashiorkor* results from a lack of protein and micro-nutrient deficiency rather than insufficient caloric intake. Symptoms include edema, skin disorders, and abdominal distention. Victims of kwashiorkor have a poorer prognosis than those of marasmus. Treatment protocols for these individuals must carefully balance carbohydrate, fat, and protein supplementation, as excessive protein refeeding can cause liver failure.

REFEEDING SYNDROME

Treating patients suffering from severe malnutrition, marasmus, and kwashiorkor requires a precise and scientific approach. Overly aggressive and unbalanced methods can cause severe electrolyte disorders (particularly phosphate, magnesium, and potassium), liver failure, altered mental status, seizures, and death.

The reintroduction of glucose after a prolonged period of starvation causes an exaggerated insulin response, which in turn causes severe shifts in intravestrus extracellular electrolytes. The physical presence of solid food in the intestines, which atrophy during starvation, causes severe irritation that manifests as poor absorption, nausea, and diarrhea.

Dietary intake should be increased in slow increments and supplemented with multivitamins, thiamine, and other micronutrients as needed. Treatment of severe malnutrition should be managed by following specific refeeding protocols in a hospital or nutrition rehabilitation center.

MICRONUTRIENT DEFICIENCY

Deficient intake of micronutrients causes a variety of diseases and worsens the symptoms of infectious pathogens. Micronutrient deficiency occurs when the volume or variety of food intake is insufficient.

Vitamin A: aka retinoic acid, Vitamin A deficiency causes xerophthalmia (an eye disorder leading to blindness); worsens the effects of measles, pneumonia, and malaria; increases maternal mortality; and slows bone development. Exam findings range from corneal xerosis (dry eye), conjunctival xerosis, night blindness, and bitot's spots to corneal ulcerations and corneal scars. Vitamin A is a fat-soluble vitamin found in meat, dairy, dark green vegetables, and certain fruits. Supplementation programs use oral tablets, fortified sugar and milk powder, or regular doses of vitamin A in areas with known prevalence of vitamin A deficiency.

Vitamin C: involved in collagen formation. Vitamin C deficiency causes scurvy and impairs wound healing. Vitamin C is a water-soluble vitamin found in many fruits and vegetables.

Vitamin D: involved in bone formation. Vitamin D deficiency causes osteomalacia and rickets. Rickets is a childhood disease classically described as "knocked knees" that causes impaired and abnormal growth of long bones. Osteomalacia is an adult disease that causes thin bones that are painful and fracture easily. There is also emerging evidence that Vitamin D plays an important role in immune response. Vitamin D is found in fish and eggs but can be obtained from sun exposure.

Folate: involved in blood formation. Folate deficiency causes megaloblastic anemia.

Iodine: a metabolic cofactor utilized in thyroid hormones. Iodine deficiency causes goiter, hypothyroidism, cretinism, and mental retardation. It is found in plants and seafood. Global health programs focus on utilizing table salt that has been supplemented with iodine.

Iron: an essential component of hemoglobin. Iron deficiency causes microcytic hypochromic anemia. Iron is found in red meat, fish, eggs, dairy products, chickpeas, black-eyed peas, leafy vegetables, and lentils. Supplementation programs use iron tablets, and iron containing multivitamins.

Niacin: a metabolic cofactor. Niacin deficiency causes pellagra, characterized by a rash, diarrhea, and neurologic symptoms.

Thiamine: a metabolic cofactor. Thiamine deficiency causes beriberi, a neurocardiac disease.

Zinc: is important for the immune system, eyesight, brain development, and wound healing. White spots on fingernails, aka leukonychia, are associated with insufficient dietary intake. Zinc deficiency increases the susceptibility to waterborne illness, worsens the effects and duration of diarrhea, and increases maternal complications of pregnancy. It is found in red meat, beans, nuts, and whole grains. Zinc tablet and fortification supplementation can reduce the incidence and mortality of gastroenteritis and pneumonia.

CONCLUSION

The solutions and treatment for malnutrition and starvation are well known in the modern context of international public health. Children should be breastfed as infants and fed with complementary foods (solid foods with high nutritional value) when they are weaned at the appropriate age. All children should eat a variety of foods rich in micronutrients. When this is not possible, micronutrient intervention programs can help by enriching or fortifying existing foods or providing oral supplements.

Hunger was recognized alongside poverty as the primary challenge of underdevelopment, as reflected by the first Millennium Development Goal declared by the United Nations Millennium Declaration in 2000. Access to food is regarded as a human right, essential to personal and community health. Numerous international organizations currently work to curtail malnutrition, including the United Nations Development Programme (UNDP), the United Nations Children Fund (UNICEF), the World Food Program (WFP), the World Health Organization (WHO), the United States Agency for International Development (USAID) and the Food and Agriculture Organization (FAO).

The ultimate responsibility for food security lies with both the global community and the nation-state. Nobel prize winning economist Amartya Sen, in his work on the subject, notes that famine is not simply a shortage of food, but also a breakdown in food distribution systems, social safety nets, and markets. He argues that many famines occur when food supplies were relatively stable, and the actual causes are economic and social trends coupled with state inaction or mismanagement.

REFERENCES

1. The Food and Agriculture Organization. *Number of Hungry People Rises to 963 Million.* Rome: The Food and Agriculture Organization; December, 2008.
2. Data from UNICEF, 2006 State of the World's Children Report. Table 2: Nutrition. Summary data from 1996 through 2004.

IV ■ RESPIRATORY DISEASES

Craig Spencer, MD

INTRODUCTION

In both developed and developing countries, the global burden of respiratory disease is vast and is the root of significant morbidity and mortality. From relatively benign viral infections to severely debilitating yet preventable and treatable chronic conditions, there exists a broad range of respiratory illnesses. When undiagnosed and undertreated, the consequences are staggering. According to the World Health Organization (WHO) World Health Report 2000, the top five respiratory diseases account for 17.4% of all deaths worldwide.[1]

The broad spectrum of disease entities and their causes complicate disease prevention and treatment. Among the top ten causes of death worldwide, four are primarily respiratory diseases, mainly lower respiratory tract infections, chronic obstructive pulmonary disease (COPD), tuberculosis (TB), and lung cancer. Even more worrisome is that as the burden of communicable diseases decreases, the prevalence of chronic respiratory disease will grow with the projected worldwide increase in tobacco use and life expectancy.

According to the latest WHO estimates (2007), 300 million people have asthma, 210 million people have COPD, while millions have allergic rhinitis and other often-underdiagnosed chronic respiratory diseases.[2] Numerous organizations are working to combat the rise in respiratory morbidity and mortality, and the WHO in combination with the Global Alliance against Chronic Respiratory Disease (GARD) has helped raise national and international awareness about the overwhelming burden of respiratory illness. Global pollution, increasing tobacco use in developing nations, and novel respiratory threats such as severe acute respiratory syndrome (SARS) and the recent H1N1 pandemic will make tackling global respiratory disease a challenging task.

ASTHMA

OVERVIEW

Asthma is defined as a chronic inflammatory pulmonary disease characterized by reversible airway obstruction to a variety of stimuli. It is manifested by a diffuse narrowing of respiratory passages with resultant coughing, wheezing, and dyspnea.

As an episodic disease, patients experience acute exacerbations interspersed with symptom-free intervals, spanning a continuum from mild to life-threatening. Asthma, although not curable, is treatable with a combination of avoidance of allergens and non-specific triggers, in addition to step-wise pharmacological management. These interventions, coupled with patient education, are often effective at achieving significant reductions in overall morbidity.

Unfortunately, asthma is both underdiagnosed and undertreated, despite its ubiquitous presence and immense social impact. Asthma affects individuals of all ages in all parts of the world, and can have staggering impacts on productivity and quality of life. According to latest WHO estimates, asthma affects about 300 million people worldwide and results in 250,000 deaths annually, the majority in low- and lower-middle income countries.[3] Many experts have speculated that the recent increase in global warming and the trend of urbanization will only increase the number of individuals suffering from asthma in the coming decades. Many patients lack access to appropriate medications and are unaware of how to manage and monitor their disease. Despite the intense efforts of groups such as the Global Initiative for Asthma (GINA), effective asthma education and treatment faces many roadblocks to success. Enhancing communication with asthma specialists, primary-care health professionals, other healthcare workers, and patient support organizations must be optimized.

Slowly we are beginning to recognize that although treating asthma may be expensive, the consequences of not treating it are even more costly.[4]

SIGNS AND SYMPTOMS

- Historical clues:
  - Personal or family history of allergic disease (allergic rhinitis, eczema, or urticaria) is frequently associated with asthma and helps in the diagnosis.
  - Occupational or environmental history.
  - Nocturnal awakening with difficulty breathing and/or wheezing as well as morning cough that relieves throughout the day.
- Presentation:
  - Patients can present with anything from a mild attack to severe respiratory distress, most classically with cough, wheezing, and dyspnea.
- Exam findings:
  - Wheezing is the most common presenting symptom, often during both phases of respiration with prolonged expiration.
  - Tachypnea, tachycardia, and increase in systolic BP.
  - Increasing severity identified by loss of adventitial breath sounds and higher-pitched wheezing.
  - Accessory muscle use and paradoxical pulse are later findings indicative of severe disease.
  - In extreme situations, wheezing may disappear, cough becomes ineffective, and respirations exhibit gasping respirations.
  - End of an episode often marked by cough productive of thick mucus.

DIAGNOSIS

- Demonstrating reversible airway obstruction
- A combination of history, physical exam, and spirometry
- Spirometry-recommended method of measuring airflow limitation and reversibility to establish a diagnosis of asthma
  - demonstrates reversibility of function abnormalities
  - Measurement of FEV1 and FVC
  - The degree of reversibility in FEV1 that indicates a diagnosis of asthma is generally accepted as a > 12% and a > 200 ml from the prebronchodilator value.[5]

TREATMENT

- Identify and minimize exposure to causative triggers
- Medication as appropriate (see Table 4-1)
- Educate individuals to provide knowledge, confidence, and skills to assume a role in the management of their condition.
- Development of a personal action plan
- Community education

GOALS OF TREATMENT

- Freedom from symptoms and lifestyle limitations
- Minimize nocturnal awakening
- Optimize lung function
- Minimize frequency of exacerbations

PNEUMONIA

OVERVIEW

Pneumonia is an acute infection of the lower respiratory tract, most commonly from a bacterial or viral source. This infectious process alters the anatomy of alveoli and distal airways with resultant fluid deposition and decreased lung function.

Pneumonia is a disease of both developed and developing countries, with staggering morbidity and mortality. However, although this is a global disease, it is individuals in developing countries and at the extremes of age that bear the majority of disease and death associated with pneumonia. For example, Africa alone may be responsible for 50% of all severe pneumonia cases and a significant proportion of pneumonia-associated mortality. It is estimated that pneumonia is responsible for one in three newborn infant deaths and up to 5000 childhood deaths every day. In their latest report, UNICEF and WHO state that pneumonia kills more children than any other illness—more than AIDS, malaria, and measles combined. Most importantly, however, is that many of these deaths are vaccine preventable and easily treated with antibiotics.

Although pneumonia can be associated with viral infections (e.g., measles, RSV), most severe infections are caused by bacteria. Of these, *Streptococcus*

Table 4-1 Classification of Asthma Severity and General Daily Treatment Guidelines[4]

	Symptoms/Day	Symptoms/Night	PEF or FEV1	PEF Variability	Treatment
Intermittent	< 1×/week	≤ 2×/month	≥ 80%	< 20%	Inhaled short-acting beta-2 agonist as required
Mild Persistent	> 1×/week but not every day Attacks may affect activity	> 2×/month	≥ 80%	20–30%	Low-dose inhaled steroid
Moderate Persistent	Daily Attacks affect activity	> 1×/week	60–80%	> 30%	Inhaled steroid + Long-acting beta-2-agonist
Severe Persistent	Continuous Limited physical activity	Often every night	≤ 60%	> 30%	High-dose inhaled steroid + Long-acting beta-2-agonist + Oral steroids (as needed)

Table 4-2 Most Common Etiology of Pneumonia by Age Group

Age Group	Organism
Neonate	Group B Streptococcus, E. coli, Klebsiella, Listeria, CMV, HSV, Chlamydia
< 5 years old	S. pneumoniae, Haemophilus influenza B, S. aureus, RSV, Adenovirus, Influenza
Youth and Young Adults	S. pneumoniae, Mycoplasma pneumoniae, Chlamydia pneumoniae, RSV, influenza
Adults	S. pneumoniae, Mycoplasma pneumoniae, Chlamydia pneumoniae, RSV, influenza

pneumoniae is the most common etiologic agent in all age groups after the neonatal period, and is the leading cause of morbidity and mortality among children worldwide. In addition to S. pneumoniae, there are numerous other viral, fungal, and chemical agents responsible for clinical disease.

■ Streptococcus pneumoniae

S. pneumoniae is responsible for the overwhelming majority of severe disease worldwide. It is a Gram positive encapsulated diplococcus whose only natural reservoir is the human nasopharynx, from where it spreads via respiratory droplets. In most healthy individuals, carriage is asymptomatic and the great majority of children around the world are believed to be reservoirs without evidence of disease. In a minority of patients, however, pneumococcus will cause otitis media, pneumonia, meningitis, and rarely, invasive disease and septicemia.

In the past, disease caused by pneumococcus was extremely sensitive to penicillins. However, recent research shows that pneumococcal resistance to essential antimicrobials including penicillins, cephalosporins, and macrolides is a serious and rapidly increasing problem worldwide. More concerning is that despite the recent development of many pneumococcal vaccines, supplies are inadequate and economic obstacles currently make widespread vaccination difficult.

■ Haemophilus influenza type B

Haemophilus influenza type B (HiB) is a common cause of epiglottitis, otitis media, pneumonia, and meningitis worldwide in children under 5 years old. It is estimated to cause up to 386,000 deaths per year and significant morbidity in disease survivors.

HiB was identified many decades ago as the etiologic cause of pneumonia and meningitis. Research lead to a very effective vaccination that has greatly reduced the disease burden on the industrialized world, where 92% of children receive the vaccination. However, vaccination rates are significantly less in the rest of the world—WHO estimates 42% for developing countries, and 8% for least-developed countries (the majority of which are in sub-Saharan Africa). Needless to say, the greatest impediment has been economic, with the HiB vaccines currently costing around US $7 per child for the recommended three doses.[6] Numerous organizations, most notably the Global Immunization Vision and Strategy (GIVS), are working to provide widespread HiB vaccinations to the poorest nations to reduce HiB-associated morbidity and mortality.

■ *Staphylococcus pneumoniae*

Staphylococcus pneumoniae classically presents as a rapidly progressing pneumonia with high mortality—more common after a preceding bout of influenza or measles infection and in patients with underlying lung disease. Less commonly, it is spread to the lungs from a distant source, such as the skin, bones, or heart. This type of pneumonia usually presents with high fevers and significant respiratory distress, and may progress to form lung abscesses or cavitary lesions.

SIGNS AND SYMPTOMS

- Pneumonia has a variable presentation depending on the age of the patient, underlying health status, infectious agent, and clinical severity.
- Classic Presentation:
  - Fever
  - Chills/rigors
  - Productive cough
  - Dyspnea
  - Tachypnea (See Table 4-3)
  - Pleuritic Chest Pain
- Classic Exam Findings:
  - Hyper- or hypothermia
  - Tachypnea
  - Crackles/egophony/dullness to percussion
  - Hypoxemia
  - Central cyanosis, nasal flaring, accessory muscle use, head nodding, and decreased level of consciousness (especially in children) all indicate impending respiratory failure and require aggressive management.
- Special Considerations:
  - Infants and children often present without classic symptoms
    - May present with abdominal pain, poor feeding, decreased activity, fever, or vomiting.
    - Often swallow secretions, so cough may appear nonproductive
  - In the elderly, classic findings are often absent and a high index of suspicion in addition to a thorough exam is required to confidently make the diagnosis. Patients may be afebrile and only nonspecific findings such as confusion may be present.

DIAGNOSIS

- In most areas, access to radiography and laboratory facilities may be limited, and pneumonia would be suspected on clinical exam. As routine chest radiography rarely changes treatment, only consider if

the diagnosis is not clear and if suspected x-ray findings will change management.
- Diagnostic Pearls in children: Respiratory rate (RR) is helpful in diagnosing pneumonia.

Table 4-3 Using Respiratory Rate to Diagnose Pneumonia in Children

Age	Severe Respiratory Distress
< 2 months	> 60
2–12 months	> 50
12 months–5 years	> 40
> 5 years	> 30

Measured over one minute in a calm, non-crying child

- Diagnostic strategies in resource poor areas
  - In children, it is always important to discern previous immunization history, as this may help with differential.

TREATMENT

- Oxygen therapy, ideally with monitoring of oxygen saturation
- Antibiotic treatment as appropriate (see Tables 4-4 and 4-5; cotrimoxazole is also known as trimethoprim-sulfamethoxazole)
- Fluids and antipyretics

Table 4-4 Recommended Antibiotic Therapy for Pneumonia in Children[7]

Severity	Antibiotic Therapy
Pneumonia: tachypnea (refer to preceding text)	Cotrimoxazole: 4 mg/kg TMP or 20 mg/kg SMX twice a day, or amoxicillin: 25 mg/kg twice a day.
Severe Pneumonia: nasal flaring, grunting, chest wall indrawing, no evidence of severe respiratory distress, able to drink	Benzylpenicillin: 50,000 units/kg IM or IV every 6 hours for at least 3 days, and if improving, switch to oral amoxicillin: 25 mg/kg twice a day for 5 days.
Very Severe Pneumonia: severe respiratory distress, central cyanosis, not able to drink	Ampicillin: 50 mg/kg IM every 6 hours and gentamicin: 7.5 mg/kg IM once a day for 5 days. If responding well, complete treatment at home or in hospital with oral amoxicillin: 15 mg/kg three times a day plus IM gentamicin once daily for a further 5 days.

- General Principles for Antibiotic Treatment
  - As microbiological confirmation of etiologic agent is unlikely available, treatment should be directed at most likely pathogen.
  - Antibiotic treatment should always take into account local resistance patterns.

Table 4-5 Recommended Antibiotic Therapy for Adults[9]

Community Acquired Pneumonia (CAP)—Infect Dis Soc Am 2007[8]	
Pneumonia—CAP **Healthy,** and no use of antibiotics in past 3 months	• azithromycin (*Zithromax*) 500 mg PO × 1, then 250 mg PO daily × 4 days (inpatient dosing— 500 mg IV q 24 h × 1–2 days, then 500 mg PO × 7–10 days) **OR** clarithromycin (*Biaxin*) 250 mg PO bid × 7–14 days **OR** *Biaxin XL* 1 g PO daily × 7 days **OR** doxycycline 100 mg PO/IV bid
Pneumonia—CAP **Outpatient** therapy if **Comorbidity** present *(heart, lung, liver, renal disease, or diabetes, alcoholism, asplenia, immunosuppression, cancer, or antibiotic use in prior 3 months)* Also see Pneumonia—CAP: Pseudomonas & MRSA	• gemifloxacin (*Factive*) 320 mg PO daily × 7 d **OR** levofloxacin (*Levaquin*) 750 mg PO/IV daily × 5 d **OR** moxifloxacin (*Avelox*) 400 mg PO/IV daily × 7–14 d • **OR** (azithromycin or clarithromycin—see pneumonia/**healthy** dose) **PLUS** β lactam (amoxicillin 1 g PO tid or *Augmentin* 2 g PO bid or cefpodoxime 200 mg PO bid or cefuroxime 250 mg PO bid) • If > 25% macrolide resistant (MIC ≥ 16 mcg/ml) *Strep. pneumonia* choose option without macrolide.
Pneumonia—CAP **Inpatient** (non-ICU) therapy	• gemifloxacin (*Factive*) 320 mg PO daily × 7 d **OR** levofloxacin (*Levaquin*) 750 mg PO/IV daily × 5 d **OR** moxifloxacin (*Avelox*) 400 mg PO/IV daily × 7–14 d • **OR** (azithromycin/*Zithromax* or clarithromycin/*Biaxin*—see pneumonia/**healthy** dose) **PLUS** (ceftriaxone 1–2 g IV q 24 h or cefotaxime 1 g IV q 12 h or ampicillin 1–2 g IV q 4–6 hours) • **OR** doxycycline 100 mp PO/IV bid **PLUS** ertapenem (*Invanz*) 1 g IV q 24 hours
Pneumonia—CAP **ICU admit** ICU Admit criteria: (1) septic shock, vasopressor use or (2) respiratory failure/ intubation, or (3) *any 3 of following*: RR ≥ 30, PaO$_2$/FiO$_2$ ≤ 250, multilobar, confusion, uremia (BUN ≥ 20), WBC < 4,000, platelets < 100,000, temperature < 36°C, ↓ BP requiring aggressive fluids	• See ICU admission criteria to left. • (ceftriaxone/*Rocephin* 1–2 g IV q 24 hours or cefotaxime/*Claforan* 1 g IV q 12 hours or ampicillin-sulbactam/*Unasyn* 1.5–3 g IV q 6 hours) **PLUS** (azithromycin/*Zithromax* or clarithromycin/*Biaxin* or gemifloxacin/*Factive* or levofloxacin/*Levaquin* or moxifloxacin/*Avelox*)— use dosing listed above for *Pneumonia healthy with outpatient comorbidity present*. • Penicillin allergy: levofloxacin (*Levaquin*) 750 mg IV daily **OR** moxifloxacin (*Avelox*) 400 mg IV daily **PLUS** aztreonam (*Azactam*) 1–2 g IV q 8–12 h

Community Acquired Pneumonia (CAP) (Continued)	
Pneumonia—CAP **MRSA** methicillin resistant *S. aureus* possible (see hospital acquired pneumonia)	• If MRSA is a concern (e.g. recent skin infection, prior MRSA, recent admission/ED visit, post-influenza, lung abscess or lung effusion, intubation/ventilator use, tracheostomy) **ADD** one of following to the inpatient regimen above (1) linezolid (*Zyvox*) 600 mg IV q 12 hours **OR** (2) vancomycin 1 g IV q 12 hours to above inpatient or ICU regimens
Pneumonia—CAP **Pseudomonas** possible (see hospital acquired pneumonia)	• If Pseudomonas is a concern (e.g. COPD, aspiration, alcoholism, chronic steroid use, structural lung disease such as bronchiectasis, tracheostomy, ventilator use, frequent antibiotic use) consider one of following regimens: • (Piperacillin-tazobactam (*Zosyn*) 3.375–4.5 g IV q 6 hours or cefepime (*Maxipime*) 1–2 g IV q 12 hours [See cefepime caution page 88] or imipenem (*Primaxin*) 1 g IV q 6–8 hours or meropenem (*Merrem*) 1 g IV q 8 hours] **AND** (2) ciprofloxacin (*Cipro*) 400 mg IV q 8–12 hours or levofloxacin (*Levaquin*) 750 mg IV q 24 hours • **OR** [Piperacillin-tazobactam (*Zosyn*) 3.375–4.5 g IV q 6 hours or cefepime (*Maxipime*) 1–2 g IV q 12 hours [See cefepime caution page 88] or imipenem (*Primaxin*) 1 g IV q 6–8 hours or meropenem (*Merrem*) 1 g IV q 8 hours] **PLUS** (gentamicin or tobramycin—see dosing on page 113) **PLUS** azithromycin (*Zithromax*) 500 mg IV q 24 h × 1–2 days, then 500 mg PO × 7–10 days • **OR** [Piperacillin-tazobactam (*Zosyn*) 3.375–4.5 g IV q 6 hours or cefepime (*Maxipime*) 1–2 g IV q 12 hours [See cefepime caution page 88] or imipenem (*Primaxin*) 1 g IV q 6–8 hours or meropenem (*Merrem*) 1 g IV q 8 hours] **PLUS** (gentamicin or tobramycin—see dosing on page 113) **PLUS** ciprofloxacin (*Cipro*) or levofloxacin (*Levaquin*) • Penicillin allergy—substitute aztreonam (*Azactam*) 1–2 g IV q 8–12 h for (1) above
Pneumonia— *aspiration or lung abscess*	• (clindamycin 600–900 mg IV q 8 h **OR** cefoxitin 2 g IV q 8 h **OR** ticarcillin-clavulanate (*Timentin*) 3.1 g IV q 6 h **OR** piperacillin-tazobactam (*Zosyn*) 4.5 g IV q 8 h) **AND** consider MRSA coverage
Pneumonia— *Pneumocystis jiroveci* (formerly *carinii*)	• *Septra* DS 2 PO q 8 h **OR** IV *Septra*—15 mg/kg of TMP if ill q 8 h × 21 days **OR** [(clindamycin 600 mg IV q 8 h or 300–450 mg PO qid) and primaquine 15–30 mg of base PO daily × 21 d] • **OR** pentamidine (*Pentam*) 4 mg/kg IV q 24 h × 21 d • **OR** dapsone 100 mg PO daily and trimethoprim (*Primsol*) 5 mg/kg PO tid × 21 days • **OR** atovaquone 750 mg PO bid × 21 days • **ADD** prednisone × 2–3 weeks if $pO_2 < 70$ mm Hg

(Continues)

Table 4-5 Recommended Antibiotic Therapy for Adults (Continued)

Hospital Acquired Pneumonia (HAP), Ventilator Associated (VAP) and Healthcare Associated Pneumonia (HCAP)—Infect Dis Soc Am 2007	
HCAP definition	Anyone hospitalized ≥ 2 days in an acute care hospital within 90 days of pneumonia, or lives in nursing home or long term care facility OR within past 30 days received recent IV antibiotics, chemotherapy, wound care, or attended a hospital or hemodialysis clinic.
HAP definition	Pneumonia occurring ≥ 48 hours after admission
VAP definition	Pneumonia arising > 48–72 hours after intubation
Early onset Pneumonia (£ 4 days of admission) with NO Multi-Drug Resistant Risk Factors (see late onset) HAP/VAP (not HCAP)	• ceftriaxone (*Rocephin*) 1–2 g IV q 24 h **OR** levofloxacin (*Levaquin*) 750 mg IV q 24 h **OR** moxifloxacin (*Avelox*) 400 mg IV q 24 h **OR** ampicillin-sulbactam (*Unasyn*) 1.5–3 g IV q 6 h **OR** ertapenem (*Invanz*) 1 g IV q 24 h
Late Onset Pneumonia ≥ 5 days from admit OR **Multi-Drug Resistant** Risk Factors present HAP/VAP/(all HCAP cases) *Recommendations are for initial empiric therapy. Streamline therapy based upon cultures and clinical response to treatment.*	• <u>Multi-Drug Resistant Risk Factors</u>: All patients defined as HCAP above or who have a family member with a multidrug-resistant pathogen, high frequency of antibiotic resistance in the community or the admission hospital unit, or immunosuppression (disease or therapy) • **Choose one of following:** Cefepime [*Maxipime*] 1–2 g IV q 8–12 h or ceftazidime (*Fortaz*) 2 g IV q 8 h or imipenem (*Primaxin*) 1 g IV q 8 h or meropenem (*Merrem*) 1 g IV q 8 h • **PLUS choose 2nd agent**—(piperacillin-tazobactam (*Zosyn*) 4.5 g IV q 6 h or *Cipro* 400 mg IV q 8 h or *Levaquin* 750 mg IV q 24 h or gentamicin 7 mg/kg/24 h or tobramycin 7 mg/kg q 24 h or amikacin 20 mg/kg q 24 h [√ aminoglycoside trough levels]) • If MRSA risk factors are present or high local incidence **ADD** linezolid (*Zyvox*) 600 mg IV q 12 h or vancomycin 15 mg/kg (max 1 g) IV q 12 h. • If ESBL+ (extended spectrum β lactamase+) organism suspected, use (1) carbepenem (imipenem or meropenem) or β-lactam/ β-lactamase inhibitor (*Zosyn*) **AND** (2) ciprofloxacin or levofloxacin or aminoglycoside • If Legionella possible, **ADD** macrolide or respiratory quinolone.

- Treatment in patients with HIV or suspected HIV-infection
  - Although *S. pneumoniae* is still the major cause of pneumonia in HIV+ patients, the healthcare worker must expand the differential to include fungal infections (cryptococcus, coccidioidomycosis, histoplasmosis) as well as pathogens not normally found in immunocompetent individuals such as *Pneumocystis jiroveci* (formerly known as *Pneumocystis carinii*). HIV patients also have a higher incidence of TB.
  - Recent recommendation by WHO and UNICEF include prophylaxis with Cotrimoxazole for HIV+ children and adults.[9]
- Complications: Due to a multitude of factors, many patients may not adequately respond to treatment and may develop secondary complications.
  - Emphysema
  - Cavitary lesions
  - Sepsis

CHRONIC OBSTRUCTIVE PULMONARY DISEASE (COPD)

OVERVIEW

COPD is an umbrella term for the diseases previously referred to as chronic bronchitis and emphysema. The Global Initiative for Chronic Obstructive Lung Disease (GOLD) describes COPD as "a preventable and treatable disease...characterized by airflow limitation that is not fully reversible. The airflow limitation is usually progressive and associated with an abnormal inflammatory response of the lung to noxious particles or gases."[10] This response will cause parenchymal tissue destruction (resulting in emphysema) and disrupt normal defense and repair mechanisms (resulting in small airway fibrosis). The end result of this pathological process is progressive air trapping in peripheral airways, which causes hyperinflation of the lungs and the clinical symptoms of dyspnea, most prominent with exertion.

COPD has received considerably more attention in the previous decade for its substantial and increasing global prevalence. Under-recognized as a significant health issue for many years, global health experts now recognize COPD as a health threat with far-reaching consequences. The WHO's Global Alliance against Chronic Respiratory Diseases (GARD) and GOLD have committed considerable research and funding to COPD prevention and treatment worldwide.

According to their reports, COPD affects up to 210 million people worldwide, and is responsible for 5% of all deaths globally,[11] the majority of which occur in low- and middle-income countries. COPD will become the third leading cause of death worldwide by 2020, as exposure to COPD risk factors and life expectancy increases globally.[12] Although COPD cannot be cured, it is important to identify individuals at risk or with the disease, as lifestyle modification and pharmacologic management can drastically slow disease progression.

RISK FACTORS

Tobacco smoking continues to be the most commonly encountered risk factor for COPD,[13] especially with the continuous increase in the number of smokers worldwide. This risk is dose-related, with age at onset of smoking, total pack years, and current smoking status all predictive of disease mortality.

COPD does develop in non-smokers however, and exposure to both indoor and outdoor air pollution from burning of wood and other biomass has been identified as a significant risk factor.[14] It is estimated that 3 billion people worldwide use biomass as an energy source for cooking and heating, representing a significant exposure risk. Moreover, it is believed that all of these independent exposures act additively to cause COPD.

Furthermore, as not all smokers or ex-smokers develop COPD, while many non-smokers do, there is believed to be a genetic component to disease development. Traditionally, severe hereditary alpha-1-antitrypsin deficiency has been associated with COPD; however, this is rare and limited to specific populations. Genetic association studies have implicated other genetic factors in COPD, though their association requires further investigation.

The role of gender as a risk factor for COPD is still contentious. Previous studies suggested that COPD was more prevalent in males than females. Recent investigations have shown the prevalence to be almost equal in men and women, reflecting recent changes in tobacco use patterns.

SIGNS AND SYMPTOMS

- Presentation
  - Frequent respiratory infections
  - Dyspnea, especially with exertion, is the hallmark symptom. Initially may only be with exertion, but progressively occurs with minimal effort and eventually at rest in many individuals.
  - Chronic sputum production—variable in amount, color, and severity; traditionally defined as regular production of sputum for 3 or more months in 2 consecutive years.
  - Chronic cough—productive or nonproductive, progressively increasing in frequency.
  - In early stages of disease, many patients will not experience significant symptoms, and may ignore cough and sputum production or credit them to increasing age. Often the initial presentation is precipitated by an acute respiratory infection.
  - Patients may also notice weight loss or anorexia, syncope after severe coughing, and ankle swelling (indicating cor pulmonale and resultant edema).
- Physical Exam
  - Many of the physical signs of COPD are nonspecific, but may help in the diagnosis
    - "Barrel-shaped" chest
    - Pursed-lip breathing
    - Tachypnea

- Wheezing and inspiratory crackles may be heard
- Paradoxical breathing or accessory muscle
- Central cyanosis

DIAGNOSIS

- Presence of dyspnea, chronic cough, or chronic sputum production, especially in the presence of significant risk factors should mandate consideration of COPD in differential.
- Diagnosis and management is based on spirometry.
  - Patients with COPD typically have decrease in FEV1 and FVC.
  - After the administration of a short-acting inhaled bronchodilator (e.g., 400 g salbutamol), FEV1/FVC < 0.70 and FEV1 < 80% predicted confirms the presence of airflow limitation that is not fully reversible.
  - In patients with FEV1 < 50% predicted or with clinical signs suggestive of respiratory failure or right heart failure, arterial blood gas measurement is recommended.
- Radiography
  - Chest x-rays for COPD are usually nondiagnostic, but may help exclude alternative diagnoses.
  - When disease is severe, may see hyperinflation, flattening of the diaphragm, and rapid tapering of vascular markings.

TREATMENT

The most important intervention after initial diagnosis is to reduce or ideally avoid exposure. Education plays a large role in smoking cessation, and all smokers with a new diagnosis of COPD should be strongly encouraged to quit. In addition, in cases where an occupational irritant is identified as a contributing factor to disease development, all attempts should be made to avoid further exposure.

Unfortunately, no existing medication for COPD treatment has been shown to modify long-term decline in lung function, but can greatly reduce symptoms. Bronchodilators are the mainstay of treatment. Beta-2-agonists, anticholinergics, and methylxanthines can be used individually or in combination to reduce symptoms and exacerbations. Inhaled, oral, or intravenous glucocorticoids are beneficial.

All patients with COPD should receive influenza (all ages) and pneumococcal vaccinations (age > 65) as appropriate, and should be encouraged to participate in exercise training programs.

Lastly, there is no current evidence that antibiotics, other than treating infectious exacerbations of COPD, are helpful and are not recommended as prophylaxis.[13]

MANAGEMENT OF COPD EXACERBATIONS

An exacerbation is defined as "change in the patient's baseline dyspnea, cough, and/or sputum that is beyond normal day-to-day variations, is acute in onset, and may warrant a change in regular medication."[13] This is most commonly caused by respiratory infections or pollution. Depending on severity, most patients respond to inhaled bronchodilators, inhaled glucocorticosteroids, and supplemental oxygen. Change in mental status or clinical signs of respiratory failure require hospitalization and stabilization.

TUBERCULOSIS

INTRODUCTION

Tuberculosis (TB) is a curable disease known to mankind for thousands of years and given numerous different names and etiologies. In 1820, J.L. Schonlein ascribed the name "tuberculosis" to the disease as we know it today. In 1882, Robert Koch discovered *Mycobacterium tuberculosis*, the causative bacilli responsible for the countless numbers of cases of TB throughout human history. Despite the intensive research into TB in the late 19th century, TB still continued to represent a significant public health issue worldwide, especially among the urban poor. Sanatoria were built, spitting and other unhygienic behaviors banned, and the eventual discovery of antibiotics to treat TB lead to a gradual decline in developed countries. TB nevertheless remains one of the biggest public health threats worldwide.

It is estimated that one-third of the world's population (2 billion people) is infected with *Mycobacterium tuberculosis*, with 9 million new cases and almost 2 million deaths reported in 2007.[15] The majority of cases occur in low-income countries and affect young adults in their most productive years. Although the etiology and treatment of TB is well-defined, multidrug resistant TB (MDR-TB), HIV, and diabetes have complicated recent treatment efforts and pose a significant challenge to meeting the global TB targets aimed at reducing incidence, prevalence, and mortality worldwide by 2015.

Table 4-6 Global Tuberculosis Treatment Goals

(i) Incidence of TB should be falling by 2015 (Millennium Development Goal Target 6.c).
(ii) TB prevalence and death rates should be halved by 2015 compared with their level in 1990.
(iii) At least 70% of incident smear-positive cases should be detected and treated in Directly Observed Short-Course (DOTS) programs.
(iv) At least 85% of incident smear-positive cases should be successfully treated.

Although many regions of the world are on track to meet some of these goals, it is likely that most will not satisfy all four goals. The rising burden of HIV has made Africa home to 13 of the 15 countries with the highest TB incidence rates. Asia, which has 55% of all global TB cases, is also witnessing an increase in HIV-associated TB.[15]

Anti-TB initiatives require a well-organized program structure to be effective. Previous experiences led to the creation in 1995 of the TB control strategy, Directly Observed Short-Course (DOTS) program, which has been shown to be very effective in treating new cases, monitoring therapy, and gaining invaluable research information. More recently, the WHO and Stop TB have expanded DOTS to include care providers and communities while recognizing the key challenges of TB/HIV and MDR-TB.

Table 4-7 WHO Directly Observed Therapy Short Course (DOTS)

1) Political commitment with increased and sustained financing
2) Case detection through quality-assured bacteriology
3) Directly observed therapy (DOT) with standardized, short-course chemotherapy (SCC)
4) An effective drug supply and management system
5) Monitoring and evaluation system and impact measurement

MICROBIOLOGY

Mycobacteria are aerobic, nonmotile bacteria with a characteristic cell wall that is described as "acid-fast" when stained. The genus contains many bacteria known to cause significant disease in humans.

The primary cause of TB, *Mycobacterium tuberculosis*, is highly aerobic and multiplies very slowly when compared to other bacteria. As such, TB normally progresses slowly and cultures for *M. tuberculosis* often require up to 6 weeks for results.

Transmission happens via tubercle bacilli in airborne droplet nuclei from patients with active pulmonary TB during coughing and sneezing. The bacilli are inhaled and cause infection in vulnerable individuals. Crowding and poor ventilation increase the risk of exposure, as does length of time in contact with infected source. TB is highly contagious, and each untreated patient with active TB will infect on average 10 to 15 people every year.

BASIC PATHOGENESIS

Most initial infections go unnoticed by the patient, as inhaled bacilli reach the pulmonary alveoli and initiate a nonspecific response. The bacilli are then ingested by alveolar macrophages, where division and replication take place. Eventual lysis of macrophages attracts lymphocytes, which ingest the bacilli. Later cell-mediated immunity results in recruitment and activation of large numbers of macrophages at the site of the primary lesion. This collection of lymphocytes and macrophages forms a granulomatous lesion that tries to isolate and limit the growth of bacilli.

In immunocompetent hosts, most lesions heal by fibrosis and later calcification. Even with healing however, bacilli may remain dormant within the granuloma, and the only indicator of infection is a positive tuberculin skin test. This is referred to as latent TB infection (LTBI) and represents 90% of all TB infections.

On average, 10% of individuals with LTBI will progress to active infection, most commonly within the first year after initial infection, but often years or decades later. It is impossible to predict which patients will progress, but there are many known risk factors associated with the development of active disease: e.g., HIV, extremes of age, diabetes, and malnutrition.

A small population of infected individuals will develop clinical illness directly following infection. This primary tuberculosis is most common in children and the immunocompromised.

SIGNS AND SYMPTOMS

- Clinical presentation
  - TB is defined as either pulmonary or extrapulmonary. Traditionally, most of the morbidity and mortality rates of TB were associated with pulmonary disease. However, the high association of HIV and TB has made extrapulmonary TB much more common. In general, TB can infect any organ in the body and present with organ-specific findings.
  - Pulmonary TB (PTB)—Primary:
    - Primarily a disease of children and the immunocompromised, primary TB presents with cough, fever, and malaise following a recent TB exposure. Chest radiography, if available, may show hilar or mediastinal adenopathy. Dissemination may occur and some patients who develop miliary TB or tuberculosis meningitis.
  - Pulmonary TB—Post primary (Secondary):
    - Reactivation of LTBI usually involves the lungs, but may involve any organ system. In pulmonary TB, the disease is usually localized to superior lung segments where oxygen concentration is greatest. Severity of pulmonary TB is highly variable, with some individuals going into remission and others following a rapidly progressive, fatal course. Others suffer from chronic disease, and present with a chronic cough that may or may not be productive. Patients may also complain of fever, night sweats, weight loss, shortness of breath, or hemoptysis.
  - Extrapulmonary TB
    - If bacilli gain entry into the bloodstream, they can travel to different end organs and develop into a disseminated disease.
    - Increasing in frequency as more individuals present with co-infection with HIV and TB. The most common sites of infection in extrapulmonary TB are listed in decreasing order in Table 4-8.
  - The physical exam in TB can be normal or nonspecific, with wasting often present and adventitious breath sounds heard on lung examination.

DIAGNOSIS

The key to diagnosis of tuberculosis is a high index of suspicion. This is especially true in resource-poor areas, where access to diagnostic modalities is limited. Ideally all patients with a chronic cough of unexplained etiology for

Table 4-8 Most Common Sites of Extrapulmonary Tuberculosis

Lymph Nodes (*Tuberculosis Lymphadenitis*)—Most frequently cervical lymph nodes
Pleural—fever and chest pain with effusion
Genitourinary—epididymitis in males
Renal
Skeletal—Spine (Pott's disease)
Meningitis—Slow course with cranial nerve symptoms
Gastrointestinal—terminal ileum, may present as small bowel obstruction
Pericardial—seen in HIV+ patients, causes effusion or tamponade

greater than 3 weeks or those with symptoms suggestive of TB should undergo diagnostic testing.

- Sputum Smears for Microscopic Examination
  - Three smears are recommended for the diagnosis of TB.
  - Collect over two days:
    - Day 1: Collect sputum sample in clinic and provide appropriate labeled sputum container for patient to collect at home.
    - Day 2 Morning: Patient collects early morning sputum at home and brings to clinic.
    - Day 2: Collect third sample when patient returns to clinic later that day.
  - It is important to instruct patient how to collect sample, explaining that the best samples come from the lungs, not the oral or nasal cavity.
  - Sputum is prepared with Ziehl-Neelsen staining and subsequently examined with microscope.
  - Sputum Smear Positive TB: Two or more initial sputum smear examinations positive for AFB; one sputum smear examination positive for AFB plus radiographic abnormalities consistent with active PTB, or one sputum smear positive for AFB plus sputum culture positive for *M. tuberculosis*.
  - Sputum Smear Negative TB: At least three negative sputum smears, chest radiography consistent with TB, and lack of response to initial broad spectrum antibiotics.

In countries with a well functioning external quality assurance (EQA) system, PTB+ can be diagnosed in a TB suspect if at least one acid fast bacilli (AFB) is visualized in at least one sputum sample. Determination of sputum status is important, as those with sputum + TB have a greater risk of treatment failure and mortality.

- Chest X-ray
  - Not required in the diagnosis or treatment of TB.
  - Useful only for patients with pulmonary TB, in whom cavitations or infiltrates may be seen.

- Not confirmatory of TB disease, cannot diagnose infection.
  - Chest X-ray may be most beneficial in patients with symptoms suggestive of TB and negative sputum smears.
  - Findings suggestive of TB on radiography require diagnostic testing with sputum smears.
- Tuberculin Skin Testing
  - Uses purified protein derivative (PPD) injected intradermally with examination 48–72 hours later and recording of area of induration. > 10 mm of induration (> 5 mm in HIV) is defined as a positive response. However, there are numerous false-positives and false-negatives. Skin testing is a good screening test, but not useful in diagnosing an active infection.
  - False Positives: Associated with exposure to nontuberculous mycobacteria, previous inoculation with BCG vaccination, incorrect interpretation.
  - False Negatives: Immunosuppression, fulminant TB, severe illness, poor technique, incorrect interpretation.

TREATMENT[16]

Patients must be educated about the importance of completing the course of treatment, as compliance often decreases as symptoms improve. Treatment can be administered either every day or in thrice-weekly dosing with comparable efficacy. Thrice-weekly dosing improves direct oversight of therapy, reduces costs, and decreases patient visits.

Table 4-9 Recommended Dosage (mg/kg) of Essential Tuberculosis Drugs

Drug Name	Daily Dose	Thrice weekly dose	Side Effects
Isoniazid	5	10	Liver toxicity
Rifampicin	10	10	Drug interactions
Pyrazinimide	25	35	Vomiting, arthralgias
Streptomycin	15	15	Ototoxicity
Ethambutol	15	30	Ocular toxicity

■ Treatment of New Cases

Treatment consists of two phases including an initial phase lasting for 2 months and a continuation phase lasting a further 4–6 months. The initial phase uses a combination of four drugs—isoniazid, pyrazinamide, rifampicin, and ethambutol—to rapidly kill tubercle bacilli. During this phase, patients symptoms improve and they are no longer infectious after 2 weeks. By the end of the initial phase, most smear-positive patients convert to smear-negative. The second stage of treatment is meant to kill any remaining bacilli, and uses fewer drugs for a longer period of time.

■ Re-Treatment Cases

Re-treatment cases are classified as those having undergone failure, relapse, or return after default. In these cases there is a higher likelihood of drug resistance and MDR-TB. The initial phase of re-treatment uses five drugs in two different phases. The continuation phase uses three drugs.

Table 4-10 Recommended Treatment for Persons Not Treated Previously, Those with HIV, and Those with Extra-Pulmonary Tuberculosis

Treatment	Initial Phase	Continuation Phase
Preferred	INH, RIF, PZA, EMB daily, 2 months; INH, RIF, PZA, EMB 3×/week, 2 months	INH, RIF daily, 4 months; INH, RIF 3×/week, 4 months
Optional	INH, RIF, PZA, EMB daily, 2 months	INH, EMB daily, 6 months

INH = isoniazid; RIF = rifampicin; PZA = pyrazinamide; EMB = ethambutol
Streptomycin may be substituted for ethambutol. Ethambutol may be omitted in the initial phase of treatment for adults and children who have negative sputum smears, do not have extensive pulmonary tuberculosis, or severe forms of extra-pulmonary disease, and who are known to be HIV negative.

Table 4-11 Recommended Approach for Re-Treatment of Tuberculosis

Treatment	Initial Phase	Continuation Phase
Preferred	INH, RIF, PZA, EMB, SM daily, 2 months followed by INH, RIF, PZA, EMB daily one month.	INH, RIF, EMB daily, 5 months.
Optional	As above, but thrice-weekly dose.	As above but thrice-weekly dose.

SM = streptomycin

■ Drug Resistant TB

Of growing concern in the international health community is the emergence of MDR-TB. Strains resistant to one or more of the standard TB drugs have been documented worldwide, and more recently, strains resistant to all major TB drugs have emerged and are referred to as extensively drug-resistant TB (XDR-TB).

Drug resistance often emerges from incomplete treatment, administration of improper treatment regimens, as well as inconsistent access to necessary medications.

MDR-TB is defined as disease with TB bacilli resistant to at least isoniazid and rifampicin, the two most powerful TB treatment drugs. Although MDR-TB is generally treatable, it requires longer treatment courses (up to two years) with more expensive medications that have more side-effects. The Green Light Committee (GLC) Initiative is a collaborative organization that helps countries gain access to second-line anti-TB drugs so they can provide treatment for people with MDR-TB. When MDR-TB treatment is mismanaged, there is an increased likelihood of XDR-TB emergence. XDR-TB is of particular importance in countries with high prevalence of HIV-TB co-infection, and will undoubtedly pose a significant threat to TB treatment around the world in the future.

■ BCG Vaccination

BCG, or bacille Calmette-Guérin, is a vaccine for tuberculosis. Used primarily in countries with high prevalence of disease, BCG is used primarily to prevent miliary disease and childhood tuberculous meningitis. In developed nations, the vaccine is rarely used since the prevalence of TB is low. The vaccine is not completely effective, and its use often interferes with PPD testing.

PERTUSSIS (WHOOPING COUGH)

Pertussis is a respiratory infection characterized by a paroxysmal "whooping" cough. Before the advent of an effective vaccine, pertussis was a significant cause of mortality and morbidity throughout the world. Although prevalence has decreased by more than 99% in developed nations with high levels of immunization, there are still frequent outbreaks in both developed and developing nations and pertussis still represents one of most common causes of vaccine-preventable death.

Pertussis is highly contagious and caused by the bacteria *Bordatella pertussis*, a gram-negative bacillus spread via droplet transmission. Humans are the sole reservoir, and infection leads to an incubation stage, most commonly presented with symptoms of a mild respiratory illness. Patients are most contagious during this catarrhal phase. Within 1–2 weeks, patients develop paroxysmal coughing with the characteristic whooping sound as air enters through a still partially closed airway. Younger patients (less than 6 months of age) often present without the high-pitched sounds, but posttussive vomiting is common and patients are at risk for fatal apneic episodes.

On physical examination, individuals with pertussis infection are usually afebrile and may only have stigmata of intense coughing (conjunctival hemorrhage or facial petechia). An acute coughing illness lasting 14 days with either paroxysmal coughing, posttussive vomiting, or inspiratory whoop is required for a diagnosis of pertussis. Ideally, nasal cultures will demonstrate *Bordatella* infection, however, previously vaccinated individuals and those that have already received antibacterial therapy may have false negative results. Although radiographic findings are nonspecific in infected individuals, chest radiography may reveal a related pneumonia or acute lung process. The last stage in the illness is the convalescent stage, where symptoms gradually diminish.

Treatment options during the various stages are minimal and largely ineffective in changing the course of illness. However, all patients with findings suggestive of respiratory distress or dehydration from vomiting require hospital admission and possible intensive care monitoring, especially premature infants and those younger than 3 months of age. Antibiotics are often prescribed during the paroxysmal phase but this has not been proven to affect the duration or severity of illness. The only benefit may be the eradication of *Bordatella pertussis* from the respiratory tract and prevention of further spread. The recommended regimen for all patients greater than 1 month old is a macrolide antibiotic (e.g., erythromycin, clarithromycin, azithromycin), whose link with hypertrophic pyloric stenosis in infants may limit its use in this age group. In addition, antibiotics may be recommended for patients during the catarrheal stage where they have been proven to reduce symptoms, and for close contacts of infected individuals.

The importance of prevention with immunization cannot be overemphasized. Every child under 7 years old should be vaccinated as childhood infections are associated with the gravest complications for infection, and boosters should be provided at later ages. The vaccine is only effective for a few years after immunization, and recent proposals have recommended revaccinating adults and the elderly as they are responsible for transmitting the bacteria to infants. Globally, pertussis vaccine is usually administered in fixed-dose combinations with diphtheria, tetanus, and other vaccines as part of primary immunization programs. Current WHO recommendations are for three doses, given at 6, 10, and 14 weeks, with a booster given 1–6 years after completion of primary sequence.[17]

DIPHTHERIA

Diphtheria is an acute bacterial disease that normally affects the tonsils, larynx, pharynx, and sometimes the skin. Diphtheria has a long history and was a worldwide health problem until the development of the diphtheria toxoid in the 1940s, after which the developed world has seen a precipitous decline in new cases. Diphtheria nevertheless continues to be prevalent in many places around the world, with occasional epidemics such as those seen in several former Soviet Republics in the 1990s.

Diphtheria is caused by an aerobic, nonencapsulated, nonmotile, gram-positive bacillus, *Corynebacterium diphtheriae*. Infection is mostly via respiratory droplets from humans and symptoms develop 2–5 days after transmission. Although many of those infected become asymptomatic carriers, some individuals will have clinical disease, presenting with non-specific symptoms such as fever, malaise, sore throat, hoarseness, and cervical lymphadenopathy. From the site of infection, inflammation of the upper respiratory tract develops and there is a characteristic formation of a dense, gray pseudomembrane covering the tonsils, soft palate, oropharynx, nasopharynx, and uvula. Displacement of the pseudomembrane with resultant airway obstruction is possible, either spontaneously or with manipulation of the airway (during oral exam or intubation). In more severe cases, inflammation can involve the majority of the tracheobronchial tree and the concomitant cervical adenopathy imparts the characteristic "bull neck" appearance of diphtheria. Infrequently, patients may develop non-healing cutaneous ulcers with a grayish membrane that can become superinfected. Late manifestations of the disease include myocarditis, endocarditis, and peripheral neuropathies.

If diphtheria is suspected, treatment should begin immediately. The treatment is an antitoxin manufactured from horse serum, so the healthcare provider should ideally perform intradermal testing to detect hypersensitivity and must be prepared for a potentially fatal anaphylactic event when administering it.

Patients should receive antitoxin immediately, the dosage depending on severity of disease. In general, mild–moderate diphtheria should receive 40,000 units IM and severe disease should receive up to 100,000 units (40,000 IM, then the rest intravenously 2 hours later). In addition, patients should be started on IV penicillin or erythromycin until they are able to swallow, at which point oral antibiotics can be given. Total treatment period of antibiotic therapy should be 14 days.

Close contacts of suspected diphtheria victim should have cultures performed and receive an age-appropriate diphtheria booster. Antibiotic therapy should be administered with benzathine penicillin (one-time dose) or oral erythromycin (7 days). If culture-positive, they should be treated as patients.

International travelers and healthcare personnel should receive either primary immunization if necessary or an appropriate booster if traveling to areas where diphtheria is common.

Infection does not confer immunity; thus, initiation or completion of immunization with diphtheria toxoid is necessary. It should be noted that even with aggressive treatment, mortality approaches 10%, and untreated patients have mortality rates of approximately 50%.

Although the worldwide incidence of diphtheria is decreasing, it remains a significant global health concern, and the most effective intervention is mass immunization. Education about disease symptoms as well as strong emphasis on immunization can help reduce diphtheria morbidity and mortality worldwide.

LUNG ABSCESS

Lung abscesses occur with localized suppuration of lung parenchyma with resultant tissue necrosis and the formation of a pus-filled cavity. There are numerous etiologic causes with different geographical distributions, however in developed countries most cases are due to impaired gag/cough, poor dental hygiene, lung cancer, or pneumonia. In developing countries, the differential is much larger and includes numerous infectious diseases, including fungal, mycobacterial, and parasitic sources.

Typical presentation includes fever, persistent cough, weight loss, malaise, and night sweats. Those with anaerobic abscesses often have foul-smelling breath and sputum, whereas patients with longer periods of symptoms often develop hemoptysis and digital clubbing. In the absence of adequate treatment, empyema may develop.

INFECTIOUS CAUSES

Bacteria: Often mixed aerobe-anaerobe infections, including Burkholderia, Nocardia, Actinomyces, *S. aureus*, Klebsiella, Bacteroides, and *E. coli.*

Fungi: Aspergillus, *Blastomyces dermatitidis, Coccidioides immitis, Cryptococcus neoformans, Histoplasma capsulatum*, and *Pneumocystis jiroveci.*

Mycobacteria: *Mycobacterium avium-cellulare*, and *Mycobacterium tuberculosis.*

Parasites: *E. histolytica* and Echinococcus.

Signs and symptoms of lung abscesses are nonspecific and may mimic pneumonia. On physical exam, signs of periodontal disease or dysphagia may be present, and amphoric or cavernous breath sounds are only rarely appreciated. Patients with *E. histolytica* infection may have right upper-quadrant pain.

Diagnosis is made with a chest x-ray showing a cavitating opacity containing an air-fluid level. In aspiration-associated abscesses, dependent areas such as the apical portions of lower lobes or posterior segments of upper lobes are commonly affected. Other sources may produce multiple abscesses (e.g., endocarditis, IV drug abuse). Ideally blood cultures and sputum are obtained for analysis. Consider other causes of cavitation, such as lung cancer, pulmonary infarct, paragonimiasis (lung parasite), and Wegener's granulomatosis.

Treatment is directed at the most likely cause and requires long-term treatment (up to 6 weeks). Anaerobic lung abscess can be treated with clindamycin 600 mg IV q8h followed by 150–300 mg PO qid, or alternatively, metronidazole combined with penicillin. Fungal and mycobacterial abscesses require treatment directed at their specific cause. *E. histolytica* infections are treated with metronidazole. Treatment can be monitored by resolution of symptoms as well as resolution of findings on the chest radiograph.

REFERENCES

1. World Health Organization. WHO Strategy for Prevention and Control of Chronic Respiratory Disorders. http://www.who.int/respiratory/publications/WHO_MNC_CRA_02.1.pdf, 2002
2. World Health Organization. http://www.who.int/respiratory/en/index.html
3. World Health Organization. Asthma Fact Sheet. 2008. http://www.who.int/mediacentre/factsheets/fs307/en/index.html. Accessed June 1, 2009.
4. Adapted from Global Initiative for Asthma. *Pocket Guide for Asthma Management and Prevention.* 2008.
5. Pellegrino R, Viegi G, Brusasco V, Crapo RO, Burgos F, Casaburi R, et al. Interpretative strategies for lung function tests. *Eur Respir J* 2005; 26(5):948–68.
6. World Health Organization. Haemophilus influenza type B (HiB) Fact Sheet. December 2005. http://www.who.int/mediacentre/factsheets/fs294/en/index.html. Accessed June 1, 2009.
7. Adapted from WHO Treatment Guidelines 2008. *Pocket Book of Hospital Care of Children.*
8. Mandell L, Wunderink R, Anzeuto A, et al. Infectious Diseases Society of America/American Thoracic Society consensus guidelines on the management of community-acquired pneumonia. *Clin Infect Dis.* 2007;44 (Suppl 2):S27–S72.
9. Rothrock, SG, ed. Tarascon Adult Emergency Pocketbook. Sudbury, MA: Jones and Bartlett Publishers; 2009:103–107.
10. Global Initiative for Chronic Obstructive Lung Disease. Global Strategy for the Diagnosis, Management, and Prevention of Chronic Obstructive Pulmonary Disease. 2008.

11. World Health Organization. Chronic Obstructive Pulmonary Disease (COPD) Fact Sheet. May 2008. http://www.who.int/mediacentre/factsheets/ fs315/ en/index.html. Accessed June 1, 2009.

12. Global Alliance Against Chronic Respiratory Disease. GARD Action Plan 2008–2013. 2008. Geneva, Switzerland.

13. Global Initiative for Chronic Obstructive Lung Disease. Global Strategy for the Diagnosis, Management, and Prevention of Chronic Obstructive Pulmonary Disease. 2008.

14. Barnes PJ. Chronic Obstructive Pulmonary Disease: A Growing but Neglected Global Epidemic. *PLoS Med*. 2007;4(5): e112. doi:10.1371/*journal. pmed*.0040112.

15. World Health Organization. *Global Tuberculosis Control: Epidemiology, Strategy, Financing : WHO Report 2009*. Geneva, Switzerland: World Health Organization. 2009.

16. World Health Organization. *Treatment of Tuberculosis: Guidelines for National Programmes*. 3rd ed. Geneva, Switzerland: World Health Organization. 2003.

17. World Health Organization. *WHO Essential Medicines Library*. Geneva, Switzerland: World Health Organization. 2009.

V ■ VECTOR-BORNE DISEASES

Clifford C. Dacso, MD, MPH, MBA

Vector-borne diseases are infectious agents that are carried to their host by either biologic or mechanical means. The history of vector-borne diseases is characterized by attempts at controlling the organism transmitting the disease. In the early days of arthropod control in North America and Europe, this strategy was successful, resulting in the disappearance of arthropod-borne diseases such as Bangui and yellow fever. Since the 1970s however, vector-borne diseases have reemerged as global public health problems.

The causes for the reemergence of vector-borne diseases are complex and include an overreliance on insect control, climate change, and intrinsic changes in the nature of the organisms. Container shipping and jet travel facilitate the spread of vector-borne diseases to places previously thought to be under control. Deaths from vector-borne diseases are widespread throughout the world, though concentrated in sub-Saharan Africa, South and Southeast Asia, and South and Central America.

MALARIA

Malaria continues to be one of the most devastating infectious diseases in developing countries. Over 40% of the world's population lives in areas where malaria transmission occurs (i.e., parts of Africa, Asia, the Middle East, Central and South America, the Caribbean, and Oceania). It is estimated that 350–500 million cases of malaria occur each year resulting in over one million deaths.[1] The Anopheles mosquito usually transmits malaria. Exceptions include congenital malaria transmitted from mother to child, direct infection via transfusion or organ transplantation, or use of shared needles. The malaria lifecycle requires a vertebrate host, so humans and mosquitoes must share the same environment for the disease to spread.

Malaria is one of the most complex vector-borne diseases. As a general rule the presence of Anopheles mosquitoes determines the spread of the disease. The Anopheles mosquito bites between dusk and dawn so prevention, including bed nets and insect repellents, is the most effective strategy.

The epidemiology of malaria is geography-specific. In areas where the virulent *Plasmodium falciparum* predominates, such as sub-Saharan Africa, morbidity and mortality from the disease will be increased. Other species of malaria, particularly *Plasmodium vivax* and *Plasmodium ovale*, may remain dormant in liver cells for extended periods of time resulting in the reintroduction of malaria to areas that were previously malaria free. Both *Plasmodium falciparum* and to a lesser extent *Plasmodium vivax* have evolved resistance to antimalarial drugs, complicating treatment in areas where these strains are endemic.

Because of the temperature, humidity, and proximity requirements, the parasite will not readily spread at high altitudes, during cool seasons, in deserts, and where the Anopheles mosquito is not present. Tropical and equatorial regions will experience intense and year-round transmission.

DIAGNOSIS

The diagnosis of malaria can be difficult, but it generally relies on microscopic identification. Rapid diagnostic tests using immunochromatographic techniques have been approved for use by hospitals and laboratories. It is still recommended however that these be confirmed by direct examination of a peripheral blood smear. A polymerase chain reaction assay is available, however its use is not yet widespread. Serology is of no use in diagnosing the acute infection.

SYMPTOMS

Following the bite of an Anopheles mosquito, malaria causes symptoms within 7–30 days. *Plasmodium falciparum* is characterized by a shorter incubation period. *Plasmodium malariae* has a longer one. The disease causes fever, chills, sweats, headaches, nausea, vomiting, body aches, and general malaise. Malaria is a common cause of splenomegaly worldwide.

Severe forms cause cerebral malaria, hemolytic anemia, hemoglobinurea from hemolysis, and pulmonary edema leading to respiratory failure and death. Severe infection with *Plasmodium falciparum* can lead to multiorgan system failure and death. *Plasmodium vivax* and *Plasmodium ovale* infections are characterized by relapse. Treatment therefore needs to be directed at eradicating the hepatic phase in the latter infections.

TREATMENT

Treatment and prophylaxis guidelines for malaria depend on regional epidemiology. Treatment of presumptive malaria, the clinical syndrome of malaria without a confirmed parasitic identification, is controversial. With the declining incidence of malaria in some sub-Saharan communities and the emergence of rapid diagnostic testing, many authorities are now recommending the end of presumptive treatment.

RABIES

Rabies can be transmitted by a variety of animals including dogs, bats, foxes, and skunks. Feral animals, particularly dogs, are common vectors of the disease. Insectivorous bats have also been known to transmit rabies. Rabies is a zoonotic disease caused by an RNA virus. The virus is typically present in the saliva of clinically ill mammals and is transmitted through a bite. After entering the central nervous system of the next host, the virus causes an acute, progressive encephalomyelitis that is almost always fatal. The incubation period in humans is usually several weeks to months, but can range from days to years. The key strategy in rabies is prevention since no specific treatment exists for the established disease.

The rabies vaccine is very effective. As opposed to previous versions made in duck embryos, the human cell-derived rabies vaccine is well tolerated. Rabies vaccination should be performed prior to entering an endemic area.

POST-EXPOSURE PROPHYLAXIS

Rabies vaccination does not preclude the need for medical evaluation following a bite by a potentially infected animal. Post-exposure prophylaxis is simplified for people who have already been immunized. Immunization is therefore recommended for travelers to rabies endemic areas and regions where post-exposure prophylaxis is not readily available.

Local wound care is critical to the early management of a bite from a potentially rabid animal. Irrigation of the wound, independent of other treatment, has been shown to decrease the incidence of rabies. Tetanus immunization status should be assessed and updated if necessary. Since the incubation period for rabies is relatively long, immunologic post-exposure prophylaxis is urgent, but not an emergency.

The combination of human rabies immune globulin (HRIG) and vaccine is recommended for exposures reported by persons not previously immunized, regardless of the interval between exposure and initiation of prophylaxis. Vaccinated individuals only need a booster vaccine course. If post-exposure prophylaxis has been initiated and appropriate laboratory diagnostic testing (i.e., the direct fluorescent antibody test) indicates that the source animal was not rabid, post-exposure prophylaxis can be discontinued.

Unvaccinated: Wound cleansing, HRIG 20 IU/KG administered around the wound and intramuscularly near the site, vaccine should be administered at a site distant for the HRIG injection on days 0, 3, 7, 14, and 28.[2]

Vaccinated: Wound cleansing, vaccine on days 0 and 3.[3]

Purified equine rabies immune globulin (ERIG) fractions have been used in developing countries where the HRIG is not available. The incidence of adverse reactions after ERIG administration has been low (0.8%–6.0%), and most of those that occurred were minor. Unpurified antirabies serum of equine origin may still be used in countries where HRIG and ERIG are unavailable. The use of this serum is associated with higher rates of serious adverse reactions, including anaphylaxis.

ARTHROPOD-BORNE DISEASES

Arthropod-borne diseases (arboviruses) comprise a large portion of vector-borne diseases. Mosquitoes are the major vectors. Birds are often the source of infection for mosquitoes, which then transmit the infection to horses, other animals, and humans. Humans are not an essential part of the life cycle for most arboviruses. The viruses are transmitted during feeding and acquisition of a blood meal and thus the key to prevention is to avoid insect bites.

CHIKUNGUNYA

Chikungunya virus (CHIKV) is an alphavirus indigenous to tropical Africa and Asia, where it is transmitted to humans by the bite of infected mosquitoes, usually of the genus *Aedes*. Chikungunya fever was first recognized in epidemic form in East Africa in 1952. The word *chikungunya* is thought to be derived from a description in the local dialect of the contorted posture of patients afflicted with the severe joint pain associated with the disease. Because CHIKV fever epidemics are sustained by human–mosquito–human transmission, the epidemic cycle is similar to those of dengue and urban yellow fever. Large outbreaks of CHIKV fever have been reported recently on several islands in the Indian Ocean and in India.

JAPANESE ENCEPHALITIS

Japanese encephalitis (JE) is a flavivirus that causes acute encephalitis progressing to paralysis, seizures, coma, and death. The majority of infections with Japanese encephalitis virus however are subclinical. JE is the leading cause of viral encephalitis in Asia with 30,000 to 50,000 cases reported annually. The case fatality rate is high as is the rate of serious neurological sequelae. The disease is transmitted by the bite of the *Culex tritaeniorhynchus* mosquito and exposure is generally limited to rural areas in endemic regions. Risk to travelers is considered to be low.

YELLOW FEVER

Yellow fever is conventionally divided into two groups: jungle yellow fever and urban yellow fever. Jungle yellow fever is primarily a disease of simians. When it infects humans it is usually limited to people who work or live in tropical rainforests. Urban yellow fever is a disease of humans. The most common mosquito carrying yellow fever is the *Aedes aegypti*. This is an urban mosquito that reproduces in standing water and usually bites at dusk and at dawn.

Yellow fever has highly variable clinical manifestations. Syndromes range from a self-limited febrile illness to severe hepatitis and hemorrhagic fever. Yellow fever of the hemorrhagic type presents with high fever, chills, headache, and muscle aches. After a brief recovery, the infection returns leading to shock and multiorgan system failure. The incubation period is generally 3–6 days from a bite by an infected mosquito. There is no specific treatment, so management is directed at supportive care.

TICK-BORNE ENCEPHALITIS

Tick-borne encephalitis (TBE) is caused by two closely related flaviviruses. The eastern subtype causes Russian spring–summer encephalitis (RSSE) and is transmitted by *Ixodes persulcatus*, whereas the western subtype is transmitted by *Ixodes ricinus* and causes Central European encephalitis (CEE).

Although the name implies geographic restriction, in reality the diseases are found throughout Europe. Of the two subtypes, RSSE is the more severe infection, having a mortality of up to 25% in some outbreaks, whereas mortality in CEE seldom exceeds 5%.

The incubation period is 7–14 days. Infection usually presents as a mild, influenza-type illness or as benign, aseptic meningitis, but may result in fatal meningo-encephalitis. Fever is often biphasic, and there may be severe headache and neck rigidity, with transient paralysis of the limbs, shoulders, or less commonly, the respiratory musculature. Some patients are left with a residual paralysis. Although the great majority of TBE infections follow exposure to ticks, infection has occurred through the ingestion of milk from infected cows or goats' milk. An inactivated TBE vaccine is currently available in Europe and Russia.

MURRAY VALLEY ENCEPHALITIS

Murray Valley encephalitis (MVE) is endemic in New Guinea and in parts of Australia and is related to the St. Louis Encephalitis and Japanese Encephalitis viruses. Subclinical infections are common, and the small number of fatalities have mostly affected children.

WEST NILE ENCEPHALITIS

West Nile virus is a flavivirus similar to Japanese encephalitis, St. Louis encephalitis, and Murray Valley encephalitis. Its name is derived from its first locus of isolation, the West Nile province of Uganda in 1937. West Nile virus is a vector-borne disease spread along modern transportation routes. It was unknown in the United States until an outbreak in 1999 and it now continues to spread throughout the U.S. The clinical manifestations of West Nile virus range from asymptomatic infection to severe encephalitis. The virus is spread principally by the *Culex* species of mosquitoes, although the *Aedes*, *Anopheles*, and other species have been also implicated in transmission.

DENGUE

Dengue fever was historically considered a mild, nonfatal disease of the tropics. Over the past two decades however, a more virulent syndrome known as dengue hemorrhagic fever has emerged as a global health problem. Dengue infects tens of millions of people each year and there are hundreds of thousands of cases of dengue hemorrhagic fever.

Dengue is transmitted primarily by species of *Aedes* mosquito. Its principal symptoms are high fever, headache, backache, joint pains, nausea, vomiting, eye pain, and rash. Its nickname "break bone fever" is very descriptive. Dengue hemorrhagic fever is characterized by fever that lasts up to a week. Following this stage, it induces hemorrhagic manifestations. "Leaky capillary syndrome" allows widespread fluid retention, circulatory failure, shock, and death. There is no effective vaccine for dengue fever. Once again, prevention of mosquito bites is the most effective means of avoiding the disease. Treatment of dengue fever is supportive.

PLAGUE

Plague is a bacterial disease caused by *Yersinia pestis*. Plague is usually spread by bites from fleas that are infected with the disease. It is typically characterized in two forms: bubonic plague and pneumonic plague. Bubonic plague consists of swollen and tender lymph nodes called *bubos*. Clinical symptoms of fever, chills, headache, and extreme exhaustion are characteristic of bubonic plague. Pneumonic plague is less common but has a higher fatality rate. It is characterized by high fever, cough, bloody sputum, and dyspnea. Pneumonic plague can be spread by droplet transmission.

Despite its notoriety, plague is generally rare in the world. The World Health Organization (WHO) reports 1000 to 3000 cases per year, the majority in Africa.[4]

Treatment of plague should include streptomycin when possible. Gentamicin, tetracycline, and chloramphenicol have also been used successfully. Consideration should be given to prophylaxis in patients with close respiratory exposure to people with confirmed or suspected plague.

VIRAL HEMORRHAGIC FEVERS

Viral hemorrhagic fevers are caused by four families of zoonotic RNA viruses. Humans are not required for the disease life cycle but infected individuals can transmit the disease to other humans.

The viral hemorrhagic fevers live in a variety of species and are generally transmitted by arthropods. Mosquitoes sometimes serve as vectors, though in some cases the reservoir and vector are unknown. Ebola virus and Marburg virus are examples of poorly understood diseases. Secondary transmission of the viral hemorrhagic fever viruses can occur once an initial human infection is established. Ebola virus, Marburg virus, Lassa fever virus, and Crimean Congo hemorrhagic fever viruses are examples of this class of disease. Transmission is likely a result of contact with contaminated bodily fluids.

Signs and symptoms of viral hemorrhagic fever vary according to type though as a general rule they are characterized by fever, fatigue, dizziness, myalgia, and exhaustion. Bleeding is a common symptom, ranging from bruising to diffuse hemorrhage. As the disease progresses, it causes central nervous system dysfunction and renal failure.

Treatment is symptomatic although ribavirin has been used in Lassa fever with anecdotal results.

Prevention remains the key to the management of the hemorrhagic fevers. Vaccines are only available for yellow fever and Argentine Hemorrhagic fever, so avoiding outbreak zones and quarantine protocols are vital.

Table 5-1 Viral Hemorrhagic Fevers

Virus	Location	Reservoir	Vector	Symptoms	Comment
Ebola	Congo, Cote d'Ivoire, Gabon, Sudan, Uganda	Unknown	Unknown	Amplified in healthcare personnel	
Marburg	Uganda, Kenya, Congo, Angola, Zimbabwe	Unknown	Unknown	Amplified in healthcare personnel	
Lassa	Sierra Leone, Guinea, Liberia, Nigeria	Rat	Unknown		Person-to-person transmission possible
Junin (Argentine)	Argentina	Rodent	Unknown		Transmission via contact with rodent secretions
Machupo (Bolivian)	Bolivia	Rodent	Unknown		Person-to-person transmission possible
Guanarito (Venezuelan)	Venezuela	Rodent	Unknown		Transmission via contact with rodent secretions
Sabia (Brazilian)	Brazil	Rodent	Unknown		Transmission via contact with rodent secretions
Rift Valley	Sub-Saharan Africa, Saudi Arabia, Yemen	Livestock	Mosquito		
Hanta	North and South America	Mouse, Rat	Unknown	Pulmonary Infection	Transmission via contact with rodent secretions
Crimean-Congo	South Africa, the Balkans, The Middle East, Russia, Pakistan, Western China	Hares, birds	Ticks		

CHAGAS' DISEASE

Chagas' disease is caused by the parasite Trypanosoma cruzi. It is sometimes also referred to as American trypanosomiasis. The disease is characterized by an acute and chronic phase. Following infection, a period of parasitemia ensues with a syndrome characterized by a mild fever and systemic symptoms. In children, the acute phase can be more severe and even lethal. The acute phase may however, be asymptomatic. Following the acute phase a chronic phase ensues that may last years. As a rule these people are initially asymptomatic and are often unaware of infection. However up to 30% of infected people will develop symptoms of chronic Chagas' disease sometime during their life. The major characteristic symptoms of chronic Chagas' disease include multiple cardiac aneurysms that may lead to heart failure, cardiac rhythm disturbances that may cause sudden death, and gut dysmotility syndromes including achalasia and megacolon.

One of the most interesting features of Chagas' disease is its lifecycle. The disease is caused by inoculation of the feces of the triatomine insect, sometimes referred to as the reduviid or "kissing" bug. The insect becomes infected through a blood meal from an infected human or animal. Following this, the lifecycle of the organism results in an infective form being excreted in the feces after it bites another victim. Inoculation occurs when the host scratches the bitten area. Transmission can occur also by transfusion of infected blood.

DIAGNOSIS

Chagas' disease is endemic with increasing frequency as one travels south of the United States through South America. Although the vector and organism are present in North America, infection is rare as a consequence of the low density of insects decreasing the opportunity for transmission. A diagnosis of acute Chagas' can be made by a peripheral smear analysis. The chronic illness can be diagnosed by serology or a PCR assay.

TREATMENT

Treatment of Chagas' disease is by nifurtimox (Lampit; Bayer) and benznidazole (LAFEPE-BENZNIDAZOLE, Laboratorio Farmacêutico do Estado de Pernambuco [LAFEPE]). In the United States, treatment should be performed in consultation with the Centers for Disease Control and Prevention (CDC). Because Chagas' disease is predominantly a disease of poverty, identifying and treating infected people remains a challenge. Vector control by decreasing the domestic infestation of the insect is a key prevention technique.

ONCHOCERCIASIS

Onchocerciasis is better known by its common name, River Blindness. It is caused by the parasite Onchocerca volvulus and spread by a bite from an infected blackfly, Simulium damnosum, that bites during the day. Its name comes from the prevalence of the fly in areas surrounding rivers. The parasite is found almost exclusively in humans. River Blindness is present in 30 African countries, in regions of 6 countries in the Americas, and in Yemen. Seventeen million people are thought to be infected worldwide. Most infected persons are in Africa, and the disease is found most frequently in rural agricultural villages that are located near rapidly flowing streams.

Adult worms live in nodules in the human body where the female worms produce high numbers of first-stage larvae known as microfilariae. They migrate from the nodules to the subepidermal layer of the skin where they can be ingested by blackflies. They further develop in the body of the insect from which more people can be infected. Eye lesions in humans are caused by the microfilariae. They can be found in all internal tissues of the eye—except the lens—where they cause eye inflammation, bleeding, and other complications that ultimately lead to blindness.

DIAGNOSIS

The diagnosis is made by finding either the microfilariae in superficial skin shavings or punch biopsy, adult worms in histological sections of excised nodules, or characteristic eye lesions.

Serologic testing is most useful for detecting infection in specific groups such as returning expatriates in who acute phase serum can be assumed to be antibody negative and in whom the microfilariae are not identifiable microscopically. The presence of antibody alone does not diagnose the disease in people with prolonged residence in endemic areas. Determination of serum antifilarial immunoglobulin (IgG) is available through the Parasitic Diseases Laboratory at the National Institutes of Health (NIH) or through the Division of Parasitic Diseases, CDC.

TREATMENT

Ivermectin (150–200 g/kg orally, once or twice per year) is the drug of choice for onchocerciasis. Repeated annual or semiannual doses may be required, because the drug kills the microfilariae but not the adult worms, which can live for many years. Its use has decreased the incidence of new cases significantly. Antibiotic trials, with doxycycline (100 mg orally per day), directed against *Wolbachia*, an endosymbiont of *O. volvulus*, have demonstrated a decrease in skin lesions with 6 weeks of therapy. Diethylcarbamazine was historically used for treatment but has been discontinued following severe and sometimes fatal reactions.

LEISHMANIASIS

Leishmaniasis is a protozoal disease that is transmitted by the bite of the phlebotomine sand fly. Although there are over 500 species of the fly, only 30 or so are known to transmit the disease. Leishmaniasis is taking its place as one of the suite of emerging infectious diseases that is changing from a rural disease of poverty to an urban threat as well. Co-infection with HIV has created new opportunities for the disease. Since there are mammalian reservoirs other than humans, overcrowding and feral animals have contributed to its spread worldwide.

Leishmaniasis is conventionally grouped into three categories: cutaneous, mucocutaneous, or visceral, also known as *kala-azar*. Cutaneous forms of the disease normally produce skin ulcers on the exposed parts of the body such as the face, arms, and legs. The disease can produce a large number of lesions—sometimes up to 200—causing serious disability and invariably leaving the patient permanently scarred, a stigma that can cause serious social prejudice in endemic areas. The mucocutaneous form of leishmaniasis produces lesions that can lead to partial or total destruction of the mucous membranes of the nose, mouth and throat cavities, and surrounding tissues. These lesions are also severely stigmatizing. Visceral leishmaniasis is characterized by recurrent fevers and severe constitutional symptoms and wasting. Anemia, splenomegaly, and hepatomegaly are common findings. Visceral leishmaniasis has a very high fatality rate if untreated.

DIAGNOSIS

The diagnosis of leishmaniasis is made based on clinical presentation and characteristic skin/mucosal findings. Unfortunately, few objective lab tests have been identified that are sufficiently sensitive and specific to confirm or negate the diagnosis. Histopathology often yields insufficient data as a result of the low parasite burden that is often found in the lesions. Parasite culture is likely the most accurate diagnostic tool, but is expensive, time-consuming, and often unavailable in resource-limited settings. PCR is a sensitive test and may be used if available. The Leishmanin Montenegro skin test is a highly specific test that detects antibody to leishmaniasis. It often yields false negatives and does not differentiate between previous and current infection.

TREATMENT

The treatment of leishmaniasis is highly variable and dependent upon which species of leishmania is suspected and whether the infection is cutaneous, mucosal, or visceral. For visceral, antimonial drugs such as sodium stibogluconate and meglumine antimonite are the mainstays of treatment where they are available. They are administered intramuscularly (IM) or intravenously (IV) for 28 days. Amphotericin B has been the subject of numerous studies given its relatively inexpensive cost and worldwide availability. Lipid-soluble amphotericin B is likely the safest option. Mucosal leishmaniasis is treated with antimonial drugs for 28 days or liposomal amphotericin B for up to 8 weeks. Cutaneous infections should be treated with antimonial drugs. Amphotericin B may be efficacious, but IV/IM pentamidine or topical paromycin are the recommended second-line agents. Fluconazole may be effective against some forms of cutaneous infections. Of course, wound care and nutrition are important elements to consider in patients with leishmaniasis to encourage wound healing and prevent secondary infections.

REFERENCES

1. Jacobsen KH. HIV/AIDS, Malaria, and TB. In: *Introduction to Global Health.* Sudbury, MA: Jones and Bartlett Publishers; 2008:158.
2. Rabies Post Exposure. The Centers for Disease Control and Prevention Web site. http://www.cdc.gov/RABIES/exposure/postexposure.html
3. Rabies Post Exposure. The Centers for Disease Control and Prevention Web site. http://www.cdc.gov/RABIES/exposure/postexposure.html
4. Plague Fact Sheet. The World Health Organization Web site. http://www.who.int/mediacentre/factsheets/fs267/en/

VI ■ MENINGITIS

Stephen Gluckman, MD

INTRODUCTION

Meningitis is an inflammation of the meninges, the dural layers that cover the brain and spinal cord. The onset can be acute, generally over hours to a day, or it can be more subacute developing over weeks to months. It is often due to infectious agents, but there are other causes of meningeal irritation such as carcinomatous meningitis or sarcoidosis. In addition, meningitis must be distinguished from *encephalitis* since though there is some overlap, the causes of meningitis are usually different from those of encephalitis. The distinction between meningitis and encephalitis is clinical; if the brain function is normal the patient has meningitis, if there is evidence of abnormal brain function the patient has encephalitis. Most people with encephalitis will have some evidence of meningeal irritation (evidence of inflammation in the cerebrospinal fluid [CSF]) and in many patients with meningitis the brain function will be compromised as the disease progresses. It is usually possible to distinguish meningitis from encephalitis based on the presenting symptoms early in the disease. This distinction is important since the causes of each syndrome are different. Typical acute bacterial meningitis has CSF findings of at least 500 white blood cells (WBCs) most of which are polymorphonuclear (PMNs), elevated protein, and low glucose. One final point of definition is the term *aseptic meningitis*. Though it is often used synonymously with viral meningitis, it is safer to think of aseptic meningitis as a description of a CSF formula that is characterized by a moderately elevated WBC count (< 500 cells/ml), more lymphocytes than polymorphonuclear leucocytes, and a normal to moderately low sugar. Table 6-1 outlines CSF findings in meningitis. Table 6-2 lists many of the, often treatable, causes of meningitis in which the CSF has these aseptic parameters.

Meningitis is seen throughout the world. Of the many causes, acute bacterial meningitis is the most urgent to diagnose and treat. Untreated bacterial meningitis is 100% fatal and even with treatment there is substantial morbidity and mortality. The causes of acute bacterial meningitis in adults are similar throughout the world; *Neisseria meningitides* and *Streptococcus pneumoniae* are the most common pathogens in normal hosts. The former tends to be the predominant cause in adolescents and young adults and the latter in adults as they get older. Other bacteria are seen with increased frequency in persons with impaired defenses. Table 6-3 outlines the common causes of meningitis.

59

Table 6-1 Cerebrospinal Fluid Findings in Bacterial and Aseptic Meningitis

	Pressure	Protein	WBCs	% PMNs	Glucose	Other
Normal	< 200 mm	< 45 mg/dl	< 5	0	< 50% blood	
Bacterial[1]	Elevated (> 200 cm H2$_0$)	Elevated	> 500	> 90%	< 2/3rd blood[2]	Gram stain is positive about 70% of the time
Aseptic[3]	Elevated	Elevated	< 500	< 50%[4]	> 2/3rd blood[2]	

[1]Listeria can have a CFS formula that is more typical of aseptic meningitis.
[2]Most bacterial meningitis is much less than 2/3rd blood. In some viral cases—mainly cryptococcal and tuberculous meningitis—the CSF glucose is low, but generally not as low as bacterial meningitis.
[3]Tuberculous, cryptococcal, and carcinomatous meningitis can have a CSF formula that is aseptic, however the onset is generally of a much longer period of time than the usual causes of aseptic meningitis.
[4]Early viral meningitis can have a predominance of PMNs, but the cell count and glucose are not typical of a bacterial infection.

Table 6-2 Treatable Causes of Aseptic Meningitis

Infectious	Noninfectious
Herpes Simplex Virus	Lymphoma
Varicella-Zoster Virus	Carcinoma
Human Immunodeficiency Virus	Drugs
Syphilis	Nonsteroidal anti-inflammatory
Rickettsial Diseases	(NSAIDs)
Cerebral Malaria	Trimethoprim-sulfamethoxazole
Para-Meningeal Abscess	Intravenous immune globulin
Leptospirosis	Sarcoidosis
	Vasculitis

CLINICAL SYNDROMES

Acute bacterial meningitis presents with headache and fever. Meningeal signs such as a stiff neck, Kernig's, and Brudzinski's are variably present. The classic findings of fever, stiff neck, and altered mental status is absent in one-third to one-half of cases. However, the absence of all three of these findings virtually rules out acute bacterial meningitis.[1] Focal neurological findings and papilledema are uncommon and should suggest a complication or an alternative diagnosis. Imaging will not help with the diagnosis of meningitis. The only way to diagnose meningitis is an examination of the CSF. In general, if the diagnosis is being considered a lumbar puncture should be promptly done. Table 6-1 outlines the typical CSF findings in bacterial and

Table 6-3 Common Causes of Meningitis

Acute
Bacterial (pyogenic)
Normal Host
Streptococcus pneumoniae (pneumococcus)
Neisseria meningitides (meningococcus)
Decreased cell mediated immunity*
Listeria monocytogenes
S/P Neurosurgery or Opened Head Trauma
Staphylococci
Gram negative bacilli
Aseptic
Viral
Acute HIV
Herpes simplex 2
Syphilis
Tuberculosis (occasionally)
Rickettsial
Subacute/Chronic
Cryptococcus
Tuberculosis
Carcinoma
Lymphoma

*Low CD 4(+) cell count HIV infection, chronic steroids, organ transplant

aseptic meningitis. Much has been written about concerns related to lumbar punctures precipitating cerebral herniation, but in fact this causation has never been established and if there is a concern about lumbar puncture it is related to masses in the brain not meningitis. If meningitis is a serious consideration a lumbar puncture should not be delayed. However, if the presentation is more suggestive of a mass and the facilities are available a brain imaging study should be performed before a lumbar puncture. Clinical parameters that increase the likelihood of a mass are focal neurological findings, papilledema, age > 50, an immunosuppressed state, and a recent seizure.[2] If both diagnoses remain on the differential, antimicrobial treatment should not be delayed while arranging for a CT scan or MRI of the brain. Antimicrobial therapy given prior to a CSF examination might make the CSF culture negative, but it will not change the spinal fluid findings sufficiently to obscure the diagnosis of bacterial meningitis.

Chronic meningitis generally presents with progressive symptoms over several weeks to months. The three major causes to consider are cryptococcus, tuberculosis, and carcinomatous (including lymphomatous). The typical presentation starts with fevers and progressive headaches. If undiagnosed and untreated, altered mental status and focal neurological findings can develop. In general, there is less urgency in making the diagnosis in a patient with chronic meningitis than with acute meningitis since the disease progresses more slowly. Therefore, imaging before a lumbar puncture is usually appropriate if it is available since mass lesions such as pyogenic brain abscesses and toxoplasmosis can occasionally present with nonfocal headache and fever. However, if imaging is not available one should not hesitate to perform CSF examination since significant morbidity and eventual mortality result if the disease remains untreated. CSF findings in chronic meningitis are expected to show a formula that is typical of aseptic meningitis with a few exceptions. Early in tuberculous meningitis there can be a predominance of polymorphonuclear leucocytes. In immunosuppressed patients, such as those with AIDS, the CSF can be surprisingly normal. In a series of almost 200 consecutive patients with culture-proven cryptococcal meningitis, 30% had no WBCs in their CSF and another 20% had less than 10 WBCs.

Although cryptococcal meningitis can occasionally develop in a person with normal immunity it is far more common in those with depressed cell mediated immunity, typically those with low CD4 positive cell count AIDS. Thus, cryptococcal meningitis is seen with high frequency in parts of the developing world with a high prevalence of HIV infection.

Tuberculosis is also common in the developing world and as with Cryptococcus is facilitated by co-infection with HIV.[3] Tuberculous meningitis usually develops in persons without evidence of active extra-CNS tuberculosis although about one-third of the time it is part of the syndrome of miliary tuberculosis. When one is considering the diagnosis of TB meningitis one should first examine the fundi for choroidal tubercles in the retina. Tuberculin skin testing is not helpful; most patients have a positive test, but this is not diagnostic of active tuberculosis and a sizable number of persons with active tuberculosis have negative skin testing at presentation.

DIAGNOSIS

The diagnosis of meningitis can *only* be made by an examination of the cerebrospinal fluid. Routine blood testing is of little help. Blood cultures are positive over 50% of the time and are especially important to obtain if antibiotics are given before a lumbar puncture is performed. When one interprets CSF findings the general goal is to place the patient's problem into one of three categories: normal CSF and therefore no meningitis, abnormal CSF that is compatible with an aseptic cause, and abnormal CSF that is compatible with a bacterial cause. Figure 6-1 outlines the approach to the diagnosis of meningitis. Once this has been done the proper initial therapy can be prescribed. It is absolutely critical to obtain an opening pressure whenever a lumbar puncture is being performed for the question of meningitis. The management of cryptococcal and tuberculous meningitis includes treatment of elevated CSF pressure. In developing countries this can be done without a manometer by attaching IV tubing to the spinal needle and measuring the height of the column of CSF in the tube. When and where available, all CSF specimens obtained for the evaluation of acute meningitis should be sent for cell count and differential, glucose, gram stain, and culture. Normal values are noted in

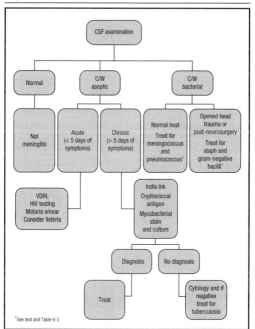

Figure 6-1 Approach to Meningitis

Table 6-1. In bacterial meningitis one expects an elevated opening pressure, elevated protein, elevated WBC count, and low glucose, though individual parameters can be quite variable and the CSF findings should be interpreted together; the clinician should not just focus on an individual value. However, a study noted that if any of the following CSF findings were present bacterial meningitis was diagnosed 99% of the time: protein > 220 mg/dl, glucose < 20 mg/dL (1.2 mmol/L), WBC count > 2000/mm.[3,4] Gram stain is a quick, inexpensive, and reasonably accurate method for identifying the causative agent.[5] Consideration should also be given to a CSF VDRL.

Table 6-4 Initial Studies

All CSF specimens
Opening pressure
WBC count
RBC count
Protein
Glucose
CSF culture and gram stain
VDRL
Subacute and chronic presentations
India ink
Cryptococcal antigen
CSF cytology
AFB stain and culture for mycobacteria
Fungal culture
Blood
Blood culture
RPR
HIV testing*

*Acute HIV syndrome can include aseptic meningitis. HIV serology may be negative early in acute HIV infection. A follow-up serology in 3–4 weeks or an HIV viral load done immediately will confirm or rule-out this diagnosis.

When evaluating a patient with a subacute or chronic presentation the fluid should be sent for cell count and differential, glucose, gram stain, and culture. In addition, the fluid should be sent for an India ink prep and cryptococcal antigen if available. See Table 6-4 for a summary of the studies to order.

The expected CSF findings in tuberculous meningitis are an elevated WBC count, though < 500/mm³. Mononuclear cells usually predominate, though early in the disease there may be a preponderance of polymorpholeukocytes. The CSF sugar is often low, though it can be normal and is rarely as low as that seen in a pyogenic bacterial infection. CSF AFB stain and culture for tuberculosis should be obtained. The larger the volume, the higher the yield; when one is considering tuberculous meningitis, three or more CSF specimens of at least 10 ml per specimen should be obtained at daily intervals.[6] Tuberculous meningitis often occurs in the absence of ongoing pulmonary tuberculosis.

Cryptococcal meningitis can be diagnosed with an India ink preparation, cryptococcal antigen testing of the CSF and/or culture of the CSF. India ink testing of the CSF is by far the least expensive. Though published sensitivity for this test has been in the 75% range, some clinicians experienced in advanced HIV patients have found it to be well over 90% sensitive and equivalent to cryptococcal antigen testing. CSF culture remains the gold standard and there are rare patients with negative India ink and cryptococcal antigen testing on the CSF who have positive CFS cultures for cryptococcus. Serum cryptococcal antigen testing is very sensitive in AIDS patients and can be used to rule out the disease where it is available, however a positive test does not eliminate the need for a lumbar puncture in order to monitor CSF pressure. If available, a cytologic examination should also be obtained on subsequent CSF examinations when the initial examination was nondiagnostic.

TREATMENT OF MENINGITIS

ACUTE BACTERIAL MENINGITIS

Treatment for acute bacterial meningitis should be initiated without delay. Studies suggest that the status of the patient at the time of the initial antimicrobial treatment predicts the outcome. Specifically, three prognostic factors have been evaluated including: altered mental status, seizures, and hypotension.[7] The presence of one, two, or three of these factors are associated with adverse outcomes in 9%, 33%, and 56% of the cases, respectively. Antibiotics often must be initiated before microbiologic information is known. The choice of empiric antibiotics depends on the expected bacteria and is determined by the clinical situation and the CSF gram stain, if available. Uncomplicated meningitis in adults is due to *Neisseria meningitidis* and *Streptococcus pneumoniae*. If the patient has problems with cell mediated immunity such as low CD4 (+) cell count HIV, *Listeria monocytogenes* should also be considered. If there has been recent neurological surgery or open head trauma, the concern should be focused on staphylococci and gram negative bacilli. Initial empiric antimicrobial choices are listed in Table 6-5.

The adjunctive use of glucocorticoids to diminish the complications and mortality of bacterial meningitis has been studied and the results are conflicting. In a randomized, prospective trial of over 301 patients from Europe a decrease in morbidity and mortality was noted for patients with pneumococcal meningitis when dexamethasone was initiated within 20 minutes of starting antibiotics.[8] In contrast, a similar study of 465 patients from Malawi showed no benefit from adjunctive treatment with corticosteroids (also no harm was observed).[9] It should be noted that 95% of patients in this latter study were HIV positive. In a study from Vietnam, a developing country with a low prevalence of HIV, dexamethasone did have some benefit.[10] Since the use

Table 6-5 Initial Antibiotic Options for Presumed Acute Bacterial Meningitis

Clinical	Antibiotic	Alternative
Normal adult	3rd generation Cephalosporin[1] plus Vancomycin	Chloramphenicol
Decreased CMI	Above plus ampicillin	Above plus Trimethoprim/ sulfamethoxazole
S/P recent neurosurgery	Antipseudomonal beta lactam[2] plus Vancomycin	Levofloxacin plus vancomycin

[1]Examples: Ceftriaxone, Ceftazidine, Cefotaxime
[2]Examples: Cefixime, piperacillin, meropenem

Table 6-6 Specific Treatment of Meningeal Pathogens

		Alternatives	Duration
Streptococcus pneumoniae	Penicillin IV 3–4 million units every 4 hours	Ceftriaxone 2 grams every 12 hours Cefotaxime 2 grams every 4 hours Chloramphenicol 25 mg/kg every 6 hours	10–14 days
Neisseria meningitides	Penicillin IV 18–24 million units in 6 divided doses daily	Ceftriaxone 2 grams every 12 hours Cefotaxime 2 grams every 4 hours Chloramphenicol 25 mg/kg every 6 hours	10–14 days
Listeria monocytogenes	Ampicillin 2 grams every 4 hours[1]		14 days
Staphylococcus aureus[2]	Nafcillin 2 grams every 4 hours	Vancomycin 15 mg/kg every 12 hours	14 days
Gram negative bacilli[3]	Ceftriaxone 2 grams every 12 hours Cefotaxime 2 grams every 4 hours	Chloramphenicol 25 mg/kg every 6 hours	14 days
Cryptococcus	Amphotericin B deoxycholate 1 mg/kg/day	Lipid preparations of Amphotericin B	2 weeks
	Fluconazole 800 mg daily × 3 days then 400 mg daily		6–8 weeks
	Fluconazole 200 mg daily[4]		Until CD 4 (+) cell count > 200
Tuberculosis[5]			

[1] Some clinicians would also add gentimicin
[2] Methicillin resistant Staphylococcal aureus use Vancomycin
[3] If pseudomonas or other resistant base treatment on sensitivity testing
[4] If HIV positive. If HIV negative and no other immunosuppression then no further treatment is necessary
[5] See chapter on the treatment of tuberculosis

of steroids has not been shown to be harmful and seems to be of benefit in HIV negative persons, they are indicated in patients likely to have pneumococcal meningitis and likely to be HIV negative. The dose used in the European study was 0.15 mg/kg every 6 hours and in the Vietnamese study 0.40 mg/kg every 12 hours; both were continued for 4 days.

CRYPTOCOCCAL MENINGITIS

Although Cryptococcal meningitis can occasionally occur in a person with a normal immune system, the vast majority occurs in persons with advanced AIDS, especially in the developing world. Treatment is not notably different in these two groups with the exception of duration. The antimicrobial treatment of subacute and chronic meningitis is not generally an emergency though relief of pressure can be. Therefore, treatment for cryptococcus is not initiated until the diagnosis is confirmed with India ink, cryptococcal antigen, or culture. The standard treatment for Cryptococcal meningitis is amphotericin B. Amphotericin B deoxycholate, at a dose of 0.7 mg/kg/day, is generally the preferred option over the lipid-associated preparations of amphotericin. Although the lipid associated preparations of amphotericin have less toxicity, amphotericin B deoxycholate is much less expensive and the standard duration of treatment is only two weeks, making side effects uncommon.[11] Adjunctive therapy with 5-FC is expensive and of modest additional benefit so it is often not included in regimens in the developing world. In addition, hematologic parameters need to be followed closely because of the concerns about bone marrow suppression with this medication. Consolidation is done with fluconazole after the initial induction phase of two weeks. A daily loading dose of 800 mg is suggested for the first three days followed by 400 mg daily for the next 6–8 weeks. Long-term suppression with 200 mg daily should be continued for at least a year in HIV patients and discontinued only if the CD 4 (+) cell count is greater than 200 cells/ml. If one is concerned about the adequacy of treatment, a repeat CSF culture should be obtained. In areas where it is available, the titer of cryptococcal antigen in the CSF can be followed. However, following India ink preparations for clearance of the organism is not useful since they may stay positive for many months even with adequate treatment.

Treatment with fluconazole alone is an option in parts of the developing world where amphotericin B may be difficult to obtain. It is not as effective as amphotericin B with response rates in the 50% range, as compared to 90% for amphotericin.[12] The doses used have been between 400 mg and 1000 mg/day. This is a reasonable treatment option in selected low-risk patients with normal mental status, WBC count in the CSF > 20/mm^3, and normal opening CSF pressure.

The aggressive management of elevated CSF pressure in patients cannot be overemphasized. Patients need a daily lumbar puncture as long as the opening pressure remains elevated. Enough CSF should be drained so that the closing pressure is about 15 cm. Even when this has been achieved, additional CSF pressure measurements should be done when there is any evidence of clinical deterioration.

TUBERCULOUS MENINGITIS

As mentioned previously, tuberculous meningitis is difficult to confirm since the diagnostic studies are insensitive and can be time consuming unless the smear is positive. In the developing world, empiric treatment for tuberculosis should be initiated in anyone with subacute meningitis where cryptococcal and cytological studies are negative. Treatment should not be delayed if there is strong clinical suspicion of tuberculous meningitis.

There are no randomized trials evaluating the best regimen for the treatment of tuberculous meningitis, however, many relevant organizations have developed consensus recommendations.[13,14] A two-month initiation phase with isoniazid, rifampin, pyrazinamide, and ethambutol or streptomycin should be followed by at least 7–10 months of continuation phase depending on clinical response and antimicrobial sensitivity of the isolate (where available). The doses of the drugs are the same as for pulmonary tuberculosis.

Adjunctive treatment of tuberculous meningitis with corticosteroids has been shown to be beneficial in a number of clinical trials. Suggested regimens for adults are either dexamethasone 12 mg/kg/day or prednisone 60 mg/day for 3 weeks and then tapered off over an additional 3 weeks.[15]

REFERENCES

1. van de Beek D, de Gans J, Spanjaard L, et al. Clinical features and prognostic factors in adults with bacterial meningitis. *N Engl J Med.* 2004;351:1849.
2. Tunkel AR, Hartman BJ, Kaplan SL, et al. Practice guidelines for the management of bacterial meningitis. *Clin Infect Dis.* 2004;39:1267.
3. Hakim JG, Gangaidzo IT, Heyderman RS, et al. Impact of HIV infection on meningitis in Harare, Zimbabwe: A prospective study of 406 predominantly adult patients. *AIDS.* 2000;14:1401.
4. Spanos A, Harrell FE, Durack DT. Differential diagnosis of acute meningitis, an analysis of the predictive value of initial observations. *JAMA.* 1989; 262:2700.
5. Fitch MT, van de Beek D. Emergency diagnosis and treatment of adult meningitis. *Lancet Infect Dis.* 2007;7:191.
6. Thwaites GE, Chau TT, Farrar JJ. Improving the bacteriological diagnosis of tuberculous meningitis. *J Clin Microbiol.* 2004;42:378.
7. Aronin SI, Peduzzi P, Quagliarello VJ. Community-acquired bacterial meningitis: risk stratification for adverse clinical outcome and effect of antibiotic timing. *Ann Intern Med.* 1998;129:862.
8. de Gans J, van de Beek D. Dexamethasone in adults with bacterial meningitis. *N Engl J Med.* 2002;347:1549.
9. Scarborough M, Gordon SB, Whitty CJ, et al. Corticosteroids for bacterial meningitis in adults in Sub-Saharan Africa. *N Engl J Med.* 2007; 357:2441.
10. Mai NT, Chau TT, Thwaites G, et al. Dexamethasone in Vietnamese adolescents and adults with bacterial meningitis. *N Engl J Med.* 2007; 357:2431.

11. Sharkey PK, Graybill JR, Johnson ES, et al. Amphotericin B lipid complex compared with amphotericin B in the treatment of cryptococcal meningitis in patients with AIDS. *Clin Infect Dis.* 1996;22:315–321.
12. Saag MS, Powdrly WG, Cloud GA, at al. Comparison of amphotericin B with fluconazole in the treatment of acute AIDS-associated cryptococcal meningitis. *N Engl J Med.* 1992;326:83–89.
13. Blumberg HM, Burman WJ, Chaisson RE, et al. American Thoracic Society/Centers for Disease Control and Prevention/Infectious Diseases Society of America: treatment of tuberculosis. *Am J Respir Crit Care Med.* 2003;167:603.
14. Tuberculosis Committee of the British Thoracic Society. *Chemotherapy and management of tuberculosis in the United Kingdom: recommendations 1998.* 1998;53:536.
15. Thwaites GE, Nguyen DB, Nguyen HD, et al. Dexamethasone for the treatment of tuberculous meningitis in adolescents and adults. *N Engl J Med.* 2004;351:1741.

VII ■ SEPSIS

Nicola Zetola, MD
Andrew Kestler, MD
Mitchell M. Levy, MD

Sepsis is one of the leading causes of morbidity and mortality worldwide. Unfortunately, due to significant under-diagnosis and under-reporting the global burden of sepsis is largely unknown. The documented incidence of sepsis is approximately 1.8 million cases per year. However, it has been estimated that with an incidence of three cases per 1000 people, over 18 million suffer from sepsis each year.[1–4] Moreover, with an average mortality rate of 30–50%, sepsis becomes a leading cause of death and disability-adjusted life years lost worldwide.[1–3,5]

Sepsis is broadly defined as the invasion of sterile tissue by one or more microbial pathogens with a resultant systemic inflammatory response.[6] Patients with a documented infection plus two or more elements of the systemic inflammatory response syndrome (SIRS) meet the criteria for *sepsis* (see Table 7-1). However, it should be noted that the offending pathogen cannot be identified in approximately 70% of cases of sepsis. The systemic inflammatory response often progresses to hypotension and end-organ failure. Patients with infection who also have hypotension and/or evidence of end-organ hypoperfusion (e.g., renal failure, hypoxemia, etc) are considered to have *severe sepsis*. Patients who develop refractory hypotension are considered to be in *septic shock* (see Table 7-1). These definitions encompass a continuum of infection severity, with progressively increased risk of end-organ failure and death that goes from sepsis, to severe sepsis, and ultimately septic shock (16%, 20%, and 46% risk of death, respectively).[7]

Over the last few decades, our understanding of the physiology and management of sepsis as a syndrome has improved significantly. New drugs and interventions for the management of sepsis have been studied and deployed in resource-rich settings. It is unclear if any of these new, typically high-cost interventions apply to patients from developing countries. Fortunately, the core of sepsis management, in rich and poor countries alike, still relies on the early implementation of simple, relatively low-cost interventions.[8–11]

Early identification and diagnosis, early initiation of appropriate antimicrobial coverage, source control, adequate fluid resuscitation, and appropriate referral remain the cornerstones of the management of sepsis. When available, the use of appropriate hemodynamic and ventilatory support is beneficial in the management of more advanced stages of sepsis. The role of other supportive measures, including invasive hemodynamic monitoring, activated drotrecogin alfa, physiological doses of corticosteroids, glycemic control,

Table 7-1 Diagnostic Criteria for Sepsis

Infection[1] documented or suspected, and some of the following[2]:
General variables[3]
Fever (core temperature >38.3°C)
Hypothermia (core temperature <36°C)
Heart rate > 90 per minute or > 2 SD above the normal value for age
Tachypnea
Altered mental status
Significant edema or positive fluid balance (> 20 mL/kg over 24 hrs)
Hyperglycemia (plasma glucose > 120 mg/dL or 7.7 mmol/L) in the absence of diabetes
Inflammatory variables
Leukocytosis (white blood cell [WBC] count > 12,000 μL^{-1})
Leukopenia (WBC count < 4000 μL^{-1})
Normal WBC count with >10% immature forms
Plasma C-reactive protein > 2 SD above the normal value
Plasma procalcitonin > 2 SD above the normal value
Hemodynamic variables
Arterial hypotension[2] (systolic blood pressure [SBP] < 90 mm Hg, mean arterial blood pressure [MAP] < 70, or an SBP decrease > 40 mm Hg in adults or < 2 SD below normal for age)
Mixed venous oxygen saturation (SvO$_2$) > 70%[2]
Cardiac index > 3.5 L min^{-1}·M^{-23}
Organ dysfunction variables
Arterial hypoxemia (PaO$_2$/FIO$_2$ < 300)
Acute oliguria (urine output < 0.5 mL kg^{-1}hr^{-1} or 45 mmol/L for at least 2 hrs)
Creatinine increase >0.5 mg/dl
Coagulation abnormalities (international normalized ratio [INR] > 1.5 or activated partial thromboplastin time [aptt] > 60 secs)
Ileus (absent bowel sounds)
Thrombocytopenia (platelet count < 100,000 μL^{-1})
Hyperbilirubinemia (plasma total bilirubin > 4 mg/dL or 70 mmol/L)
Tissue perfusion variables
Hyperlactatemia (> 1 mmol/L)
Decreased capillary refill or mottling

[1]Infection is defined as a pathologic process induced by a microorganism.

[2]SvO$_2$ sat > 70% is normal in children (normally, 75–80%), and CI 3.5–5.5 is normal in children; therefore, NEITHER should be used as signs of sepsis in newborns or children.

[3]Diagnostic criteria for sepsis in the pediatric population are signs and symptoms of inflammation plus infection with hyper- or hypothermia (rectal temperature < 38.5 or −35°C), tachycardia (may be absent in hypothermic patients), and at least one of the following indications of altered organ function: altered mental status, hypoxemia, increased serum lactate level, or bounding pulses.

Definitions from Levy et al. Crit Care Med. 2003;31(4):1250–1256.

blood transfusions, stress ulcer prophylaxis, DVT prophylaxis, and dialysis will depend on the resources available. In many cases, the added benefit of these supportive interventions is controversial or small in proportion to the cost.

This chapter will review basic concepts on the initial approach and management of patients with sepsis in developing countries and other resource-limited settings. Guidelines are proposed for the most appropriate management of sepsis depending on the level of resources available. It is interesting to note that most research on sepsis in very low-resource areas has focused on children, specifically in the diagnosis and management of neonatal sepsis in the community setting.[12] Although, we will focus on adults, the same core principles apply in the treatment of pediatric sepsis. Specific differences in the management of sepsis between adults and children will be addressed in the relevant sections that follow.

SIGNS AND SYMPTOMS

The presentation of sepsis is nonspecific and depends on the type and severity of the underlying infection. The signs and symptoms of sepsis also depend to a large extent on the host response.[13] At least two of the signs and symptoms listed in Table 7-1 are required for the diagnosis of sepsis. A decline in a patient's level of consciousness can be one of the first manifestations of sepsis, particularly among the elderly population and/or patients with underlying central nervous system pathology (e.g., patients with HIV dementia and/or HIV encephalopathy).[14,15] An altered mental status has been associated with worse clinical outcomes.[16,17] As the systemic inflammatory response progresses, it affects multiple organ systems: low vascular tone and decreased cardiac contractility lead to hypotension, brain hypoperfusion leads to altered mental status, renal hypoperfusion leads to oliguria and renal failure, acute lung injury leads to acute respiratory distress syndrome, and mucosal hypoperfusion leads to ulceration and gastrointestinal bleeding.

DIAGNOSIS

Two major challenges in the management of sepsis are making the diagnosis quickly and then identifying the cause.[11,18,19] Early recognition and diagnosis of sepsis are crucial to achieving successful outcomes since they expedite the treatment that is associated with improved survival.[10] Therefore, sepsis should be considered in any patient presenting with elements of the systemic inflammatory response syndrome, even if infection has not yet been established or documented.

A thorough history and physical examination is paramount in the initial approach of any patient with sepsis. The history and physical examination should focus on distinguishing sepsis from other noninfectious conditions that may mimic sepsis on presentation (e.g., pancreatitis, drug toxicities, cardiogenic shock, thyrotoxicosis). If infection is considered possible, the history (e.g., diabetes, liver failure, HIV/AIDS, travel history, exposures, indwelling lines, valvular disease, heart failure, renal failure, prosthetic devices) will focus the search for the etiology and source of the infection, and may well alter management. Worldwide, it is particularly important for clinicians to know the seasonal and regional prevalence of other pathogens that cause sepsis, or sepsis-like syndromes—notably malaria, dengue fever, melioidosis, and typhoid. (These will be discussed further in this chapter.) The physical exam will then help the clinician determine the severity of the infection and the presence of end-organ damage (e.g., altered mental status, heart failure due to cardiac function impairment, acute lung injury).

The use and selection of laboratory tests and imaging will depend on the resources available. If a microbiology laboratory is available, direct microscopy and culture of any potential source of infection should be performed. Blood cultures should be collected—ideally before the initiation of antibiotics. However, blood cultures should not delay the initiation of antibiotics. When blood cultures are drawn, two sets should be collected.[20] Invasive procedures such as bronchoscopy, lumbar punctures, thoracentesis, paracentesis, soft tissue aspirations, and biopsies should be performed as indicated and as resources permit to localize the infection. Even if microscopy and cultures are not available, an aggressive search for the source of infection is advised: Finding pus or other signs of infection in a usually sterile body cavity may lead to the implementation of life-saving interventions (placement of chest tube, exploratory laparotomy, drainage of abscesses, appropriate antibiotics for meningitis, etc.) and may narrow the differential diagnosis.

The role of imaging studies in identifying the infection is growing. Ultrasound, computed tomography (CT), and magnetic resonance imaging (MRI) can provide clues to the etiologic pathogen based on radiographic patterns, can identify targets for aspiration or biopsy, and can lead to the timely diagnosis of complications such as bowel ischemia and thrombosis. The selection of the imaging technique will depend on its availability, institutional experience, and clinical scenario.

Although determination of HIV status has not been traditionally included in the workup of patients with sepsis, it may provide important information on potential etiology and prognosis. Bacterial infections are more common and more likely to progress to sepsis among HIV-infected patients than in the general population.[21] Sepsis also carries a higher mortality rate in HIV-infected patients.[22,23] In areas with a high prevalence of HIV infection, HIV testing should be performed during the initial approach to septic patients.

In most developing countries, a peripheral blood smear should be ordered (and repeated) for malaria, although a negative result does not conclusively rule out the diagnosis. Other important tests will vary by region, but rarely provide immediate answers: Dengue serology may be useful for public health purposes, but acute serology may be negative early in disease. Although imperfect and time consuming, blood cultures still remain the best test for typhoid that is widely available, since the commonly used Widal test is not reliable. The diagnosis of many regional causes of sepsis, such as melioidosis, plague, scrub typhus, yellow fever, and leptospirosis, require culture or other diagnostic modalities that either do not produce immediate results or are not available in low-resource settings. Initial diagnosis (and therefore appropriate empiric therapy) of typhoid, melioidosis, dengue, other tropical causes of sepsis, and even malaria rely on syndromic recognition and basic epidemiology rather than laboratory testing.

TREATMENT

The cornerstones of the management of sepsis are:
- Early recognition of the syndrome and identification of the source of infection
- Early initiation of effective antibiotics
- Early fluid resuscitation
- Appropriate referral
- Appropriate hemodynamic and/or ventilator support, when available

Other interventions have also proved to be efficacious in certain populations and will be discussed in this section. However, the fact that the management of sepsis still relies on the early implementation of simple, inexpensive interventions, likely to be available in most healthcare settings, rather than on the use of costly, resource-intensive interventions cannot be overemphasized.

EARLY RECOGNITION OF THE SYNDROME AND IDENTIFICATION OF THE SOURCE OF INFECTION

Sepsis should be considered in any patient with at least two elements of SIRS and a possibility of infection. As mentioned previously, the initial approach to the patient should attempt to confirm the presence of infection and determine its source and etiology. Some patients cannot be successfully treated without removing or draining the site of infection.

Any foreign body known to be the source of the infection should be removed immediately (catheters, prosthetic joints, pacemakers, etc.). Foreign bodies with a high chance of being the source of the infection should also be removed or changed when possible (urinary catheters, central venous access catheters, etc.). Collections of purulent fluid must be drained surgically or by needle aspiration in most situations.

EARLY INITIATION OF EFFECTIVE ANTIBIOTIC

Empiric broad spectrum antibiotics should be started as early as possible. The choice of the empiric regimen should be determined by the suspected pathogen, local epidemiology and resistance patterns, the site of infection, and the host's immune status. Delays in the initiation of antimicrobials and/or the selection of an inappropriate initial regimen have been associated with worse outcomes. Therefore, clinicians should select a regimen that targets the antibiotic sensitivities of the likely pathogens. When choosing the initial antibiotic regimen, clinicians should evaluate the risk for infections caused by resistant bacteria (particularly MRSA, pseudomonas, and resistant gram-negative organisms), fungal infections (particularly candida or endemic fungi), and atypical/infrequent pathogens (rickettsial diseases, melioidosis, malaria, etc.). Similarly, antibiotics that reach appropriate levels at the site of infection should be selected (meningitis, abscesses, etc.).

Once the pathogen has been identified, the antibiotic regimen should be narrowed. Although relatively infrequent, the potential of polymicrobial infections or multiple, concomitant infections (particularly among HIV-infected patients) should be given consideration at the time of narrowing the antibiotics. Although still controversial, there is no evidence supporting the use of bactericidal antibiotics over bacteriostatic antibiotics in sepsis (except in endocarditis). Similarly, there is no evidence to support the use of double coverage for gram-negative infections.

EARLY FLUID RESUSCITATION

All patients with sepsis require fluid resuscitation to maintain an adequate perfusion of the organs. These fluids should be given as boluses with a goal to maintain a mean arterial pressure of $\geq$ 65 mmHg or a systolic blood pressure of $\geq$ 90 mmHg. Given their availability and lower cost, crystalloids are usually the fluid of choice. A bolus of 20 cc/kg of normal saline (approximately 1500 cc for a person that weighs 75 kg) should be administered over no more than 30 minutes. The determination of the need for further resuscitation should be guided by hemodynamic monitoring (preferably with an arterial line and a central venous catheter), and evidence of end-organ perfusion (e.g., urine output > 0.5 ml/kg/hr, mental status). Patients with septic shock average a fluid deficit of 6–10 liters.[24] The same mean arterial blood pressure target applies to children over the age of 2, but the urine output target is higher at > 1 ml/kg/hr. Children differ from adults in that the hypovolemia proportional to body weight may be even greater, and > 60 cc/kg (up to 200 cc/kg!) may safely be given *within the first hour*.

APPROPRIATE REFERRAL

In the lowest-resource settings, referral should be considered as soon as sepsis is identified. Widely disseminated guidelines such as the WHO's (World Health Organization) Integrated Management of Childhood Illness (IMCI) and Integrated Management of Adult Illness (IMAI for HIV-infected adults) help community providers recognize patients who need immediate referral. Where possible, antibiotics and fluids should be given before transfer. The decision to refer is more complicated in intermediate facilities that can provide fluid resuscitation and antibiotics but lack the more advanced modalities that follow. Long transfers without proper equipment or staff may put the patient in greater danger than staying in place.

APPROPRIATE HEMODYNAMIC SUPPORT

Vasopressor therapy should be initiated in any patient that remains hypotensive or develops evidence of pulmonary edema after fluid resuscitation. Ideally, vasopressors should be administered through a central line. The selection of the initial vasopressor remains controversial and, given that the benefits of one vasopressor over another are likely to be marginal, it should be guided by availability. In general, norepinephrine is the vasopressor most commonly recommended for septic shock.[25] The use of low-dose vasopressin offers some theoretical advantages over other vasopressors in septic shock but it has failed to show improvements in mortality in clinical trials.[26,27] Dopamine and epinephrine are likely to be more readily available in resource-limited settings and should be considered excellent alternatives if norepinephrine is not available.[24] Relative to adults, septic children are more likely to have preserved vascular tone, but impaired contractility. Pediatric experts have thus emphasized inotropic support before vasopressor support, a function better served by dopamine and epinephrine than norepinephrine.[28]

VENTILATORY SUPPORT

Respiratory failure and progression to acute respiratory distress syndrome are frequent complications of sepsis. In developed countries, ventilatory support using low tidal volumes has proven to improve survival in patients who develop acute respiratory distress syndrome. However, when mechanical ventilation is available and used in the management of acute respiratory distress syndrome in developing countries, it has been associated with very high mortality.[29] Although the reasons behind this association are unclear, the use of older ventilators and lack of highly trained staff are likely to play a role. Although only useful in patients in the early stages of respiratory failure who are also able to maintain an adequate mental status, noninvasive positive-pressure ventilation has been successfully utilized in developing countries.[30,31]

SPECIAL SCENARIOS

- *Dengue*: Dengue hemorrhagic fever (DHF) and dengue shock syndrome (DSS) are associated with severe but slowly developing capillary leakage. In the right epidemiological scenario, empiric antibiotics for possible bacterial sepsis are not indicated. Appropriate fluid resuscitation is the mainstay of therapy, but because of pulmonary vascular leakage and cardiac dysfunction, guidelines call for less aggressive rescuscitation: 15 cc/kg of crystalloid over the first hour, followed by 10 cc/kg over the second hour, and rescue colloid solutions thereafter.
- *Malaria*: In many ways, severe malaria is not different than sepsis—SIRS and infection coexist. However, some evidence points to less or no hypovolemia (intravascular), and less capillary permeability in malaria when compared to bacterial sepsis. This would argue for more cautious fluid resuscitation.
- *Typhoid*: Empiric therapy often begins with third-generation cephalosporins or azithromycin. Resistance patterns vary by country, and often include fluoroquinolone resistance. In the specific case of typhoid septic shock, corticosteroids (dexamethasone) may reduce mortality but increase the risk of intestinal perforation.
- *Melioidosis*: In Southeast Asia, melioidosis (caused by the bacteria *Burkholderia pseudomallei*) is a relatively common cause of sepsis with fatal outcomes, especially during the rainy season. Ceftazidime or imipenem improve survival as compared to the usual first-line empiric antibiotics for sepsis.
- *Other tropical sepsis syndromes*: Relapsing fever, scrub typhus, plague, or leptospirosis may be regionally and seasonally important pathogens.

In the right place and the right time, one may consider adding doxycy-cline, which is inexpensive and readily available, to the first-line empiric antibiotics for sepsis.

OTHER ADJUNCTIVE THERAPIES

■ DVT prophylaxis

Critically ill patients commonly develop DVT, with rates that vary from 22% to almost 80%, depending on patient characteristics.[32] Ten to thirty percent of medical and surgical intensive care unit (ICU) patients develop DVT within the first week of ICU admission. The use of subcutaneous low-molecular-weight heparin reduced the rate by 50% compared with no prophylaxis. Use of unfractionated heparin appears to decrease the incidence of DVT by only 20%, whereas low-molecular-weight heparin decreases the incidence by a further 30%.[33,34] Both therapies are associated with very low rates of adverse events and complications. Although no rigorous trials evaluating the efficacy of DVT prophylaxis in septic patients have been conducted in developing countries, it seems likely that this intervention will confer similar benefits to this popula-tion. Given its availability and lower cost, the use of unfractionated heparin in most settings is recommended. The use of DVT prophylaxis may be particu-larly beneficial to HIV-infected patients with sepsis given the higher risk for thrombosis among HIV-infected patients.[35]

■ Ulcer prophylaxis

Stress ulcers are a common complication of sepsis leading to upper gas-trointestinal bleeding in up to 1.5% of patients admitted to the ICU.[36] Prophylactic agents with proven benefit include H2-receptor blockers and proton pump inhibitors. Although the use of proton pump inhibitors is con-sidered the gold standard in most developed countries, more extensive data supports the use of H2-receptor blockers for ulcer prophylaxis in sepsis.[37–39] Given the cost, availability, and data supporting their use in sepsis, the use of H2-receptor blocker for ulcer prophylaxis in resource-limited settings is recommended.

■ Glucocorticoids

The use of glucocorticoids in the management of sepsis in developed coun-tries remains controversial. The use of physiologic doses of glucocorticoids for the management of sepsis is based on the assumption that a signifi-cant proportion of critically-ill patients have relative adrenal insufficiency. A meta-analysis showed that patients with septic shock and relative adre-nal insufficiency got a marginal but significant mortality benefit from the administration of physiologic doses of glucocorticoids (hydrocortisone 200 to 300 mg daily for 5–7 days).[40] However, more recent trials have failed to confirm these findings.[41] In some studies, corticosteroids have sped time to resolution of hypotension without giving a clear mortality benefit. In hypoten-sion that is refractory to maximum doses of the available vasopressor (espe-cially if just one vasopressor is available), it may be reasonable to give a trial of physiologic steroid.[40] Pediatric experts continue to recommend steroids for catecholamine-resistant septic shock in children with suspected adrenal insufficiency (e.g., chronic steroid therapy, purpura fulminans), and testing for adrenal insufficiency with a stimulation test, whenever possible.[28]

▄ Intensive insulin therapy

The benefit of intensive insulin therapy (serum glucose maintained between 80–110 mg/dl) was initially proposed after it showed survival benefit in critically ill postoperative surgical patients. However, two subsequent trials on severe septic patients showed no mortality benefit and high rates of severe hypoglycemia (< 40 mg/dl).[42,43] Given the lack of proven survival benefit, high rates of adverse events, and high cost, intensive insulin therapy should not be routinely recommended in resource-limited setting. That said, as it is recommended in resource-rich settings, it would be prudent to maintain a patient's blood glucose below 180 mg/dl, provided the patient's levels are not exceedingly labile.

▄ Renal replacement therapy

Renal replacement therapy is frequently utilized in developed countries to support severely ill patients with acute renal failure. Unfortunately, the cost and availability of this intervention limits its use in resource-limited settings. Recently, some data suggests that high-volume peritoneal dialysis may offer an alternative for the management of patients with acute renal failure in developing countries.[44,45] However, due to the high rates of complications and paucity of data, renal replacement therapy should not be considered standard in the management of sepsis in developing countries.

▄ Drotrecogin alpha (activated protein C)

Activated protein C is a vascular protein that has an important role orchestrating many of the normal regulatory endothelial responses to inflammation. In severe sepsis and septic shock, levels of activated protein C are often reduced, with coincident procoagulation, failure of normal fibrinolysis, leaky capillaries, and other correlates of inflammation. The use of activated protein C as an adjunctive therapy for the management of sepsis was approved based on the results of a single randomized controlled trial, that showed a survival benefit only among the sickest patients (patients with a severity of illness score [APACHE II] greater than 25 within 24 hours of the onset of shock).[46] Two subsequent randomized controlled trials failed to confirm these results and were stopped early on the grounds of futility.[47,48] Given the cost of this drug and the limited data available to support its use in developing countries, its use should be considered only when resources are available and patients fail to respond to other measures.

▄ Transfusion

To improve oxygen carrying capacity, early goal-directed therapy guidelines recommend transfusion for hematocrit < 30 if the SvO_2 < 70 after maximal treatment with fluids and vasopressors. In settings without access to SvO_2 monitoring, one may consider transfusion in anemic patients who fail to improve despite maximal therapy and optimization of measurable parameters, such as MAP, oxygenation, and urine output. Of course, in areas of high HIV prevalence and/or in areas with uncertain safety of the blood supply, one must weigh the potential benefits of transfusion versus the definite risks.

Table 7-2 Recommended Interventions for the Appropriate Management of Sepsis Depending on the Resources Available

Intervention	Very limited resources	Some resources	Considerable resources	Standard of care in developed countries
		Minimal intervention recommended		
Diagnosis and initial approach	• Early recognition • Early referral	• Early recognition • Early referral	• Early recognition • Early referral	• Early recognition
Source control	• Complete clinical assessment and needle drainage of potential collections	• Complete clinical and radiologic assessment and needle or surgical drainage of collections	• Complete clinical and radiologic assessment and needle, surgical, or radiologic drainage of collections	• Complete clinical and radiologic assessment and needle, surgical, or radiologic drainage of collections
Antibiotic therapy	• Early initiation of antibiotics (IV if available)	• Early initiation of IV antibiotics • Gram stain of potential sources	• Early initiation of IV antibiotics • Culture and microscopy of all potential sources • Advanced diagnostics	• Early initiation of IV antibiotics • Culture and microscopy of all potential sources • Advanced diagnostics
Fluid resuscitation	• Fluid challenge (1000 cc over < 30 min) if hypotensive • Oral rehydration if IV fluids not available • Fluid resuscitation guided by urine output and clinical assessment*	• Fluid challenge (1000 cc over < 30 min) if hypotensive • Fluid resuscitation guided by urine output and clinical assessment*	• Fluid challenge • Fluid management guided by central venous monitoring • Electrolyte monitoring and replacement	• Fluid challenge • Fluid management guided by central venous monitoring • Electrolyte monitoring and replacement

Vasopressors	Not applicable	• Epinephrine or dopamine (ideally through central venous access) to maintain MAP > 65	• Central venous access • Continuous arterial pressure monitoring • Norepinephrine or vasopressin to maintain MAP > 60	• Central venous access • Continuous arterial pressure monitoring • Norepinephrine or vasopressin to maintain MAP > 60
Ventilatory support	• Supplemental oxygen when available	• Supplemental oxygen guided by SaO_2 • Noninvasive ventilation (if available)	• Arterial blood gas monitoring • Noninvasive ventilation • Mechanical ventilation	• Arterial blood gas monitoring • Noninvasive ventilation • Mechanical ventilation
Ulcer prophylaxis	• H2-receptor blocker (if available)	• Oral or parenteral H2-receptor blocker	• Parenteral H2-receptor blocker	• Proton pump inhibitor
DVT prophylaxis	• SQ unfractionated heparin (if available)	• SQ unfractionated heparin	• SQ unfractionated or low-weight heparin	• SQ unfractionated or low-weight heparin
Low-dose steroids	Not applicable	Not recommended	Not recommended	
Renal replacement therapy	Not applicable	Peritoneal dialysis (if available)	Peritoneal dialysis, Intermittent HD, or CVVHD	Intermittent HD or CVVHD if unstable
Activated protein C	Not applicable	Not applicable	Not recommended	Recommended for patients with APACHE score > 25

*Recommendation in septic children: Repeated boluses of 20 cc/kg of intravenous crystalloid, usually > 60 cc/kg within the first hour and as much as 200 cc/kg within the first hour if no pulmonary edema.

FURTHER READING

Surviving Sepsis Campaign: http://www.survivingsepsis.org

Cheng AC, West E, Limmathurotsakul D, Peacock S. Strategies to reduce mortality from bacterial sepsis in adults in developing countries. *PLoS Medicine*. 2008;5(8):e175. http://www.plosmedicine.org/article/info:doi/10.1371/journal.pmed.0050175

Dellinger RP, Levy MM, Carlet JM, Bion J, Parker MM, et al. Surviving Sepsis Campaign: International guidelines for management of severe sepsis and septic shock: 2008. *Crit Care Med*. 2008;36:296–327.

Rivers E, Nguyen B, Havstad S, Ressler J, Muzzin A, et al. Early goal-directed therapy in the treatment of severe sepsis and septic shock. *N Engl J Med*. 2001;345:1368–1377.

Brierley J, Carcillo JA, Choong K, et al. Clinical practice parameters for hemodynamic support of pediatric and neonatal septic shock: 2007 update from the American College of Critical Care Medicine. *Crit Care Med*. 2009; 37:666–688.

WHO and UNICEF, Integrated Management of Childhood Illness (IMCI) Chart booklet, 2008, available at http://www.who.int/child_adolescent_health/documents/imci/en/index.html

WHO, Integrated Management of Adult Illness (IMAI), Acute Care Module, WHO/CDS/IMAI/2004.1 Rev. 2, available at http://www.who.int/hiv/pub/imai/primary/en/index.html

REFERENCES

1. Hoyert DL, Anderson RN. Age-adjusted death rates: trend data based on the year 2000 standard population. *Natl Vital Stat Rep*. 2001;49(9):1–6.
2. Angus DC, Linde-Zwirble WT, Lidicker J, Clermont G, Carcillo J, Pinsky MR. Epidemiology of severe sepsis in the United States: analysis of incidence, outcome, and associated costs of care. *Crit Care Med*. 2001;29(7):1303–1310.
3. Cheng AC, West TE, Peacock SJ. Surviving sepsis in developing countries. *Crit Care Med*. 2008;36(8): 2487; Author Reply: 2487–2488.
4. Cheng AC, West TE, Limmathurotsakul D, Peacock SJ. Strategies to reduce mortality from bacterial sepsis in adults in developing countries. *PLoS Med*. 2008;5(8):e175.
5. Surviving Sepsis. http://wwwsurvivingsepsisorg.
6. American College of Chest Physicians/Society of Critical Care Medicine Consensus Conference: definitions for sepsis and organ failure and guidelines for the use of innovative therapies in sepsis. *Crit Care Med*. 1992; 20(6):864–874.
7. Rangel-Frausto MS, Pittet D, Costigan M, Hwang T, Davis CS, Wenzel RP. The natural history of the systemic inflammatory response syndrome (SIRS). A prospective study. *JAMA*. 1995;273(2):117–123.
8. Balk RA. Pathogenesis and management of multiple organ dysfunction or failure in severe sepsis and septic shock. *Crit Care Clin*. 2000;16(2):337–352, vii.

9. Balk RA. Severe sepsis and septic shock. Definitions, epidemiology, and clinical manifestations. *Crit Care Clin*. 2000;16(2):179–192.

10. Rivers E, Nguyen B, Havstad S, Ressler J, Muzzin A, Knoblich B, et al. Early goal-directed therapy in the treatment of severe sepsis and septic shock. *N Engl J Med*. 2001;345(19):1368–1377.

11. Wheeler AP, Bernard GR. Treating patients with severe sepsis. *N Engl J Med*. 1999;340(3):207–214.

12. Bang AT, Bang RA, Baitule SB, Reddy MH, Deshmukh MD. Effect of home-based neonatal care and management of sepsis on neonatal mortality: field trial in rural India. *Lancet*. 1999;354(9194):1955–1961.

13. Levy MM, Fink MP, Marshall JC, Abraham E, Angus D, Cook D, et al. 2001 SCCM/ESICM/ACCP/ATS/SIS International Sepsis Definitions Conference. *Crit Care Med*. 2003;31(4):1250–1256.

14. Bolton CF, Young GB, Zochodne DW. The neurological complications of sepsis. *Ann Neurol*. 1993;33(1):94–100.

15. Papadopoulos MC, Davies DC, Moss RF, Tighe D, Bennett ED. Pathophysiology of septic encephalopathy: a review. *Crit Care Med*. 2000; 28(8):3019–3024.

16. Bleck TP, Smith MC, Pierre-Louis SJ, Jares JJ, Murray J, Hansen CA. Neurologic complications of critical medical illnesses. *Crit Care Med*. 1993; 21(1):98–103.

17. Sprung CL, Peduzzi PN, Shatney CH, Schein RM, Wilson MF, Sheagren JN, et al. Impact of encephalopathy on mortality in the sepsis syndrome. The Veterans Administration Systemic Sepsis Cooperative Study Group. *Crit Care Med*. 1990;18(8):801–806.

18. Angus DC, Wax RS. Epidemiology of sepsis: an update. *Crit Care Med*. 2001;29(7 Suppl):S109–S116.

19. Vincent JL. Sepsis definitions. *Lancet Infect Dis*. 2002;2(3):135.

20. O'Grady NP, Barie PS, Bartlett JG, Bleck T, Carroll K, Kalil AC, et al. Guidelines for evaluation of new fever in critically ill adult patients: 2008 update from the American College of Critical Care Medicine and the Infectious Diseases Society of America. *Crit Care Med*. 2008;36(4):1330–1349.

21. Proctor RA. Bacterial sepsis in patients with acquired immunodeficiency syndrome. *Crit Care Med*. 2001;29(3):683–684.

22. Rosenberg AL, Seneff MG, Atiyeh L, Wagner R, Bojanowski L, Zimmerman JE. The importance of bacterial sepsis in intensive care unit patients with acquired immunodeficiency syndrome: implications for future care in the age of increasing antiretroviral resistance. *Crit Care Med*. 2001; 29(3):548–556.

23. Huang L, Quartin A, Jones D, Havlir DV. Intensive care of patients with HIV infection. *N Engl J Med*. 2006;355(2):173–181.

24. Practice parameters for hemodynamic support of sepsis in adult patients in sepsis. Task Force of the American College of Critical Care Medicine, Society of Critical Care Medicine. *Crit Care Med*. 1999;27(3):639–660.

25. Martin C, Viviand X, Leone M, Thirion X. Effect of norepinephrine on the outcome of septic shock. *Crit Care Med*. 2000;28(8):2758–2765.

26. Landry DW, Levin HR, Gallant EM, Ashton RC, Jr., Seo S, D'Alessandro D, et al. Vasopressin deficiency contributes to the vasodilation of septic shock. *Circulation.* 1997;95(5):1122–1125.

27. Russell JA, Walley KR, Singer J, Gordon AC, Hebert PC, Cooper DJ, et al. Vasopressin versus norepinephrine infusion in patients with septic shock. *N Engl J Med.* 2008;358(9):877–887.

28. Brierley J, Carcillo JA, Choong K, Cornell T, Decaen A, Deymann A, et al. Clinical practice parameters for hemodynamic support of pediatric and neonatal septic shock: 2007 update from the American College of Critical Care Medicine. *Crit Care Med.* 2009;37(2):666–688.

29. Tanriover MD, Guven GS, Sen D, Unal S, Uzun O. Epidemiology and outcome of sepsis in a tertiary-care hospital in a developing country. *Epidemiol Infect.* 2006;134(2):315–322.

30. Hussain SF, Haqqee R, Iqbal J. Non-invasive ventilation in the management of acute respiratory failure in Pakistan. *Trop Doct.* 2004;34(4):238–239.

31. George IA, John G, John P, Peter JV, Christopher S. An evaluation of the role of noninvasive positive pressure ventilation in the management of acute respiratory failure in a developing country. *Indian J Med Sci.* 2007;61(9):495–504.

32. Attia J, Ray JG, Cook DJ, Douketis J, Ginsberg JS, Geerts WH. Deep vein thrombosis and its prevention in critically ill adults. *Arch Intern Med.* 2001;161(10):1268–1279.

33. Cade JF. High risk of the critically ill for venous thromboembolism. *Crit Care Med.* 1982;10(7):448–450.

34. Geerts WH, Jay RM, Code KI, Chen E, Szalai JP, Saibil EA, et al. A comparison of low-dose heparin with low-molecular-weight heparin as prophylaxis against venous thromboembolism after major trauma. *N Engl J Med.* 1996;335(10):701–707.

35. Saif MW, Greenberg B. HIV and thrombosis: a review. *AIDS Patient Care STDS.* 2001;15(1):15–24.

36. Cook DJ, Fuller HD, Guyatt GH, Marshall JC, Leasa D, Hall R, et al. Risk factors for gastrointestinal bleeding in critically ill patients. Canadian Critical Care Trials Group. *N Engl J Med.* 1994;330(6):377–381.

37. Messori A, Trippoli S, Vaiani M, Gorini M, Corrado A. Bleeding and pneumonia in intensive care patients given ranitidine and sucralfate for prevention of stress ulcer: meta-analysis of randomised controlled trials. *BMJ.* 2000;321(7269):1103–1106.

38. Shuman RB, Schuster DP, Zuckerman GR. Prophylactic therapy for stress ulcer bleeding: a reappraisal. *Ann Intern Med.* 1987;106(4):562–567.

39. Cook D, Guyatt G, Marshall J, Leasa D, Fuller H, Hall R, et al. A comparison of sucralfate and ranitidine for the prevention of upper gastrointestinal bleeding in patients requiring mechanical ventilation. Canadian Critical Care Trials Group. *N Engl J Med.* 1998;338(12):791–797.

40. Minneci PC, Deans KJ, Banks SM, Eichacker PQ, Natanson C. Meta-analysis: the effect of steroids on survival and shock during sepsis depends on the dose. *Ann Intern Med.* 2004;141(1):47–56.

41. Sprung CL, Annane D, Keh D, Moreno R, Singer M, Freivogel K, et al. Hydrocortisone therapy for patients with septic shock. *N Engl J Med*. 2008; 358(2):111–124.

42. Van den Berghe G, Wilmer A, Hermans G, Meersseman W, Wouters PJ, Milants I, et al. Intensive insulin therapy in the medical ICU. *N Engl J Med*. 2006;354(5):449–461.

43. Brunkhorst FM, Engel C, Bloos F, Meier-Hellmann A, Ragaller M, Weiler N, et al. Intensive insulin therapy and pentastarch resuscitation in severe sepsis. *N Engl J Med*. 2008;358(2):125–139.

44. Gabriel DP, Caramori JT, Martin LC, Barretti P, Balbi AL. Continuous peritoneal dialysis compared with daily hemodialysis in patients with acute kidney injury. *Perit Dial Int*. 2009;29 Suppl 2:S62–S71.

45. Gabriel DP, Caramori JT, Martim LC, Barretti P, Balbi AL. High volume peritoneal dialysis vs. daily hemodialysis: a randomized, controlled trial in patients with acute kidney injury. *Kidney Int Suppl*. 2008 (108):S87–S93.

46. Bernard GR, Vincent JL, Laterre PF, LaRosa SP, Dhainaut JF, Lopez-Rodriguez A, et al. Efficacy and safety of recombinant human activated protein C for severe sepsis. *N Engl J Med*. 2001;344(10):699–709.

47. Nadel S, Goldstein B, Williams MD, Dalton H, Peters M, Macias WL, et al. Drotrecogin alpha (activated) in children with severe sepsis: a multicentre phase III randomised controlled trial. *Lancet*. 2007;369(9564):836–843.

48. Abraham E, Laterre PF, Garg R, Levy H, Talwar D, Trzaskoma BL, et al. Drotrecogin alpha (activated) for adults with severe sepsis and a low risk of death. *N Engl J Med*. 2005;353(13):1332–1341.

VIII ■ WOMEN'S HEALTH, REPRODUCTIVE HEALTH, AND CONTRACEPTION

Jacqueline Firth, MD, MPH

Women's health topics in the global context include gender rights, violence against women, breast/uterine/cervical malignancy, maternal health, contraception, and reproductive rights. Two millennium development goals specifically address these topics: Goal 3, the promotion of gender equality of women's empowerment; and Goal 5, improving maternal health by 2015 by reducing maternal mortality and providing universal access to reproductive health care.[1] This chapter will specifically focus on maternal health and contraception.

It is estimated that over 500,000 women die annually during pregnancy or childbirth.[2] More than 80% of maternal deaths worldwide are due to five causes: hemorrhage, sepsis, unsafe abortion, obstructed labor, and hypertensive disease of pregnancy.[1] Complications of labor can also be devastating. Vaginal fistulas and incontinence following birth trauma are difficult to treat and the affected women are often ostracized from their families and communities. Women in developing countries are particularly at risk for complications when they do not have access to prenatal care or trained birth attendants. Early age at first pregnancy and lack of access and empowerment to choose contraception exacerbates these factors.

Over 200 million women who want to delay or avoid childbearing lack access to safe and effective methods of contraception.[1] Eighty million unintended pregnancies worldwide result in 42 million induced abortions and 34 million unintended births.[3] Of these, 19 million unsafe abortions are conducted in the developing world, resulting in 68,000 deaths.[1] Some sources estimate that more than 55% of abortions in developing countries are unsafe.[4]

Demand for contraception is growing, and contraceptive use among married women in less developed countries has increased from 9% in the 1960s to over 60% in the late 1990s.[5] In the developing world, 268 million women are using some form of reversible birth control that requires trained providers and regular continuous supplies, as opposed to surgical options and intra-uterine devices (IUDs).[6] Some estimate that over US $7.1 billion per year is spent on family planning services in the developing world (as of 2003).[6] Health providers practicing in developing countries should familiarize themselves with locally available methods of contraception, their cost, and their side effect profiles.

CONTRACEPTION AND MATERNAL HEALTH

Table 8-1 Contraceptive Methods

Method	Non-contraceptive benefits	Absolute Contraindications* *Disadvantages in italics*	Failure rate ideal use *(typical use)*

Combined Oral Contraceptive Pills (OCPs)	• Regular menses
	• Decreased menstrual flow
	• Decreased acne
	• Decreased endometriosis
	• Decreased risk of:
	  ◦ Ovarian CA/cysts
	  ◦ Endometrial CA
	  ◦ Fibrocystic changes of the breast
	  ◦ Dysmenorrhea
	  ◦ Ectopic pregnancy
		• Smoker > 35 years;
		• Uncontrolled HTN;
		• H/O stroke, TIA, CAD;
		• Thrombotic disorder; h/o VTE
		• DM w/end organ damage, other cardiovascular risk factors;
		• Migraine w/focal neurological symptoms;
		• Breast or endometrial CA;
		• Hepatic adenoma/CA;
		• Severe cirrhosis
			3 per 1,000 patients per year *(8% for typical use)*

Micronor	• No ↓ breast milk • Decreased dysmenorrhea and menstrual flow • Preferred for smokers	• Undiagnosed vaginal bleeding • *Irregular bleeding* • *Can increase acne and ovarian cysts* • *Must use at same time daily*	5 per 1,000 patients per year *(8% typical use)*
Ortho Evra	• Compliance weekly • Cycle regularity • Noncontraceptive benefits as OCPs	• Same OCP contraindications • *Unrecognized detachment* • *Skin irritation* • *Increased VTE risk*	3 per 1,000 pts per year *(8% typical use)*
NuvaRing (etonogestrel/ ethinyl estradiol vaginal ring)	• Less nausea than OCPs • Same noncontraceptive benefits as OCPs • Lasts for 3 weeks	• Contraindications same as OCPs • *Requires vaginal insertion/removal* • *No STD protection* • *Unrecognized ring loss*	3 per 1,000 patients per year *(8% typical use)*
Condoms	• STD protection • Readily available • No delay in fertility once discontinued	• *Less spontaneity* • *Can break or fall off* • *Can decrease sexual sensitivity*	2% ideal failure rate *(15% typical failure rate)*
Diaphragm	• No delay in fertility once discontinued • Can remain in place for 4–5 hours	• *Requires vaginal insertion* • *Less spontaneity* • *Physician visit for fitting* • ↑ *Vaginal/bladder infections*	6% ideal failure rate *(16% typical failure rate)*

(Continues)

Table 8-1 Contraceptive Methods (Continued)

Method	Non-contraceptive benefits	Absolute Contraindications* *Disadvantages in italics*	Failure rate ideal use (typical use)
Natural Family Planning	• Free • No side effects • Self awareness	• *Requires motivation* • *No STD protection* • *Periodic abstinence*	2–9% ideal use (25% typical use)
Spermicide	• Readily available • Some ↓ STD risk	• *Nonoxynol 9 may increase HIV transmission* • *High failure rate* • *Less spontaneity*	18% ideal use (29% typical use)
Implanon (etonogestrel implant)	• 4 cm implant. Lasts 3 years • ↓ bleeding, anemia, dysmenorrhea & HA	• Irregular bleeding • *Insertion requires training*	0.2% ideal failure rate
Intrauterine Device (IUD) Mirena (M) ParaGard (P)	• Prolonged efficacy ○ 5 yr–Mirena ○ 10 yr–ParaGard • Decreased menstrual flow (Mirena) • Decreased dysmenorrhea (Mirena) • Lactation not disturbed • Fewer ectopic pregnancies	• Uterine anomalies; active PID; postpartum endometritis or septic abortion in last 3 mo; uterine or ovarian or cervical cancer; unresolved abnormal pap smear; genital bleeding of unknown etiology; AIDS; high risk sexual behavior; genital infection; cirrhosis; history of ectopic pregnancy. **(Only Mirena)** acute hepatitis **or** hepatoma **or** breast cancer	**ParaGard:** 0.6% ideal use (0.8% typical use) **Mirena:** 0.1% ideal use (0.1% typical use)
Tubal ligation (TL)	• Permanent • No compliance needed	• Ambiguous about decision • *High initial cost* • *Risks of surgery* • *No STD protection* • *Post-TL regret*	0.5% ideal failure rate (0.5% typical failure rate)
Vasectomy (V)	• Permanent • Office procedure	• Ambiguous about decision • *Sexual dysfunction* • *Anxiety about their virility* • *High initial cost* • *No STD protection* • *Post-vasectomy regret*	0.1% ideal failure rate (0.15% typical failure rate)
Medroxy-progesterone acetate	• Quarterly injections • ↓ sickle cell crises, PID risk, endometrial CA **and** ovarian cysts	• Undiagnosed vaginal bleeding • Breast CA • Liver disease or tumor • H/O stroke or CAD • DM with end-organ disease	0.3% ideal failure rate (3% typical failure rate)

(Continues)

Table 8-1 Contraceptive Methods (Continued)

Method	Non-contraceptive benefits	Absolute Contraindications* Disadvantages in italics	Failure rate ideal use (typical use)
Essure	• Hysteroscopic sterilization • Office procedure • No change in menses	• *Hysterosalpingogram needed 3 months after procedure* • *More than 1 procedure is required*	0.5% ideal failure rate
Plan B (levo-norgestrel)	• Emergency contraception • Can take within 72 hrs of unprotected sex • ↓ side effects vs OCP • Take 2 tablets (0.75 mg each) × 1	• *Less available than OCPs* • *Spotting is common* • *Not as readily available in some states*	1.1% ideal failure rate

CA = cancer, STD = sexually transmitted disease, VTE = venous thromboembolic event, PID = pelvic inflammatory disease, trans. = transmission and poss. = possible, wt = weight, d/o = disorder, IUP = intrauterine pregnancy, TIA = transient ischemic attack, CVA = stroke, CAD = coronary artery disease

*Pregnancy and history of hypersensitivity is contraindication to all methods except natural family planning

Reference: Managing Contraception, 2007 ed., available at www.managingcontraception.com and Esherick JS. *Tarascon Primary Care Pocketbook*. 3rd ed. Sudbury, MA: Jones and Bartlett Publishers; 2010:55–56.

Table 8-2 Worldwide Fertility, Contraceptive Use, and Maternal Mortality by Region[7]

Region	Births per 1000 population	Average # children per family	% Married women using modern contraception	Lifetime risk of dying from maternal causes, 1 in
Latin America	21	2.5	64%	290
Eastern Europe	11	1.4	44%	3500
Sub-Saharan Africa	40	5.4	16%	22
Asia	19	2.4	61%	120
US	14	2.1	68%	4800

• Approximate prices are given for the Indian market as India supplies many other developing countries with pharmaceuticals and condoms. Many of these methods are heavily subsidized by governments, often with international assistance (e.g., the female condom is subsidized by the Government of India to cost only $0.10, especially for female commercial sex workers).[13]

Table 8-3 Usage and Cost of Contraceptive Methods in the Developing World

Type of contraceptive (overall % among contraceptive users[d])	Specific type/name	Percentage of use by region[g]			Approximate cost in India* (manufacturing cost)
		LAm	SsA	Asia	
Sterilization (29–39%)	Tubal ligation (female)	43.4%	6.5%	42.1%	$22.20–$155[9]
	Vasectomy (male)	2.2%	0.3%	5.1%	Less than tubal[9]
IUD (20%)	Copper IUD	9.9%	2.9%	22.8%	$2.75–$5.50 ($0.25)[10]
Hormonal Oral Contraceptives (12%)	Many different combinations	18.1%	18.6%	8.2%	$0.78–$4.90/cycle ($0.01 each)[10]
Nonhormonal oral contraceptive	Ormeloxifene 30 mg (Centchroman—SERM)	Limited use in LDCs			$0.80/cycle[10]
Emergency contraception	Hormonal OCP sold in two-pill packet	Available in 140 countries, OTC in 44[11]			$0.45 ($0.01)[10]
Injectable hormonal contraceptive (8%)	Medroxyprogesterone acetate (Depo-Provera)	6.3%	25.7%	5.8%	$3.80/each ($0.83)[10]
Barrier (5–7%)	Male condom	7%	8.3%	6.5%	$0.10–$0.19 each[12]
	Female condom	Limited use in LDCs			$2.80 ($1.00)[13]
Induced abortion (rate/1000 women 15–44 yrs[f])	Dilation and curettage (D&C) or vacuum extraction (surgical abortion)	31	29	29	$10–$23.50[14]
	mifepristone/misoprostol (medical abortifacients)	Limited use in LDCs			$23.30[15]

*Approximate conversion of Rupees to Dollars (US $): US $1; Dollars = R4S; US $1; IUD = Intra-Uterine Device; LAm = Latin America; SsA = Sub-Saharan Africa, LDCs = Less Developed Countries; OTC = Over the Counter (i.e., not requiring a doctor's prescription).

SPECIAL CONSIDERATIONS FOR DEVELOPING COUNTRIES

- Cost/pricing of contraceptives:
  - Developing world manufacturers of pharmaceuticals and medical devices/condoms are growing to meet the needs of their own populations and those of other developing countries with generic products.[10]
  - India in particular has a strong pharmaceutical industry that supplies much of the developing world's medications, including contraceptives; however, 80% of Indian couples opting for contraception choose male or female sterilization,[10] likely related to the government incentive program (more information follows).
- Government support for family planning:
  - Many developing countries, recognizing the financial burden of larger families and unintended pregnancies on society, heavily subsidize family planning programs and receive international funding to provide contraceptive commodities.
  - Some heavily populated countries even offer financial incentives for longer-lasting methods of contraception. In India, the national government gives money to each state for the following: R300 (US $7.50) per tubal ligation procedure, R200 (US $5) per vasectomy, and R20 (US $0.50) per IUD insertion.[16] Tubal ligations and vasectomies are then provided to qualifying members of the population at no charge.

TIPS ON STARTING PATIENTS ON CONTRACEPTIVES

- Ensure that the patient (and partner, if involved in the decision) are aware of all the available options including their efficacy, side effects, advantages, disadvantages, and costs.
- Obtain a full personal and family medical history, including history of breast or gynecological cancers, coagulation disorders, or blood clots.
- Ensure that the patient is not currently pregnant, infected with a sexually transmitted infection (STI) or smoking (if the patient is a smoker, educate patient regarding risks and consider a nonhormonal form of contraception).
- Do a baseline vitals check and physical exam, paying particular attention to blood pressure and breast abnormalities.
- Have the patient start oral contraceptives on the first day of the next period or on a convenient day close to the start of the period (for example, the Sunday after menses start).
- IUDs are generally placed during menstruation as the cervix is more open and insertion will be less painful, although there is a slightly higher risk of expulsion of the device because the os is open. Additionally, they can be placed immediately after dilation and curettage (D&C).

- Have the patient return 2 weeks after beginning any hormonal form of contraception for a blood pressure check.
- Ensure that the patient receiving injectable contraception understands the date on which she must return for the next dose, and the risk of pregnancy if she delays. Continue monitoring blood pressure and weight gain at these subsequent visits, even if the patient is seen only by a nurse.

POSSIBLE COMPLICATIONS OF CONTRACEPTIVE USE

- Elevated blood pressures (with hormonal contraceptives)
- Deep vein thrombosis (with estrogen-containing contraceptives)
- Headaches
- Irregular or absent menses (occasionally with breakthrough bleeding)
- Weight gain (especially with injectables)
- Decreased sexual libido or change in mood
- Rare incidents of endometritis or pelvic inflammatory disease (PID) with IUDs (usually due to STI prior to or within 20 days after placement of device)

FURTHER READING

Planned Parenthood—programs in 17 countries outside the United States—http://www.plannedparenthood.org
United Nations Population Fund (UNFPA): http://www.unfpa.org
Alan Guttmacher Institute: http://www.guttmacher.org
Population Reference Bureau: http://www.prb.org
CDC Reproductive Health Surveys: http://www.cdc.gov/Reproductivehealth/Surveys/index.htm

REFERENCES

1. United Nations. Millennium Development Goal 5: Improve Maternal Health Facts Sheet, September 25, 2008. http://www.un.org/millenniumgoals/ 2008highlevel/pdf/newsroom/Goal%205%20FINAL.pdf. Accessed July 12, 2009.
2. United Nations Population Fund. 2008. UNFPA Annual Report. New York, UNFPA. 2008. http://www.unfpa.org/about/report/2008/en/pdf/UNFPA_Annual_Report_2008.pdf. Accessed July 12, 2009.
3. Wulf D, Hollander D, Johnson J, Henshaw S, Bankole A, Haas T, Singh S. New York and Washington: Alan Guttmacher Institute. 1999. www.guttmacher.org/pubs/sharing.pdf. Accessed July 21, 2009.
4. Sedgh G, Henshaw S, Singh S, Ahman E, Shah I. Induced abortion: estimated rates and trends worldwide. *Lancet*. 2007;370:1338–1345.
5. Haub C, Herstad B. Family planning worldwide 2002 datasheet. 2002. Washington, DC. Population Reference Bureau. http://www.prb.org/pdf/FamPlanWorldwide_Eng.pdf. Accessed July 14, 2009.

6. Singh S, Darroch J, Vlassoff M, Nadeau J. 2003. Adding it up: the benefits of investing in sexual and reproductive health care. New York and Washington: Alan Guttmacher Institute and UNFPA. http://www.guttmacher.org/pubs/addingitup.pdf. Accessed July 12, 2009.

7. Reprinted with permission from Haub C, Kent MM. 2008. World population data sheet 2008. Washington, DC: Population Reference Bureau. http://www.prb.org/Publications/Datasheets/2008/2008wpds.aspx. Accessed July 12, 2009.

8. Seiber E, Bertrand J, Sullivan T. Changes in Contraceptive Method Mix in Developing Countries. *Int Fam Plann Perspect.* 2007;33(3):117–123.

9. Lionel J. Personal communication with Dr. Jessie Lionel, Associate Professor of Obstetrics and Gynecology at Christian Medical College, India. Vellore, Tamil Nadu, India. July 21, 2009.

10. Beer K, Armand F. 2006. Assessment of India's locally manufactured contraceptive product supply. Bethesda, Maryland: Private Sector Partnerships-One Project, Abt Associates. http://pdf.usaid.gov/pdf_docs/PNADF989.pdf. Accessed July 14, 2009.

11. International Consortium for Emergency Contraception. 2009. Availability of emergency contraception. http://www.cecinfo.org/index.php. Accessed July 26, 2009.

12. Hindustan LLC. http://www.moodsplanet.com. Accessed July 19, 2009.

13. Indo-Asian News Service. 2006. Hindustan Latex launches first female condom. *Times of India.* May 6, 2006.

14. Duggal R, Barge S. 2004. Abortion services in India: Report of a multi-centric enquiry. Mumbai: Center for Enquiry into Health and Allied Themes (CEHAT) and Health watch. http://www.cehat.org/go/uploads/AapIndia/national.pdf. Accessed July 12, 2009.

15. Srinivasan S. 2003. Problem pill. *The Tribune Online Edition.* http://www.tribuneindia.com/2003/20031123/herworld.htm#3. Accessed July 19, 2009.

16. Department of Health and Family Welfare, Government of India. 2008. Manual for Family Planning Insurance Scheme. http://mohfw.nic.in/dofw%20website/FP_Manual_2008-Final.pdf. Accessed July 15, 2009.

IX ■ HIV/AIDS IN THE DEVELOPING WORLD

Premal Patel, MD, MSc
Matthew Dacso, MD, MSc
Nicola Zetola, MD, MPH

INTRODUCTION

Since the 1980s, the term *global health* has been nearly synonymous with the HIV/AIDS pandemic. Thirty years following the discovery of HIV/AIDS, hundreds of organizations, thousands of healthcare workers, and billions of dollars are committed to HIV/AIDS research and clinical practice. In 2008 alone, over $8.7 billion were committed to the funding, prevention, diagnosis, and treatment of HIV in low- and middle-income countries.[1]

The past three decades have seen numerous achievements. Many national governments have developed country-specific HIV/AIDS guidelines in parallel with the World Health Organization's (WHO) standards (though implementation is often fraught with challenges). Non-governmental organizations (NGOs) and local organizations are active in promoting the rights of people living with HIV as well as encouraging destigmatization. Many people living with HIV have become outspoken regarding issues of education, policy, legislation, and advocacy.

Though the mobilization of support and funds for global HIV/AIDS issues has been unparalleled to any other disease in our lifetimes, the disparities between the developed and developing world have only worsened. The global burden of disease provides staggering statistics: by 2007, HIV had infected 59 million people and claimed the lives of an estimated 35 million.[3,2] At that time, 33 million people were living with HIV with over 22 million of those residing in sub-Saharan Africa (SSA), comprising 67% of all patients in the world with HIV. Of the 2 million children affected, 1.8 million were from SSA. In 2007 alone, HIV/AIDS claimed the lives of 2 million people worldwide (1.5 million of those in SSA) and at the same time 2.5 million individuals were diagnosed with new infections. HIV/AIDS has torn apart families and orphaned 15 million children.[4] The burden of disease has disproportionately fallen on resource-limited countries in the regions of SSA and South and Southeast Asia.[3]

INEQUALITIES

A gap between the developed and developing world has emerged. In certain regions of developed countries, knowledge regarding prevention, availability of diagnostics/treatment for HIV, and public awareness have all resulted in a decreased incidence of HIV infection Mortality has decreased, life expectancy has increased, and in many ways the management of HIV has become that of a chronic illness. In some non-resource poor settings, policy makers are even calling for an end to AIDS exceptionalism as HIV/AIDS competes for healthcare funding with diseases of greater incidence and mortality such as cancer and heart disease.[4]

Meanwhile, the developing world has not enjoyed similar results. Though many organizations and programs such as the Gates Foundation, the President's Emergency Program for AIDS Relief (PEPFAR), UNAIDS, and various NGOs are providing funding and advocating the targets exemplified in the Millennium Development Goals (MDGs), the HIV pandemic continues to claim millions of lives a year. HIV is reducing life expectancy in meaningful ways in heavily affected regions.[3] Only 31% of HIV positive individuals in middle- to low-income countries received Highly Active AntiRetroviral Therapy (HAART) in 2007 and over 9.7 million people still await treatment.[2]

Numerous obstacles contribute to the aforementioned inequalities. In resource-limited settings, external donor funding is necessary but not sufficient to expand and sustain HIV/AIDS programs. Ineffective or inadequate healthcare infrastructure, excess bureaucracy, lack of political will, and a scarcity of healthcare workers are often cited as obstacles to building capacity. Despite the augmentation in donor funding for HIV/AIDS-related activities, testing for HIV and access to HAART remains a barrier to effective care. On the community level, social and cultural factors are of extreme importance and often result in stigmatization and discrimination.

HIV is a social disease—violence, education, poverty, and asymmetric gender relationships are at the heart of the pandemic. Marginalized groups are disproportionately affected. Violence and conflict create special circumstances that exacerbate both international and local inequalities. Complex emergencies, resulting from political instability, ethnic tension, civil/international war, or lack of entitlements (in the case of famine), impose pressures on the population. Migration, whether forced or voluntary, can transform individuals into refugees and internally displaced persons (IDPs) overnight. The interactions among migration, poverty, and sexual violence can disrupt social norms and kinship patterns, producing easier avenues for virus transmission.

Women are especially vulnerable and account for well over 50% of cases worldwide.[2] Numerous community-specific social factors play a role in their experience including sexual violence, oppressive societal norms, limited control over their sexual life, lack of reproductive rights, and inferior status in society.

Children are a particularly vulnerable group as they are dependent upon adult caregivers for testing and treatment. Many caregivers are also infected and ultimately succumb to the virus, leaving children susceptible to poverty and premature death. In addition, many HIV-infected children face unique medical challenges such as malnutrition and impaired growth and development.

PATHOGENESIS

HIV is an RNA retrovirus with a predilection for CD4+ lymphocytes. By importing a reverse transcriptase, HIV can transcribe its RNA into DNA, which directs viral replication. The virus escapes detection by directing its activities within the host cell's nucleus. CD4 (helper) T-cells stimulate both cell-mediated and humoral immunity. As HIV replication occurs over time, the CD4 cells are destroyed and cell-mediated immunity is impaired. The subsequent immune dysfunction increases the risk for opportunistic infections and certain malignancies. Paradoxically, there is also an immune *activation* phenomenon that predisposes HIV-infected individuals to conditions associated with a hyperinflammatory state. For that reason, myocardial infarction, stroke, and venous thromboembolism may be seen with greater frequency in the HIV population. HIV is also highly adaptable and capable of developing mutations that confer resistance to certain antiretroviral medications.

MODES OF TRANSMISSION

HIV is transmitted by direct contact with blood and/or bodily fluids. The most common routes of transmission are via sexual contact, needle use, and mother to child. Any sexual contact can lead to infection, though unprotected receptive anal intercourse has the highest risk of transmission, followed by receptive vaginal penetration. Burden of virus, sexually transmitted co-infection, and the presence of mucosal ulcers or lesions elevate the risk of transmission. In the intravenous drug abuse population, HIV infection commonly occurs from sharing contaminated needles. Similarly, reusing needles in a healthcare setting also confers risk. Improved blood screening techniques have drastically reduced the incidence of HIV acquired from blood transfusions. With regard to infants and children, the transmission of HIV can occur at various times during pregnancy, at delivery, or after birth with breastfeeding.

STAGES/ NATURAL COURSE

The natural progression of untreated HIV follows six stages: viral transmission, acute HIV infection, seroconversion, symptomatic HIV infection, symptomatic HIV/AIDS, and death.[5] In developed countries, the average time course from initial infection to death is approximately 10 years, but with wide individual variation (from < 3 to > 30 years). Data from developing countries is sparse, but suggests a much shorter time course (possibly related to the high prevalence of other infectious agents such as tuberculosis).

Following transmission, the virus gains entry into CD4 cells via recognition and attachment to gp41 and gp120 surface proteins as well as other coreceptors. An acute retroviral syndrome, which is often mistaken for an influenza-like illness, may occur 3 to 4 weeks following viral transmission. Prior to antibody formation, the only evidence of infection at this time may be a detectable HIV viral load (VL). During this stage, the virus replicates, spreads, and CD4 counts start to decline. *Patients are most infectious during this replication stage and may only manifest flu-like symptoms.* Viral load, which is initially high, declines and stabilizes at a new set point. As antibodies form against the virus, a brief "recovery" of CD4 count occurs. The next phase is clinical latency, which is marked by a relative lack of overt symptoms. Though the patient is asymptomatic, this phase is accompanied by a steady increase in VL and subsequent drop in CD4 count. Symptomatic HIV infection includes a wide range of conditions and complications not meeting criteria for AIDS. AIDS typically occurs when the CD4 count reaches < 200/mm^3 (<14% or AIDS defining category). Severe immunodeficiency results in increased risk of opportunistic infections and malignancies. The precipitous rise in VL and decline in CD4 count characterizes this stage. Advanced AIDS occurs as CD4 falls < 50/mm^3 and is associated with high mortality.[6]

CLINICAL SIGNS AND SYMPTOMS

The clinical signs and symptoms will differ depending on the stage of HIV, specific complications, and opportunistic infections that are present. HIV affects virtually every organ system. A detailed sexual history should be obtained and HIV risk factors assessed. In all regions of the world, there should be a low threshold for considering and testing for HIV, even for atypical presentations.

ACUTE RETROVIRAL SYNDROME

The acute retroviral syndrome occurs 3–4 weeks after viral transmission and, *in most cases is asymptomatic.* Among the patients presenting with symptoms, the acute retroviral syndrome is often dismissed as an influenza or infectious mononucleosis-like illness. From a clinical perspective, the presence and severity of symptoms during this acute phase correlates with a more rapid progression of disease during the chronic phase of the HIV infection. Acute retroviral syndrome is usually associated with nonspecific symptoms such as fever, chills, rash, weight loss, nausea, vomiting, diarrhea, ulcers, malaise, pharyngitis, lymphadenopathy, myalgia, arthralgia, and headache. Fever is the most common presenting symptom occurring in 97% of symptomatic patients.[6] A maculopapular rash has been noted in 77% of symptomatic patients especially on the face and trunk but it can also affect the palms and soles.[6] The physical exam should be thorough with special attention to the presence of fever, skin exam for rash, lymphadenopathy, and oropharynx exam for thrush or pharyngitis.[5] Symptoms of fever with headache, nuchal rigidity, or altered mental status could represent aseptic meningitis from acute HIV infection.

The period surrounding the acute retroviral syndrome is one of extremely high infectivity. It is believed that most transmissions of HIV take place during this period.[7] *From a public health perspective, there should be a low threshold to counsel regarding safe sex measures and testing patients with these symptoms as they are most infectious during this time.*

The following symptoms should raise suspicion for acute retroviral syndrome and necessitate immediate testing:

- flu-like symptoms
- fever
- new dermatologic findings
- headache
- lymphadenopathy
- genital ulcers

DIAGNOSIS

Patients with recent exposure to HIV should always receive an antibody test first, though false negative antibody testing can occur if seroconversion has not taken place. If there is a high clinical suspicion for HIV and the ELISA is negative, an HIV RNA PCR or fourth generation ELISA should be used, as acute HIV is associated with a high VL. The sensitivity of HIV RNA PCR is 95–98%.[6]

Antibody testing is the standard screening test for HIV. Antibodies are usually present at 6–8 weeks after acquisition of HIV, though 50% of patients will be positive within 3–4 weeks.[6] Antibody testing has a 99% sensitivity rate. There are different types of enzyme-linked immunosorbent assays (ELISAs), the newer of which are able to detect antibodies at earlier intervals. The types of ELISAs used worldwide vary in their abilities to detect HIV-1 and HIV-2 as well.

The rapid HIV is an antibody test that makes results available in 20 minutes or fewer. Samples can be from blood (whole or plasma) or oral mucosa exudate. In situations that require quick decisions, such as during birth or after a needle stick, the rapid HIV test may be preferred.

The CDC recommends screening for HIV with a conventional ELISA or rapid HIV test. If the initial test is positive, it is confirmed by performing a more specific western blot, which uses electrophoresis to identify HIV-specific glycoproteins (such as p24 and gp41). A positive Western blot confirms HIV. In the case of an intermediate Western blot, a VL is performed to assess whether HIV virus particles are present.[5] Western blot technology is not readily available in many parts of the world, so the WHO guidelines recommend drawing two ELISAs instead, either in sequence or in parallel. Two positive ELISAs confirm the diagnosis of HIV. In some countries, two rapid tests are performed instead. Discordant studies are repeated at regular intervals.

Specific guidelines for the diagnosis of HIV vary greatly between countries. State-sponsored HIV programs may have different preferences and limitations.

PRETEST AND POSTTEST COUNSELING

Ideally, pretest and posttest counseling should be performed at the point of care. Pretest counseling provides an opportunity to identify HIV risk factors, promote awareness, and encourage behavioral modification. Patients should be screened for other sexually transmitted infections (STIs) such as herpes, syphilis, chlamydia and gonorrhea,. Assessing social support and identifying impediments to treatment are crucial. Patients should also be assured that all testing and diagnoses are strictly confidential.

A patient whose test returns negative should be counseled on reducing HIV risk factors. For those found to be HIV positive, assessing baseline understanding of HIV is important. A new diagnosis of HIV should be accompanied by education on HIV as well as safe sex practices, the need for laboratory and symptom surveillance, and most importantly, the treatable nature of the disease. Any possible obstacles to adherence should be identified.

Social support in the form of a clinic, hospital, support group, or family member/friend facilitates improved outcomes. Disclosure should be culture- and age-appropriate. The issue of disclosure is complicated and should be directed by the patient on his or her own terms. Discordant couples may require extra counseling. Every effort to reduce stigma and discrimination should be attempted.

STAGING OF HIV

Once the diagnosis of HIV is made, staging is the next step. The WHO classification system is generally utilized in resource-restricted regions. In high-income countries, the staging of HIV and decision to initiate HAART both rely heavily on laboratory testing that may not be available in many parts of the world. For resource-limited settings, the WHO has developed a clinical staging system based on symptoms. This staging system does not rely on CD4 count or VL and serves as the international standard of care in many countries where laboratory testing is not readily available. (See Appendix 1 for WHO staging for adults and children.) The new 2009 Rapid Advice Revision to the WHO HIV guidelines emphasizes the need for patients to have CD4 monitoring.

TREATMENT

INDICATIONS FOR ANTIRETROVIRAL TREATMENT

The decision to initiate HAART can be based solely on clinical stage, but CD4 count (if available) should be used in conjunction with clinical staging to guide treatment decisions.

Current recommendations for the initiation of HAART have recently changed in both the developing and developed world with the new 2009 revisions to the WHO and DHHS guidelines respectively. It is important to be familiar with both the new and old guidelines as many countries may lack the resources to implement these changes. Prior to December 2009, the recommendation through the industrialized world was to initiate antiretroviral therapy at CD4 counts < 350/mm^3 to decrease VL, reduce susceptibility to opportunistic infections/malignancies, and mitigate long-term complications. The US Department of Health and Human Services (DHHS), International AIDS Society (IAS-USA), Centers for Disease Control and Prevention (CDC), and all European nations previously recommended initiation of HAART before the CD4 count falls below 350/mm³. However, the new 2009 United States DHHS guidelines are more far-reaching by recommending HAART for any patient with a CD4 below 500/mm³. While these recommendations will become mainstream in the United States, most practitioners in the developing world follow WHO and country-specific guidelines.

The new Revised 2009 WHO guidelines also reflect the trend towards earlier initiation of HAART. The 2009 and older 2006 WHO clinical and immunologic guidelines for initiating therapy are found in Table 9-1a and b. According to the 2009 WHO revised guidelines, the following individuals meet criteria for the initiation of HAART:

Any patients who meet classification of WHO Clinical Stage 3 or 4 regardless of CD4 value or CD4 < 350/mm³ (CD4<200 in the 2006 WHO guidelines) irrespective of clinical staging. Ideally patients should have access to CD4 and VL monitoring as needed.

TREATMENT STRATEGY

The treatment of HIV is complex and involves consideration of individual, medical, social, and economic factors. Comprehensive counseling regarding the significance of HIV is essential to empowering patients who are infected. Screening for ongoing risk factors such as commercial sex work, domestic

Table 9-1a 2006 WHO Clinical and Immunologic Guidelines for Initiating Therapy

WHO Clinical staging	CD4 testing not available	CD4 testing available
1	Do not treat	Treat if CD4 count is below 200/mm³ ª
2	Do not treat ᵇ	
3	Treat	Consider treatment if CD4 count is below 350/mm³ ª,ᶜ,ᵈ and initiate antiretroviral therapy (ART) before CD4 count drops below 200/mm³ ᵉ
4	Treat	Treat irrespective of CD4 cell count ª

Adapted from World Health Organization. Antiretroviral Therapy for HIV infection in adults and adolescents. Geneva, Switzerland: WHO. 2006.

ªCD4 count is advisable to assist with determining the need for immediate therapy in situations such as pulmonary TB and severe bacterial infections, which can occur at any CD4 level

ᵇA total lymphocyte count (TLC) of 1200/mm³ or less may be substituted for the CD4 count when a CD4 count is not available and mild HIV disease exists. It is not useful in asymptomatic patients. Thus, in the absence of CD4 cell counts and TLCs, patients with WHO adult clinical stage 2 should not be treated

ᶜThe initiation of ART is recommended in all HIV-infected pregnant women with WHO clinical stage 3 disease and CD4 counts below 350/mm³

ᵈThe initiation of ART is recommended for all HIV-infected patients with CD4 counts below 350/mm³ and pulmonary TB or severe bacterial infections

ᵉThe precise CD4 cell level above 200/mm³ at which ARV treatment should be started has not been established

Table 9-1b 2009 Revision to WHO HIV Guidelines

WHO Clinical staging	CD4 testing not available	CD4 testing available
1	Do not treat	Treat if CD4 count is below 350/mm³
2	Do not treat	
3	Treat	Treat irrespective of CD4 cell count
4	Treat	Treat irrespective of CD4 cell count

abuse, multiple sexual partners, sexually transmitted infections, and intravenous drug abuse should take place on a regular basis. Those in relationships will need counseling regarding reducing the risk of transmission through safe sex techniques. Often, HIV is associated with malnutrition and wasting—multivitamins and encouragement of nutrition are crucial parts of a comprehensive treatment strategy. Prevention of opportunistic infections (OIs) using such methods as the initiation of co-trimoxazole, even where HAART is not available, can affect mortality. Finally, initiation of treatment and ARV selection will depend on each country's particular guidelines.

Generally, HIV treatment involves the following elements:
1. Counseling regarding risk factors and prevention of transmission
2. Nutritional optimization and encouragement of a healthy diet
3. Evaluation of risk factors for nonadherence
4. Initiating an appropriate HAART regimen
5. Providing prophylaxis and treatment of OIs or malignancies
6. Monitoring response to HAART treatment
7. Management of side effects and interactions of ARVs
8. Managing HIV complications and co-infections

Treatment regimens often depend on country guidelines, the presence of international organizations, and available pharmaceuticals. Single-drug therapy has long been known to breed resistance, so ARV regimens utilize a complimentary combination of drugs and classes. The types of ARVs most widely utilized are nucleoside reverse transcriptase inhibitors (NRTIs), non-nucleoside reverse transcriptase inhibitors (NNRTIs), and protease inhibitors (PIs). See Appendix 2 for a list of agents and common side effects. Newer classes such as fusion inhibitors, CCR5 antagonists, and integrase inhibitors are not commonly available or indicated for first line treatment.

The backbone of most regimens are NRTIs that can be used in various combinations:
- Two NRTI with one NNRTI
- Two NRTIs with one to two PIs
- Three NRTIs (not a typical 1st line regimen)

The durability of a regimen depends on the potency, adherence, tolerability, and convenience along with the patients' baseline immunologic and virologic status.[8] It is important to consider relative effects and possible toxicities when choosing combinations of ARVs. Patients with underlying renal and/or liver disease require special regimens and/or dosing adjustments.

Of note, potentially lethal side effects include Stevens-Johnson syndrome (NVP), hypersensitivity reactions (ABC), hepatitis (NVP, d4T, ddI, AZT), anemia (AZT), and pancreatitis (ddI).[8] The nonlethal longer term side effect of lipodystrophy has been associated with prolonged d4T, ddI, AZT and PI use. Patients with lower CD4 counts have considerable mortality, even after initiating HAART, and should be closely followed.

LABORATORY TESTING

If laboratory testing is available, baseline CD4 and VL should be obtained and followed every 3–6 months for monitoring. If labs are unavailable, adherence should be emphasized and the patient should be followed clinically. Depending on the regimen, liver function tests (LFTs) should be drawn at regular intervals. Evidence of liver failure (jaundice, bleeding, etc.) or increase in LFTs necessitates closer monitoring. LFTs up to five times the upper limit of normal may be followed clinically, but levels greater than those or acute hepatic failure necessitate cessation of treatment. Renal function should be periodically assessed with regimens containing tenofovir such that dose adjustments can be made based on creatinine clearance. Lipid panels, if available, are useful for patients on PI-based regimens. Latent and active TB should be ruled out and warrant a purified protein derivative (PPD) or chest x-ray (CXR) depending on the presence of symptoms.

TREATMENT FAILURE

Failure of treatment is divided into three categories: immunologic, virologic, and clinical (the definitions of which may vary).

Immunologic failure is defined as any of the following:

- CD4 declining below baseline after 6 months
- 50% reduction of highest CD4 value while on treatment
- CD4 that never exceeds 100/mm³ after 6 months[9]

Virologic failure is defined as a VL exceeding 10,000 copies for 6 months after sufficient evaluation for adherence.[9]

The WHO defines clinical failure as the development of a new or recurrent WHO Stage 4 condition.[9] Confounders such as immune reconstitution inflammatory syndrome (IRIS), an inflammatory condition caused by ARVs, should be excluded in the appropriate clinical context. If there is discordance among VL and CD4 or clinical symptoms, lab tests should be repeated.

The most common cause of treatment failure is nonadherence and usually centers on a complex array of psychosocial issues. *Adherence cannot be overemphasized as missing 1–2 doses/month of some ARVs can lead to viral mutations that can render an entire class of ARV ineffective.* An adherence rate of 95% or greater is encouraged.[9] Commonly used simple and low-cost technologies such as cell phones have been utilized in innovative ways to increase adherence. If adherence is an issue, it is important to identify and remedy patient-specific barriers in a culturally sensitive, nonjudgmental manner.

Resistance testing may be obtained to help guide an ARV regimen in a patient with virologic failure. A few governments have protocols for first and second line ARV treatment after which resistance testing may be performed.

However, the cost of resistance testing is prohibitive in many areas and it is not widely available.

OPPORTUNISTIC INFECTIONS—PROPHYLAXIS AND TREATMENT

Opportunistic infections (OI) are infections that exploit depressed immune systems. Though they are unlikely to cause serious disease in healthy hosts, OIs in persons with advanced immunodeficiency are associated with severe disease and high mortality rates (especially if untreated). In fact, many OIs are considered AIDS-defining illnesses. The risk of developing particular OIs increases as the CD4 count decreases. Therefore, prophylaxis is determined by CD4 count. It is important to note that HIV-infected patients are more susceptible to common pathogens as well. Table 9-2 demonstrates conditions associated with the CD4 counts at which they commonly occur.

■ *Pneumocystis jiroveci (carinii)*

PCP (now called *Pneumocystis jiroveci*) is a common cause of pneumonia in the HIV population. The risk for PCP increases as the CD4 count drops below 200/mm^3 (or 14%). Most patients presenting with PCP are unaware of their HIV status and therefore not on appropriate prophylaxis. PCP typically presents with cough, fever, and dyspnea on exertion, often occurring over a period of weeks. Diagnosis requires a high clinical suspicion. Physical exam is usually notable for hypoxia especially during ambulation. Patients may present in respiratory distress and require mechanical ventilation. LDH, a nonspecific

Table 9-2 Opportunistic Infections Correlated with CD4 Count[6]

CD4 (cells/mm^3)	Associated Conditions
> 500	Most illnesses are similar to those in HIV-negative patients. Some increased risk of bacterial infections (pneumococcal pneumonia, sinusitis); herpes zoster, tuberculosis, skin conditions
200–500*	Bacterial infections (especially pneumococcal pneumonia, sinusitis), cutaneous Kaposi's sarcoma, vaginal candidiasis, ITP
50–200*	Thrush, oral hairy leukoplakia, classic HIV-associated opportunistic infections (e.g., *P. jiroveci [carinii]* pneumonia, cryptococcal meningitis, toxoplasmosis). For patients receiving prophylaxis, most opportunistic infections do not occur until CD4 cell counts < 100/mm^3 (Ann Intern Med 1996;124:633–642)
< 50*	"Final common pathway" opportunistic infections (disseminated *M. avium* complex, CMV retinitis), HIV-associated wasting, neurologic disease (neuropathy, encephalopathy)

*Patients remain at risk for all processes noted in earlier stages

marker of inflammation, is typically elevated. CXR and CT findings are often nonspecific and vary greatly, ranging from normal to the presence of interstitial infiltrates, cysts, and pneumothoraces. Blood gas analysis may be helpful to assess the degree of hypoxia and need for steroid administration. Definitive diagnosis depends on PCP-direct fluorescent antibody (DFA) in sputum or bronchoscopy samples (likely unavailable in resource limited settings).

First line treatment is co-trimoxazole DS—oral for mild disease and IV for severe disease.[5] For patients with sulfa allergies or side effects from bactrim, pentamidine or dapsone can be used. For patients with a PaO$_2$ of < 70 mmHg or an A-a gradient of > 35, there is mortality benefit from steroid treatment.[5] In the developing world, most decisions are made based on the prevalence of HIV, clinical presentation, available radiography, and labs. Patients are commonly empirically treated for both bacterial pneumonia and PCP while establishing HIV status and ruling out tuberculosis.[10] It is important to remember that bacterial pneumonias such as *S. pneumoniae* are also highly prevalent in the HIV population and are more associated with bacteremia.

PCP should be suspected and empirically treated if:
- HIV positive
- Insidious onset (over ~2 weeks)
- Dry cough
- Interstitial infiltrates
- Hypoxic

Patients with a CD4 count of < 200/mm^3 or < 14% should be initiated on cotrimoxazole for primary prophylaxis.

■ Cryptococcus

Cryptococcus neoformans is a fungus that can cause meningitis in immunocompromised patients. The risk increases as CD4 falls below 200/mm^3 and becomes particularly prevalent at CD4 < 50/mm^3.[11] Presenting symptoms include altered mental status, headache, fever, and neurologic deficits. The physical exam may reveal signs of elevated intracranial pressure (ICP), but findings of papilledema are rare. Lumbar puncture is a crucial procedure in these patients—it typically reveals elevated opening pressure. CSF fluid should be sent for India ink preparation, which yields 80% sensitivity in HIV positive patients. CSF cryptococcal antigen is > 90% sensitive, but may not be available.[11] Frequently an elevated opening pressure (OP) in a patient with HIV can provide a presumptive diagnosis. Once cryptococcal meningitis is diagnosed, treatment is divided into induction, consolidation, and maintenance phases. In the induction phase, amphotericin (can be lipid-based) and (if available) flucytosine are used for 2 weeks. The consolidation phase consists of high-dose fluconazole for 8 weeks.[6] Patients are then switched to low-dose fluconazole for maintenance therapy. *If opening pressures are elevated, patients should have daily lumbar punctures to remove CSF.* The goal is to reduce opening pressure by 50% or to less than 200 mmH$_2$O.

Lumbar puncture is a highly safe and *essential* diagnostic and therapeutic procedure in patients with HIV and headache, especially if the CD4 count is < 100/mm^3.

There is no recommended primary prophylaxis for Cryptococcus.

■ Toxoplasmosis

Cerebral toxoplasmosis is caused by *Toxoplasma gondii*, a parasite that causes encephalitis in the immunocompromised patient. Toxoplasma is seen predominately at CD4 < 100/mm^3.[10] Presenting symptoms include fever, headache, seizures, and focal neurologic deficits affecting motor, speech, or sensory loss.[5] Diagnosis is supported by characteristic radiographic findings such as head CT evidence of cerebral edema, mass effect, and classic ring enhancing lesions. Clinical response to empiric treatment also supports the diagnosis as 90% of patients should have clinical improvement at 2 weeks.[5] Serologic testing for toxoplasma titers is not readily available in the resource-constrained setting and results have not been validated for diagnosis.[10] Treatment is composed of a three drug regimen: pyrimethamine (with folinic acid supplementation), sulfadiazine, and leucovorin for acute therapy for 6–8 weeks followed by suppressive treatment doses.

Other space-occupying lesions may present similarly to toxoplasmosis. When patients do not respond to treatment for toxoplasmosis, consider empiric treatment for tuberculosis while evaluating for other etiologies such as brain abscess and CNS lymphoma.

Though primary prophylaxis is not indicated, PCP prophylaxis with co-trimoxazole also confers some protection against toxoplasmosis.

■ *Mycobacterium-avium complex (MAC)*

MAC is a mycobacterium that causes a variety of clinical syndromes. The risk for MAC increases with a CD4 count < 100/mm^3, especially as CD4 falls below 50/mm^3. Presenting symptoms can be diverse and require a high index of suspicion in the context of severe immunosuppression. For disseminated MAC, patients may complain of fever, chills, night sweats, wasting from weight loss, watery diarrhea (often copious), and/or abdominal pain.[12] Localized MAC can also cause lymphadenitis, osteomyelitis, or abscesses as well.[12] Differentiating MAC from other infections, such as TB, on a clinical basis can be difficult. Anemia and elevated alkaline phosphatase may be present and usually indicate bone marrow and asymptomatic liver involvement respectively.[12] Diagnosis is made by culture from an infected site: blood, stool, sputum, lymph node, or bone marrow. Treatment is complicated but usually consists of clarithromycin and ethambutol +/- rifabutin.[6] Duration of treatment is dependent on control of HIV and should be reassessed frequently.

Pimary prophylaxis for MAC is recommended for patients with a CD4 < 50/mm^3. Commonly used agents are azithromycin and clarithromycin.[6]

■ *Mycobacterium tuberculosis (TB)*

The co-infection of HIV and TB presents a unique and challenging clinical dilemma. TB and HIV have synergistic deleterious effects. There is a high incidence of tuberculosis among patients with HIV (eight times greater), and HIV is found in up to 40% of patients with TB in Africa.[10] Co-infected patients are more likely to manifest extrapulmonary TB, often with atypical presentations (especially in the setting of CD4 < 50/mm^3). TB accounts for the highest cause of mortality among HIV-infected patients.[10] In effect, *patients with HIV should be tested for TB and patients with TB should be tested for HIV.*

Newly diagnosed TB in an untreated HIV-positive patient is a complicated clinical quandary. Antituberculous therapy (ATT) and ARV treatment may cause significant drug interactions and toxicities that necessitate careful monitoring. IRIS can also confuse the clinical picture when both ATT and ARVs are initiated together. As a general rule, it is prudent to start ATT prior to ARVs. The timing of ARV initiation is still an issue of much debate. In the past, the decision depended on the patient's clinical status. If a patient is stable, ARVs can be started after completion of ATT with careful monitoring, although newer evidence suggests a mortality benefit with earlier initiation of ARVs.[13] If a patient has advanced immune deficiency, simultaneous treatment for both HIV and TB may be indicated. In such a circumstance, ATT should be started first, followed by a 2-week delay before starting ARVs. The WHO officially recommends starting ATT first followed by ARVs as soon as possible.[14] Country specific guidelines will determine when ARVs are initiated after ATT.

The benefits of Isoniazid Preventative Therapy (IPT) in reducing the incidence of active TB disease in HIV-infected individuals are well described.[15,16] Since 1998, the WHO has recommended IPT as an important strategy to reduce the burden of TB in the HIV population. However, IPT has not been universally accepted, largely due to concerns about its inadvertent use in patients with active TB disease, rather than latent infection, which promotes drug resistance. Despite some evidence that a symptom screen alone can accurately detect active TB disease,[17] the diagnosis of TB in HIV-infected patients remains challenging, particularly at low CD4 counts. Currently, only Botswana has formally adopted IPT as a component of national HIV/AIDS strategy. Other unanswered questions include the duration of IPT effect, the optimal timing of ART and IPT, and the best strategies for adherence.

THE IMMUNE RECONSTITUTION INFLAMMATORY SYNDROME (IRIS)

The immune reconstitution inflammatory syndrome (IRIS) is a condition that sometimes occurs after starting HAART in severely immunocompromised patients. As the CD4 count rises, the recovering immune system creates a substantial inflammatory response to previously acquired opportunistic infections, resulting in paradoxically worsened symptoms. IRIS can involve many pathogens, but the most common etiologies are TB, CMV, herpes zoster, MAC, and PCP. A similar IRIS has been described in patients not on HAART who initiate treatment for TB as well.

IRIS is often confused with treatment failure and thus should always be considered in patients being evaluated for inadequate response to HAART. Treatment for IRIS centers on supportive care, although some data advocate for the use of steroids in severe cases.

HIV-ASSOCIATED MALIGNANCIES

HIV increases the risk of malignancies such as Kaposi's sarcoma (KS), lymphoma, and cervical cancer. These malignancies in the context of HIV seropositivity confer a diagnosis of AIDS.

KS is caused by human herpesvirus-8 (HHV-8). It typically presents as a purplish cutaneous eruption with macules and erythematous, violacous patches most commonly seen on the lower extremities and torso. Up to 40% of patients with KS also have gastrointestinal involvement at presentation.[18] Pulmonary KS may present as shortness of breath with nonspecific interstitial airspace disease on CXR. Treatment centers on initiation of HAART and is aimed at symptomatic relief. In cases refractory to HAART, chemotherapeutic agents can be used but are still under investigation.

HIV is also associated with non-Hodgkin's lymphoma (NHL), which presents with nonspecific "b-type" symptoms such as fevers, chills, and weight loss. When lymphadenopathy occurs, excisional biopsy or fine needle aspiration is indicated. Treatment of NHL depends on the stage and type. It often includes a regimen of cyclophosphamide, hydroxydoxorubicin (adramycin), onchovin (vincristine), and prednisone (CHOP).[18]

Central Nervous System (CNS) lymphomas present with brain masses in patients with AIDS and are treated with ARVs and methotrexate-based chemotherapeutics with or without radiation. They are strongly associated with Epstein-Barr virus. Steroids are indicated for patients with elevated intracranial pressure.[10]

Cervical carcinoma is caused by infection with certain strains of human papilloma virus (HPV). The incidence is greater among HIV-infected women than the general population. This association may be even greater in the African population.[19] Depending on stage, cervical cancer can be managed with minimally invasive techniques such as LEEP, cryotherapy, or surgery in advanced stages. The papanicolau (PAP) smear is the mainstay of screening for cervical cancer.

SPECIAL CONSIDERATIONS: MTCT AND PEP

PREVENTING MOTHER TO CHILD TRANSMISSION (MTCT)

Transmission of HIV from mother to child can occur during the following phases: during pregnancy, at labor and delivery, or after birth with breastfeeding. Perhaps the most pronounced contrast between the developed and developing world is in the incidence of mother to child transmission. In 2007, there were 400,000 cases of vertical transmission worldwide, 90% of which were in sub-Saharan Africa. In contrast, only 1000 cases took place in the United States and Western Europe.[2]

Ideally, HIV-infected women should have undetectable VLs prior to becoming pregnant and be offered contraception if they do not wish to become pregnant. Women already on a suppressive ARV regimen should continue it with few exceptions.. Those on a regimen with inadequate viral suppression should undergo resistance testing (if available) and consider treatment changes.[9] In practice, however, many women may have undiagnosed HIV infection at the time of pregnancy.

Interventions aimed at PMTCT center on testing pregnant women, initiating ARV treatment or prophylaxis, providing reliable delivery practices, and educating patients about sensible breastfeeding strategies.[20] Refer to country-specific guidelines as variations in the provision of drugs and resources available for PMTCT are great. The PMTCT changes in the revised 2009 WHO HIV guidelines reflect the incorporation of new data and unprecedented expansion of PMTCT. In the new guidelines, if a woman meets an indication to initiate ARVs based on the aforementioned criteria (CD4<350, WHO Stage 3 or 4), she should be started on treatment. If a patient does not meet criteria for her own health, prophylaxis should be initiated for PMTCT in the form of daily AZT or a three drug regimen depending on resources available. Prophylaxis should be initiated at 14 weeks (instead of 28 weeks) and extend for the duration of breastfeeding.[21]

The WHO recommends safe delivery practices. C-sections are associated with lower HIV transmission rates compared to vaginal deliveries for women with higher viral loads; however, the risks and benefits of c-section must be weighed in a country-specific context according to local capacity, resources, and safety. These factors may ultimately make vaginal delivery a more appropriate decision, especially if the patient is receiving PMTCT.

The issue of breastfeeding is a complex one. The risk of HIV transmission from breastfeeding must be weighed against early childhood mortality from diarrheal diseases, pulmonary infections and malnutrition in the non-breastfeeding population (ref 21). Breastfeeding is essential for infant nutrition and survival, but confers a 10–16% risk of HIV transmission from HIV-infected mothers.[6] Previously, in the developed world, exclusive formula use was the recommendation, especially for mothers with detectable VLs. The recommendation was exclusive breastfeeding for HIV-infected mothers for the first six months of life unless replacement feeding meets the following criteria (AFASS):[10]

Acceptable, **F**easible, **A**ffordable, **S**ustainable, **S**afe.

The 2009 Rapid Advice WHO guidelines depart from this paradigm. New research has shown significant reductions in HIV transmission through breastfeeding from mother's on ARVs for treatment or prophylaxis. In such circumstances, mothers can breastfeed for the first year. For infants who are found to be HIV infected, breastfeeding can continue until 2 years of age or older.[22,23] National recommendations will be determined by the availability of resources and capacity to scale up existing PMTCT programs.

Above all, preventing MTCT relies on preventing HIV infection in adults and providing adequate contraception to those infected.

POSTEXPOSURE PROPHYLAXIS (PEP)

PEP is the short-term use of a combination of ARVs in an attempt to destroy the virus before it becomes fully entrenched in a patient who is occupationally exposed.[24]

Occupational exposure to HIV via needle stick injuries, scalpels, sutures, and exposure to mucous membranes are concerning. The risk of transmission from these injuries depends on a number of factors, namely:

- HIV status of the patient
- Timing of exposure[25]
- Depth of injury
- Presence of visible blood on the instrument
- Physical contact to a vein or artery
- Diameter of the needle[6]

The risk of transmission is 0.33% for needle stick injuries,[6] which is lower than other infectious diseases such as hepatitis. Whenever resources permit, a patient with unknown HIV status should be tested for HIV and hepatitis serology. Upon contact, the area of injury should be thoroughly cleaned and flushed with soap and water. For smaller wounds, a local antiseptic can be used. Depending on the type and risk of exposure, PEP should be initiated *immediately*. Standard treatment is with two NRTIs. However, if drug resistance is suspected, a regimen of two NRTIs and a PI are preferred. The WHO recommends zidovudine and lamivudine as first line therapy for PEP.[25] Countries may have different protocols regarding PEP, including use in victims of rape. Repeat HIV testing is indicated at the onset and at regular intervals usually every 3–6 months.[25]

CONCLUSION

The HIV/AIDS pandemic remains a challenge to local and international health communities. Regardless of the location or setting, it is important to be familiar with national guidelines for HIV testing and treatment as considerable variation exists and can have far reaching implications for patients. Understanding the socioeconomic, political and cultural milieu, and history of HIV in the region in which you are providing health care will greatly enhance your ability to identify and address barriers to diagnosis and treatment.

The pandemic is in various phases in different countries. Some nations lack a national strategy for the prevention, testing and treatment of HIV. Others are in the process of scaling up their national programs and access to testing and treatment. Many middle- income nations are faced with the chronic nature of HIV infection and the great cost of 2nd line and salvage medications for treatment experienced patients. Even the implementation of the revisions to the WHO guidelines will require the commitment of more resources, capacity and political will superimposed on already fragile healthcare systems, governments and donor networks.

Table 9-3 HIV Clinical Strategy Based on Level of Resource Limitation[a]

Intervention	Minimal Intervention Recommended			
	Limited Resources (no labs or HAART)	Some resources (limited labs, HAART)	Considerable resources (some labs, HAART)	Standard of care in the developed world
Prevention of transmission (non-pregnant)	• Early recognition of risk factors • Counseling regarding abstinence and/or limitation of sexual partners • Domestic abuse screening	• Early recognition of risk factors • Counseling regarding abstinence, limitation of sexual partners, and condom use • Domestic abuse screening	• Early recognition of risk factors • Counseling regarding abstinence, limitation of sexual partners, and condom use • Domestic abuse screening	• Early recognition of risk factors • Counseling regarding abstinence, limitation of sexual partners, and condom use • Domestic abuse screening • Postexposure prophylaxis (still being studied)
Diagnosis	• History, physical exam • Clinical suspicion • Presence of WHO Stage 3 or 4 conditions	• History/Physical • Clinical suspicion • Presence of WHO Stage 3 or 4 conditions, or • Double rapid testing or ELISA (if available, parallel or serial)	• History/Physical • Clinical suspicion • Presence of WHO Stage 3 or 4 conditions, or • Double rapid testing or ELISA (parallel or serial) • Fourth generation ELISA for the diagnosis of acute HIV infection	• History/Physical • Clinical suspicion • Antibody testing (ELISA or rapid) • Western blot for confirmation • HIV viral load for diagnosis of acute HIV infection

(Continues)

111

Table 9-3 HIV Clinical Strategy Based on Level of Resource Limitation[a] (Continued)

| Intervention | Limited Resources (no labs or HAART) | Minimal Intervention Recommended | | |
		Some resources (limited labs, HAART)	Considerable resources (some labs, HAART)	Standard of care in the developed world
Staging	**Clinical:** • WHO staging criteria	**Clinical:** • WHO clinical staging, treat for any Stage 3 or 4 condition **Immunologic:** • CD4 (if available)—treat for < 350/mm^3	**Clinical:** • WHO clinical staging, treat for any Stage 3 or 4 condition **Immunologic:** • CD4—treat for < 350/mm^3	**Clinical:** • CDC or WHO clinical staging, treat for any "AIDS-defining" illness **Immunologic:** • CD4—treat for < 500/mm^3
Baseline evaluations	• Clinically evaluate for TB • Evaluate for clinical signs of other STIs, jaundice, or renal failure	• Clinically evaluate for TB • Evaluate for clinical signs of other STIs, jaundice, or renal failure • Blood count • Chemistry/renal function (if available) • LFTs (if available)	• Clinically evaluate for TB • Evaluate for clinical signs of other STIs • Blood count • Chemistry/renal function • LFTs • Lipid/glucose testing	• Resistance testing (RA) • Blood count • RPR • PPD • Chest x-ray • LFTs • Chemistry/renal function • Hepatitis serologies • Toxoplasma serology • GC/Chlamydia • Lipid/glucose testing

Treatment	• Optimize nutritional status • Syndromic treatment of STIs	• Optimize nutritional status • Syndromic treatment of STIs • NNRTI-based HAART	• Optimize nutritional status • Syndromic treatment of STIs • NNRTI-based HAART	• Optimize nutritional status • Syndromic treatment of STIs • NNRTI or PI-based HAART depending on RA
Monitoring	• Ongoing counseling for risk factor modification	• Ongoing counseling for risk factor modification • Adherence monitoring • Evaluation for side effects (Stevens-Johnson, renal failure, liver failure) • PAP smear yearly (if available)	• Ongoing counseling for risk factor modification • Adherence monitoring • Clinical evaluation for side effects (Stevens-Johnson, renal failure, liver failure) • LFTs, renal function yearly depending on regimen • CD4 every 3-6 months • HIV RNA when failure is suspected • Lipid panel (if on PIs) • Yearly PAP smear	• Ongoing counseling for risk factor modification • Adherence monitoring • Clinical/lab evaluation for side effects (Stevens-Johnson, renal failure, liver failure) • CD4 and HIV RNA every 3-6 months • PAP smear every 6 months for the first year, then yearly
Failure	• Referral	• Adherence evaluation • Alteration of regimen • Referral for continued failure	• Adherence evaluation • Alteration of regimen • Resistance testing (if available) • Referral for continued failure	• Adherence evaluation • Alteration of regimen • Resistance testing

(Continues)

113

Table 9-3 HIV Clinical Strategy Based on Level of Resource Limitation[a] (Continued)

		Minimal Intervention Recommended		
Intervention	Limited Resources (no labs or HAART)	Some resources (limited labs, HAART)	Considerable resources (some labs, HAART)	Standard of care in the developed world
PMTCT	• Counseling and early recognition of HIV status • Optimize clean delivery techniques • Exclusive breastfeeding	• Counseling and early recognition of HIV status • Optimize clean delivery techniques • HAART for women who meet indication for treatment for their own health • 2006 Guidelines: AZT from 28 weeks. High dose AZT during delivery + single dose nevirapine (sdNVP) with sdNVP for child/+7 day AZT tail • 2009 Revised Guidelines: Daily AZT for the mother starting at 14 weeks and infant prophylaxis for 6 weeks after birth.	• Counseling and early recognition of HIV status • HAART for women who meet indication for treatment for their own health • 2006 Guidelines: AZT from 28 weeks. High dose AZT during delivery+ sdNVP, sdNVP with 7 day AZT tail for child • 2009 Revised Guidelines: Daily AZT for the mother starting at 14 weeks and infant prophylaxis for 6 weeks after birth. Infant prophylaxis expanded until completion of breastfeeding OR • 3 drug regimen given to mother starting at 14 weeks and throughout the pregnancy until completion of breastfeeding Infant prophylaxis for 6 weeks Optimize clean delivery techniques, c-section if VL elevated (if available)	• Counseling and early recognition of HIV status • CD4 count • Initiation of 3-drug ARV regimen (AZT should be a component) • Clean delivery techniques, c-section if VL elevated • Exclusive formula feeding • HAART for women who meet indication for treatment for their own health

| | | • Infant prophylaxis expanded until completion of breastfeeding
• If the mother received AZT during pregnancy, daily nevirapine should be given to the child until the completion of breastfeeding. | • Breastfeeding:
If the mother received AZT during pregnancy, daily nevirapine should be given to the child until the completion of breastfeeding.
OR
• If the mother received a 3 drug regimen, continue until the completion of breastfeeding | |
| Prevention of OIs | • Co-trimoxazole for PCP (if available) | • Co-trimoxazole for PCP | • Co-trimoxazole for PCP | • Co-trimoxazole for PCP
• Weekly azithromycin for MAC |

[a]Please consult national guidelines for details regarding available ARVs, diagnostics, PMTCT protocols, and baseline laboratories as these items are highly variable.

REFERENCES

1. Kates J, Lief E, Avila C. *Financing the Response to AIDS in Low- and Middle-Income Countries: International Assistance from the G8, European Commission and Other Donor Governments in 2008*. Menlo Park, CA: Kaiser Family Foundation; 2009.

2. UNAIDS. *2008 Report on the Global AIDS Epidemic*. Geneva: Joint United Nations Program on HIV/AIDS; 2009.

3. Quinn T. The global human immunodeficiency virus pandemic. *Lancet*. 1996;348:99.

4. Piot P. AIDS: Exceptionalism Revisited. Public lecture given at London School of Economics. May 15, 2008.

5. Bartlett J, Gallant J. *Medical Management of HIV Infection*. Baltimore: Johns Hopkins Medicine Health Publishing Business Group; 2007.

6. Sax P, Cohen C, Kuritzkes D. *HIV Essentials*. Sudbury, MA: Jones and Bartlett Publishers; 2008.

7. Center for the AIDS Programme of Research in South Africa, Important new research findings on treatment of TB-HIV co-infection [press release]. Durban, South Africa: Sep 19 , 2008. http://www.caprisa.org/joomla/index.php/memberaccess/95-pressrelease17092008, accessed December 29, 2009.

8. Gulick R. Adherence to antiretroviral therapy: How much is enough? *Clin Infect Dis*. 2006;43:942–944.

9. World Health Organization. Antiretroviral Therapy for HIV infection in Adults and Adolescents: Recommendations for a Public Health Approach. Geneva, Switzerland: World Health Organization; 2006.

10. Hoffman C, Rockstroh J, Kamps B, eds. *HIV Medicine 2007*. 15th ed. http://www.flyingpublisher.com. 2007.

11. Perfect J, Casadevall A. Cryptococcosis. *Infect Dis Clin North Am*. 2002;16:837–874.

12. Crowe S, Hoy J, Mills J. *Management of the HIV-Infected Patient*. New York: Cambridge University Press; 1996.

13. P Tabarisi *et al*, Early initiation of antiretroviral therapy results in decreased morbidity and mortality among patients with TB and HIV, *Journal of the International AIDS Society*. 2009; 12(14).

14. World Health Organization. Rapid Advice: Antiretroviral therapy for HIV infection in adults and adolescents. Geneva, Switzerland: World Health Organization 2009.

15. Wilkinson D, Squire SB, Garner P. Effect of Preventive Treatment for Tuberculosis in Adults Infected with HIV: Systematic Review of Randomized Placebo Controlled Trials. *BMJ*. 1998;317:625–629.

16. Woldehanna S, Volmink J. Treatment of Latent Tuberculosis Infection in HIV Infected Persons. *Cochrane Database Syst Rev*. 2006;(3):CD000171.

17. Mosimaneotsile B, Talbot EA, Moeti TL. Value of Chest Radiography in a Tuberculosis Prevention Programme for HIV-Infected People, Botswana. *Lancet*. 2003;362:1551–1552.

18. Dezube B, Groopman J. AIDS-related Kaposi's sarcoma: Epidemiology and pathogenesis. http://www.uptodate.com/patients/content/topic.do?topicKey=~UOtfEmAP69rx4M

19. Holmes R *et al.* HIV Infection as a Risk Factor for Cervical Cancer and Cervical Intraepithelial Neoplasia in Senegal, *Cancer Epidemiology, Biomarkers & Prevention*, September 2009 (18); 2442.

20. World Health Organization. Antiretroviral Drugs for Treating Pregnant Women and Preventing HIV Infection in Infants in Resource-Limited Settings: Towards Universal Access. Geneva, Switzerland: World Health Organization; 2006.

21. World Health Organization. Key Messages:New WHO recommendations: Preventing mother-to-child transmission. Geneva, Switzerland: World Health Organization 2009.

22. World Health Organization. Key Messages: New WHO recommendations: Infant feeding in the context of HIV. Geneva, Switzerland: World Health Organization 2009.

23. World Health Organization. HIV and infant feeding Revised Principles and Recommendations: Rapid Advice. Geneva, Switzerland: World Health Organization 2009.

24. Bartlett J. Management of healthcare workers exposed to HIV. http://www.uptodate.com/patients/content/topic.do?topicKey=~NBEyE8fawhDzFJB

25. World Health Organization. Post-Exposure Prophylaxis to Prevent HIV Infection: Joint WHO/ILO Guidelines on Post-Exposure Prophylaxis (PEP) to Prevent HIV Infection. Geneva, Switzerland: World Health Organization; 2007.

X ■ TOXICOLOGY AND ENVIRONMENTAL HEALTH

Amit K. Gupta, MD

Gar Ming Chan, MD

Poisoning is a global concern and toxicologic exposures vary across different parts of the world. Inadequate federal regulations, improper packaging, and limited access to healthcare facilities make poisoning in developing countries particularly dangerous. Limited access to certain life-saving resources such as mechanical ventilation, antidotes, and antivenom complicates the treatment of poisoning in resource-poor areas.

Federal regulations play an important role in the prevention of toxic exposure. Lead paint is a prime example. In the United States, since 1978, household paint cannot contain more than 0.06% lead.[1] However, in some countries such as India, China, Nigeria, Egypt, and Equador, lead concentrations of enamel household paint remain extremely high and pose a risk to developing children in those homes.[2]

Unintentional poisonings kill an estimated 350,000 people globally each year.[3] Suicide (by intentional poisoning) accounts for an additional estimated 877,000 deaths every year.[3] In addition to ingestion, toxins may be emitted directly into soil, air, and water—from industrial processes, pulp and paper plants, tanning operations, mining, and unsustainable forms of agriculture—at levels or rates well in excess of those tolerable to human health.[4] As evident, toxicologic concerns vary depending across different parts of the world. This chapter will divide common issues of global toxicologic concern and each category will be discussed. The categories include pesticides, animal envenomations, plants, herbal medications, global disasters, medications, and adulterations.

PESTICIDES AND AGRICULTURAL COMPOUNDS

A pesticide is any substance or mixture of substances intended for preventing or destroying a pest. Though often misunderstood to refer only to insecticides, the term pesticide also applies to herbicides, fungicides, and rodenticides. Studies in developed countries have demonstrated the annual incidence rate of acute pesticide poisoning (APP) in agricultural workers to be as high as 18.2 per 100,000 full-time workers and 7.4 per million among school children.[5,6] An estimated 300,000 annual deaths per pesticide self-poisoning in Asia alone establishes this as a major global health problem.[7] Developing countries face a higher incidence of APP due to insufficient regulation, lack of surveillance systems, inadequate access to information systems, and poorly maintained or nonexistent personal protective equipment. The use of highly toxic pesticides, many that are banned in industrialized countries, are still greatly used in larger agriculturally-based countries.[8] About 60% of suicides in Sri Lanka are caused by intentional self-poisoning and, of these, 90% are due to deliberate pesticide ingestion.[9] Studies from Sri Lanka regarding self-poisoning reveal an APP incidence rate of approximately 180 per 100,000.[10]

Organic phosphorous compounds and carbamates are the two groups of cholinesterase-inhibiting pesticides that commonly produce human toxicity. Both are well absorbed across skin and mucous membranes, and by inhalation and ingestion.[11] Clinical findings of toxicity from these compounds derive from excessive stimulation of muscarinic and nicotinic cholingeric receptors. Excessive muscarinic activity is characterized by several mnemonics, including SLUDGE (salivation, lacrimation, urination, defecation, GI distress, and emesis) and DUMBBELS (defecation, urination, miosis, bronchospasm/bronchorrhea, brady-cardia, emesis, lacrimation, and salivation). Bronchorrhea can be so profuse that it mimics pulmonary edema. Nicotinic signs include muscle fasciculations that lead to muscle weakness and ultimately paralysis of respiratory muscles.

Currently, the only practical diagnostic study for verifying cholinesterase inhibitor poisoning is a measurement of cholinesterase activity in plasma and red blood cells.[11] Treatment includes airway management, GI decontamination, and escalating doses of atropine, beginning with 1–5 mg for adults and 0.05 mg/kg for children, until the patient has resolution of pulmonary secretions. Some adults have required over 1000 mg of atropine in 24 hours.[12] Controversy still exists regarding the use of the pralidoxime (2-PAM) therapy for organophosphate and carbamate toxicity. It is most effective if started early before an irreversible bond is formed between the compound and the ACHase (termed *aging*) that is more common with OPs.[13] The initial dose of pralidoxime for adults is 1–2 grams intravenously over 10–15 minutes and 20–40 mg/kg IV for children. Maintenance infusion is 250–500 mg/hr.

Table 10-1 shows toxic pesticides commonly used throughout the world.

Table 10-1 Toxicology of Commonly Used Pesticides

Class	Pathophysiology	Toxicity	Antidote
Organic Phosphorus Compounds	Irreversibly inhibits acetylcholinesterase	Cholingeric crisis: DUMBBELS (defecation, urination, miosis, bronchospasm/ bronchorrhea/bradycardia, emesis, lacrimation, and salivation); muscle fasciculations, or weakness	Atropine and Pralidoxime (2-PAM)
Organic Chlorine (DDT, Lindane)	CNS hyperexcitability	Seizures, respiratory failure	Benzodiazepines for seizures; supportive care
Carbamates	Reversibly inhibits acetylcholine	Cholingeric crisis: DUMBBELS, muscle fasciculations, or weakness	Atropine and Pralidoxime (2-PAM)

(Continues)

Table 10-1 Toxicology of Commonly Used Pesticides (Continued)

Class	Pathophysiology	Toxicity	Antidote
Dipyridyl herbicides: Paraquat and Diquat	Superoxide radical formation	Pulmonary Toxicity; GI caustic injury, CNS depression	supportive care
Aluminum Phosphide	Inhibit oxidative phosphorylation; similar to cyanide	Diffuse cellular toxicity and hemodynamic collapse	supportive care

INDUSTRIAL DISASTERS

Recent toxic disasters have come to symbolize our increasingly industrialized world. Globalization has led to the proliferation of toxic chemicals in the developing world.[14] Table 10-2 lists a few examples of major disasters in the recent years.

Table 10-2 Recent Industrial Disasters

Area	Year(s)	Toxicity	Outcome
Bhopal, India Union Carbide Plant	1984	Methyl isocyanate from carbaryl-producing plant	2500 deaths and 200,00 injuries due to dispersion.
Minamata Bay, Japan	1950s	Methyl mercury discharged from vinyl chloride factory dumped mercury into bay	Congenital defects, chronic brain damage, tunnel vision, and deafness in the offspring of the local people.
Japan	1939–1954	Cadmium runoff from mine into local water supply	Approximately 200 people developed Itai-Itai (ouch-ouch) disease due to extreme bone pain and osteomalacia.
Japan	1968	Polychlorinated biphenyls (PCBs) leaked from a heating pipe into rice oil	Yusho (rice oil disease). More than 1600 people developed chloracne, hyperpigmentation, and increased incidence of cancer and reproductive effects.
Bangladesh	1990s–2000s	Arsenic leakage from rocks into drinking water	At least 220,000 diagnosed with arsenic poisoning, cancer, skin lesions, cardiovascular, and pulmonary disease.

ANIMAL ENVENOMATIONS

The WHO estimates that there are 5 million snakebites each year that are responsible for at least 125,000 deaths annually.[15] The majority of deaths occur in the Asia-Pacific region. In contrast, fewer than 100 snakebite deaths occur yearly in Europe, the United States, Canada, and Australia combined.[16] In developing countries a large proportion of snakebites occur while farming on plantations. The severity and clinical manifestations of envenomation depend on a number of factors, including number of strikes, depth, size of snake, potency and amount of venom injected, location of bite, and underlying health of the victim.[17] Intravenous envenomation may occur and lead to rapid development of life-threatening complications.

Venom consists of numerous proteolytic enzymes, procoagulants and anticoagulants, neurotoxins, cardiotoxins, and hemotoxins, making it very complex to analyze.[18]

Clinical manifestations of snakebites include asymptomatic ("dry" bite), local tissue destruction, and systemic toxicity such as anaphylaxis, hypotension, altered mental status, muscle paralysis, and disseminated intravascular coagulation (DIC) picture. The mainstay of effective therapy for snake envenomation is antivenom.[19] However, the currently available antivenoms are either expensive or have a high rate of adverse reactions.

Scorpion stings are the second most common cause of mortality and morbidity via envenomation in the world. The role of antivenom therapy is widely accepted in many countries as the treatment for many forms of scorpion envenomation. Other venomous creatures include Arachnida (spiders) and Hymenoptera (bees, ants, and wasps).

Table 10-3 lists common venomous animals throughout the world.

Table 10-3 Common Venomous Animals

Animal	Area	Toxin
Fat-tailed Scorpion (*Androctonus* spp)	Africa, Middle East	Neurotoxin
Deathstalker Scorpion (*Leiurus quinquestriatus*)	Africa, Middle East	Neurotoxin
Recluse, "Fiddle-back" Spider (*Loxosceles* spp)	North America	Cytotoxin, local tissue necrosis
Black Widow Spider (*Lactrodectus*)	North America, Australia, Europe	Neuroexcitability
Brazilian Armed Spider (*Phoneutria* spp)	Central and South America	Neurotoxin
Austrian Funnel Spider (*Atrax robustus*)	Australia	Neuroexcitability
Cobra (*Naja* spp)	Africa, Asia, Middle East	Neurotoxin, hemotoxin

(Continues)

Table 10-3 Common Venomous Animals (Continued)

Animal	Area	Toxin
Pit Viper (*Crotalus* spp)	North, Central, and South America	Cytotoxin, hemotoxin, myotoxin
Black Mamba (*Dendroaspis polylepis*)	Africa	Hemotoxin, neurotoxin
Russel Viper (*Vipera russelli*)	Asia	Hemotoxin, septicemia
Carpet Viper (*Echis carinatus*)	Africa, Asia, Middle East	Hemotoxin
Malaysian Pit Viper (*Calloselasma rhodostoma*)	Asia	Hemotoxin

PLANTS

Plant compounds have been used therapeutically and for harm throughout human history. They can be used for recreational intoxication, self-harm, homicidal acts, or to induce abortions. Table 10-4 lists commonly encountered poisonous plants.

Table 10-4 Commonly Encountered Poisonous Plants

Plant	Area Found	Toxin	Treatment
Yellow oleander (*Thevetia peruviana*)	Sri Lanka, Latin America	Cardioactive Steroid Digoxin-like	Digoxin-specific antibody fragments (high doses may be required)
Ackee tree fruit (*Blighia saphia*)	Caribbean and Africa	Hypoglycin— hypoglycemia, hepatitis, and seizures	Glucose; benzodiazepines for seizures
Superb lily (*Gloriosa superba*) and Meadow saffron (*Colchicum autumnale*)	Sri Lanka	Colchicine toxicity— GI symptoms and bone marrow suppression	Supportive care
Castor beans (*Ricinus communis*)	Mexico, Central and South America	Ricin—Ribosomal toxin. Diffuse cellular toxicity	Supportive care
Jimson weed/Thorn apple (*Datura stramonium*)	Africa, Asia, and Latin America	Atropine/scopolamine/ hyosamine. Anticholingeric toxidrome	Physostigmine

(Continues)

Table 10-4 Commonly Encountered Poisonous Plants (Continued)

Plant	Area Found	Toxin	Treatment
Monkshood (*Acontium napellus*)	Asia	Aconitine. Cardiac sodium channel opener	Supportive care
Poison Hemlock (*Conium maculatum*)	Europe, Africa	Coniine-similar to nicotine. Muscle fasciculations and paralysis	Supportive care, benzodiazepines for seizures

HERBAL MEDICATIONS

The WHO estimates that 80% of the world's population presently uses herbal medicine for some aspect of primary health care.[20] Commercial pharmaceuticals are prohibitively expensive for most of the world's population, while herbal medicines can be grown from seed or gathered from nature for little or no cost. Herbal treatments are the most popular form of traditional medicine, and are highly lucrative on the international marketplace, generating annual revenues in Western Europe that reached US $5 billion in 2003–2004. In China, sales of herbal products exceeded US $14 billion in 2005.[21] Herbal products can be marketed without any proof of testing for efficacy or safety. Therefore, adverse drug reactions are very commonly reported with their use.

Table 10-5 Common Herbal Medications

Herbal	Area Found	Traditional Use	Toxicity	Treatment
Khat (*Catha edulis*)	East Africa	Depression, fatigue, obesity	Contains Stimulant and dysphoria	Benzodiazepines for sedation
Valerian (*Valeriana officinalis*)	Europe, United States	Anxiety, Insomnia	Sedative	Supportive care
Japanese star anise (*Illicium anastum*)	Asia	Culinary, URI symptoms	Seizure	Benzodiazepines for seizures
Ch'an Su "Love Stone" "Rock Hard" (*Bufo bufo* spp)	Asia	Aphrodisiac	Bufadienolides: digoxin-like cardioactive Steroid	Digoxin FAB products: high doses may be required
Ayurvedic remedies	India	Various medical conditions	Gold, silver, copper, zinc, iron, lead, arsenic, tin, and mercury toxicity	Various depending on metal
Comfrey Tea (*Symphytum* spp)	Europe	Gastric ulcers, bronchitis, burns, bruises, swelling	Pyrrolizidine Alkaloids; Hepatic Venoocclusive disease	Supportive care

MEDICATIONS

Overall, medications are the most common products used to self-poison in the developing world. Medications such as benzodiazepines are commonly ingested as a method of self-poisoning due to increasing availability and perception by lay people that they are dangerous in overdose.[22]

Due to easy accessibility, analgesics, such as acetaminophen (paracetamol or APAP), are commonly ingested in overdose levels.[23] In an overdose, whether acute or chronic, a large ingestion of acetaminophen overwhelms the liver's ability to conjugate and detoxify APAP, leading to the production of the toxic electrophile N-acetyl-p-benzoquinoneimine (NAPQI). NAPQI goes on to cause centrilobular hepatic necrosis. The treatment for APAP toxicity is N-acetylcysteine, orally or intravenously, which reduces NAPQI and regenerates glutathione stores in the liver to aid in APAP metabolism.

People intentionally overdose on medications for similar reasons around the world, emotional distress combined with economic hardship.[24]

ADULTERATIONS AND MEDICINAL DRUG DISASTERS

Historically, the use of adulterants has been common in societies with inadequate legal controls on food quality and poor monitoring by authorities; sometimes it has extended to dangerous chemicals and poisons. Intentional or unintentional medication disasters have occurred following poor safety testing and drug contamination. In 1937, more than 100 deaths were associated with diethylene glycol toxicity which was used as a diluent for an early sulfa drug preparation.[25] This led to the US Food, Drug, and Cosmetic Act of 1938 that required more stringent drug testing and more marketing to the general public.

Table 10-6 lists recent adulterant disasters.

Table 10-6 Recent Adulterant Disasters

Countries	Year(s)	Toxin	Consequence
Africa, India, Haiti, and China		Diethylene Glycol	Medical diluent for toothpaste and acetaminophen elixir
United States	1990s	Heroin	Heroin tainted with fentanyl and scopolamine
India	1980s–1990s	Methanol	Over 500 deaths due to methanol which was substituted for ethanol.
China	2008–Current	Melamine	Melamine intentionally added as a protein substitute in infant's formula. 12,800 hospitalizations and four infant deaths due to melamine renal stones.

REFERENCES

1. American Academy of Pediatrics, Committee on Environmental Health. Lead Poisoning: From screening to primary prevention. *Pediatrics*. 1993; 92:176–183.

2. Clark CS, Rampal KG, Thuppil V, Roda SM, Succop P, Menrath W, Chen CK, Adebamowo EO, Agbede OA, Sridhar MK, Adebamowo CA, Zakaria Y, El-Safty A, Shinde RM, Yu J. Lead levels in new enamel household paints from Asia, Africa and South America. *Environ Res*. 2009.

3. World Health Organization. The World Health Report 2003—Shaping the Future. Geneva: World Health Organization; 2003.

4. Yáñez L, Ortiz D, Calderón J, Batres L, Carrizales L, Mejía J, Martínez L, García-Nieto E, Díaz-Barriga F. Overview of human health and chemical mixtures: problems facing developing countries. *Environ Health Persp*. 2002; 110(6):901–909.

5. Calvert GM, Plate DK, Das R, Rosales R, Shafey O, Thomsen C, Male D, Beckman J, Arvizu E, Lackovic M. Acute occupational pesticide-related illness in the US, 1998–1999: surveillance findings from the SENSOR-pesticides program. *Am J Ind Med*. 2004;45:14–23.

6. Alarcon WA, Calvert GM, Blondell JM, Mehler LN, Sievert J, Propeck M, Tibbetts DS, Becker A, Lackovic M, Soileau SB, Das R, Beckman J, Male DP, Thomsen CL, Stanbury M. Acute illnesses associated with pesticide exposure at school. *JAMA*. 2005;294:455–465.

7. Gunnell D, Eddleston M. Suicide by intentional ingestion of pesticides: a continuing tragedy in developing countries. *Int J Epidemiol*. 2003; 32:902–909.

8. Buckley NA, Roberts D, Eddleston M. Overcoming global apathy in research on organophosphate poisoning. *BMJ*. 2004;329:1231–1233.

9. Mode of Suicide 2005. *Sri Lankan Police Services, Crime Trends*. 2005.

10. Eddleston M, Sudarshan K, Senthilkumaran M, Reginald K, Karalliedde L, Senarathna L, de Silva D, Rezvi Sheriff MH, Buckley NA, Gunnell D. Patterns of hospital transfer for self-poisoned patients in rural Sri Lanka: implications for estimating the incidence of self-poisoning in the developing world. *Bull World Health Organ*. 2006;84:276–282.

11. Gallo MA, Lawryk NJ. Organic phosphorus pesticides. In Hayes WJ, Laws ER, eds. *Handbook of Pesticide Toxicology*. San Diego, CA: Academic Press; 1991:917–1090.

12. Du Toit PW, Muller FO, Van Tonder WM, Ungerer MJ. Experience with intensive care management of organophosphate insecticide poisoning. *S Afr Med J*. 1981;60:227–229.

13. Segall Y, Waysbort D, Barak, D. Direct observation and elucidation of the structures of aged and nonaged phosphorylated cholinesterases by 31P spectroscopy NMR. *Biochemistry*. 1993;32:13441–13450.

14. OECD environmental outlook for the chemicals industry. Paris: Organization for Economic Cooperation and Development, Environment Directorate; 2001.

15. Chippaux JP. Snake-bites: Appraisal of the global situation. *Bull World Health Organ.* 1998;76:515–524.

16. Currie BJ. Snakebites in Tropical Australia, New Guinea, and Iranian Jaya. *Emerg Med.* 2000;12:285–294.

17. Lewis JV, Portera CA. Rattlesnake bite of the face: Case report and review of the literature. *Am Surg.* 1994;60:681–682.

18. Iyaniwura TT. Snake venom constituents: Biochemistry and toxicology, Part 1&2. *Vet Hum Toxicol.* 1991;33:468–480.

19. Chippaux JP, Goyffon M. Venoms, antivenoms, and immunotherapy. *Toxicon.* 1998;36:823–846.

20. World Health Organization. Web site. http://www.who.int/mediacentre/factsheets/fs134/en/

21. Ko RJ. Causes, epidemiology, and clinical evaluation of suspected herbal poisoning. *J Toxicol Clin Toxicol.* 1999;37:697–708.

22. Khan MM, Reza H. Benzodiazepine in Pakistan: Implications for prevention and harm reduction. *J Pak Med Assoc.* 1998;48:293–295.

23. Chan TY, Chan AY, Critchley JA. Paracetamol poisoning and hepatotoxicity in Chinese-the Prince of Wales Hospital experience. *Singapore Med J.* 1993;34:299–302.

24. Hettiarachichi J, Kodithuwakku GC. Self poisoning in Sri Lanka: Motivational aspects. *Int J Soc Psych.* 1989;35:204–208.

25. Geiling EHK, Cannon PR. Pathological effects of elixir of sulfanilamide (Diethylene glycol) poisoning: A clinical and experimental correlation-Final report. *JAMA.* 1938;111:919–926.

26. Bertolote JM,Fleischmann A,Eddleston M,Gunnell D. Deaths from Pesticide Poisoning: Are we lacking a global response? *Br J Psychiatry.* 2006; 189:201–203.

XI ■ EXTREMES OF TEMPERATURE

PART 1 HIGH TEMPERATURE AND DESERT MEDICINE

Sanjey Gupta, MD

Modern mankind's activities are altering the world's climate. During the 20th century, the average surface temperature of the Earth increased approximately 0.6%, and two-thirds of the warming has occurred since 1975.[1] According to the UN's Intergovernmental Panel on Climate Change, the global average temperature will rise by several degrees centigrade this century.[2] Extremes of heat will cause thermal stress on local populations in the form of heat waves. Rising global temperatures and localized urban heat island effect may increase temperatures 5–12°C.[3] Temperature modulation by ecological processes and social conditions will increase temperature-related death and morbidity and increase the negative health effects of food and water shortages.

Most deaths during times of thermal extreme occur in people with preexisting disease, especially cardiovascular and respiratory disease.[4] The very young or elderly, the frail, and the poor are most susceptible. Some predict that by 2050, excess summer heat-related mortality related to climate change in New York City will increase sevenfold.[5] Currently, 60,000 people per year die from weather-related natural disasters.[6] Furthermore, as a consequence of climate change and human activity, "desertification" of arid and semi-arid land is occurring on all inhabited continents.[7] It is estimated that 10–20% of these lands and their populations are threatened with desertification. A global health crisis is looming with the lack of sustainable food, fresh water, and shelter in these areas.

Medical professionals are challenged to increase their fund of knowledge in treating diseases associated with thermal stress like heat stroke and dehydration. Further, knowledge of desert medicine will quickly become requisite on the global stage.

HEAT ILLNESS

In August 2003, a record summer heat wave in Europe caused 35,000 deaths in a 2-week period.[8] These deaths were likely due to the effects of hyperthermia: heat illness, heat stroke, and dehydration. Risk factors for heat illness include extremes of age (> 75 or < 4), medication use that interferes with heat loss, dehydration, alcohol or illicit drug use, exertion in the heat without proper acclimatization, continual heat stress, and rare medical conditions.

PATHOPHYSIOLOGY

The body regulates heat through four mechanisms: radiation, conduction, convection, and evaporation. In higher temperatures, evaporation is the primary mechanism for body cooling. Conduction and convection are ineffective above 32°C and 35% humidity.[9] Radiation is only effective in cooler environments. The body's response to heat stress is through four mechanisms: dilatation of blood vessels, increased sweating, decreased heat production in brown fat (ineffective in adults), and behavioral control to seek cooler environments. The body acclimatizes to heat stress over 1–2 weeks with an increase in sweating at a lower core temperature, improvement in cutaneous vascular flow, and reduction of the thermoregulatory set point.[10] Heat illness often occurs in two settings: prolonged periods of high environmental heat stress, as may occur in a heat wave, or by exertional heat injury under conditions of high heat stress, as may occur with aid workers, laborers, fire fighters, or military personnel.

MINOR HEAT RELATED ILLNESSES

Minor heat related illnesses are easily recognizable and treated.[11] These conditions are typically nonlethal.

■ Heat Cramps

Heat cramps are involuntary, painful spasms of skeletal muscles involving primarily the lower extremities, especially the calves. This condition often occurs in nonacclimatized or poorly conditioned individuals working or exercising in hot environments. The individuals typically sweat profusely (high sodium loss) and replace fluids with water or hypotonic solutions. This relative deficiency in electrolytes and fluids causes a cellular hyponatremia and muscle spasm due to calcium-dependent muscle relaxation. Hypokalemia may also contribute.

Prevention involves adequate acclimatization and physical conditioning, maintaining proper dietary salt intake, and rehydrating during activity with electrolytes or salt-rich solutions.

Treatment involves oral or intravenous fluid and salt replacement and immediate rest in a cool, sheltered environment. Commercial electrolyte replacement drinks or a 0.1–0.2% oral saline solution can be given to replace fluids and salt. In less developed areas, a 0.1% saline solution can be made by dissolving two 10-grain (650 mg) salt tabs in 1 quart of water. Alternatively, an oral saline solution can be made by dissolving one-quarter to one-half teaspoon table salt in 1 quart of water.[12] More severe cases may require intravenous rehydration with normal saline. Pain control may have to be administered with opiates.

■ Heat Tetany

Heat tetany occurs secondarily to hyperventilation during exposure to short periods of intense heat stress. This results in respiratory alkalosis, circumoral and extremity paresthesia, and carpopedal spasm. Other heat cramps are not present. Treatment includes removing the individual from the heat and decreasing the breathing rate.

■ Heat Syncope

Heat syncope results from postural hypotension and relative volume depletion from venous pooling, peripheral vasodilatation, and reduced vasomotor tone in nonacclimatized individuals often early in heat exposure. These patients are generally not significantly volume-depleted.

Treatment involves removing the individual from the heat, oral or intravenous rehydration, and rest. Evaluation for other causes of syncope must be considered, especially in the elderly.

■ Heat Exhaustion

Heat exhaustion is an acute, stress-related illness characterized by body water volume depletion and variable body temperature from normal to 40°C.[13] The symptoms are nonspecific: weakness, fatigue, dizziness, lightheadedness, headache, nausea, vomiting, and muscle pain. Clinical signs include sinus tachycardia, orthostatic hypotension, tachypnea, sweating, and core temperature increase up to 40°C, syncope, and normal mental status. Laboratory studies reveal electrolyte disturbances, evidence of dehydration with an increased blood urea nitrogen (BUN), CR ratio or hypernatremia, hemoconcentration, and elevated creatine kinase (CPK) if rhabdomyolysis occurs.

Treatment of heat exhaustion includes removal from heat, rest, and rapid volume and electrolyte replacement. Oral salt or electrolyte solutions may be used in mild cases. In more severe cases of volume depletion, rapid infusion of several liters of normal saline may be necessary. Other electrolyte abnormalities like hypokalemia or hypophosphatemia should be addressed individually.

SEVERE HEAT RELATED ILLNESS

These conditions have multiorgan system involvement and high mortality rates if untreated.

■ Heat Stroke

The classic definition of heat stroke is a core temperature above 40°C, CNS dysfunction, and anhidrosis.[12] There are two types of heat stroke: (1) classic heat stroke and (2) exertional heat stroke. Classic heat stroke affects those with underlying medical conditions that impair thermoregulation or prevent removal from hot environments. Exertional heat stroke occurs generally in young, healthy people who engage in exercise in high heat and humidity.[13]

The presence of anhidrosis may be variable, so anyone with CNS dysfunction and high body temperature should be considered to have heat stroke. Heat stroke is caused by the complete failure of the body to thermoregulate.

Sweating in classic heat stroke is present early on, but then the individual develops anhidrosis by the time of the medical evaluation due to hypovolemia or sweat gland dysfunction. In exertional heat stroke, sweating is observed in 50% of patients during medical assessment.

The clinical signs and symptoms of CNS dysfunction include irritability, confusion, agitation, combativeness, hallucinations, bizarre behavior, seizures, focal weakness, posturing, lethargy, or coma. Seizures and status epilepticus are common. Central nervous system dysfunction is universally present at core temperatures above 42°C.

Initial resuscitation should include assessment of airway, breathing, circulation, oxygenation, and cardiac rhythm monitoring. Intravenous access should be obtained and high volume normal saline or lactated ringer's solution should be started at 250 ml/hr. Diagnostic tests including a complete blood count, chemistry, coagulation studies, hepatic panel, CPK, urinalysis, myoglobin, toxicology screen, and EKG should be obtained.

Treatment of heatstroke should be focused on immediate cooling of the core body temperature to below 40°C. A delay in cooling increases mortality. The following is a list of cooling techniques.

(1) Evaporative cooling: spray tepid water on the naked individual and use electric fans for convection. Ice packs should be placed to neck, axilla, and groin in close proximity to large blood vessels which may facilitate in heat exchange.
(2) Immersive cooling: place undressed individual in an ice water bath that covers the trunk and extremities.
(3) Cooling blankets
(4) Cold water catheter lavage: gastric, bladder, and rectal
(5) Cold water peritoneal or thoracic lavage
(6) Cardiopulmonary bypass

These techniques should be discontinued when the individual's temperature approaches 40°C as overshoot hypothermia may occur. Shivering may be suppressed with intravenous benzodiazepines, e.g., diazepam 5 mg or lorazepam 1–2 mg intravenously as needed.

Once the patient is stabilized, monitor for signs of fluid overload or congestive heart failure due to aggressive fluid rehydration. Electrolytes should be monitored and replaced accordingly. The CPK, myoglobin, renal function, and lactic acid should be monitored for evidence of rhabdomyolysis. Hematologic and coagulation studies often become abnormal due to thermal injury to cells and endothelium. Signs of abnormal bleeding, thrombocytopenia, and coagulopathies may take several days to develop. Thermal injury to the liver causes elevations in liver enzymes, peaking 24–72 hours after heat stroke. Renal failure is also common due to volume depletion, rhabdomyolysis, and direct thermal injury. Renal function and urine output should be monitored.

PREVENTION OF HEAT RELATED ILLNESS

(1) Increase fluid intake, even when not thirsty
(2) Maintain proper electrolyte and carbohydrate intake for the level of activity
(3) Decrease activity in the warmer parts of the day

(4) Wear loose and light colored clothing
(5) Avoid alcohol or illicit drugs
(6) Avoid direct sun exposure
(7) Utilize shade and breaks from the heat
(8) Promote acclimatization to hot environments

DESERT MEDICINE

Deserts are areas that receive < 10 inches of rain per year and are often located on the leeward (dry) side of mountain ranges. About 15% of the Earth's land mass is desert. Regionally, 50% of Africa is desert, but only 8% of the United States is desert. Desertification is occurring worldwide due to climate changes, over-grazing and over-planting in semi-arid border areas, and socioeconomic-driven human activities. Large temperature variations characterize desert climate, reaching 49°C during the day and 5°C at night. Water is sparse, often found in dispersed "oases," supplied by underground springs and wells.[14] Desert plants are often toxic, adapting to their harsh environment by growing thorns, spines, needles, or producing toxins to prevent foraging by animals. Desert terrain is rough, comprised of grainy sand dunes, loose rocks, steep grades, and perpetually hot surfaces.

Preparation for the desert environment is paramount for survival and to prevent injury. First, acclimatization and conditioning geared toward the desert is important. Acclimatization for the hot environment takes 1–2 weeks, and involves an increase in volume of sweat and active sweat glands, a decrease in electrolytes in sweat, and sweating at a lower body temperature. Clothing should be lightweight, light colored, and made from a breathable fabric like cotton. Long sleeves, long pants, and sturdy boots are recommended to protect against thorns, splinters, insects, blowing sand, and the rough terrain. Foot care is very important, socks should not be cotton, they should be wool or polypropylene and gaiters should be used to prevent sand and rocks from entering shoes. Leather gloves are recommended to protect hands from splinters, spines, or bites. A wide brimmed hat and sun goggles are recommended to protect the head, face, and eyes from the sun and sand.[15] Preparation is important as closed injuries like sprains, contusions, fractures, and open injuries like cuts, blisters, abrasions, and bites, stings, or toxin exposure will reduce the ability to walk to shade and will intensify dehydration and heat illness.[16]

Behavior while in the desert is equally as important and is often what determines the chance for developing a heat related illness. The desert is hot and dry, strenuous activity is necessary to pass the expansive environment, the availability of water is spotty, and it is often impossible to carry enough water to sustain hydration (1 gallon of water weighs 8 lbs). One should rest in shade or cover during the day, and travel in the evening or night during cooler temperatures and limited sunlight. Found water should be filtered or boiled as it may be contaminated with bacteria or parasites. Unknown plants and animals should be avoided.

PART 2 COLD RELATED ILLNESSES (FROSTBITE AND HYPOTHERMIA)

Daniel Irving, MD

In contrast to heat related illnesses, the global health burden of cold related illnesses may be expected to decline in the coming decades if global warming continues at its current pace. However, conflicting research exists regarding climate change. For example, one study postulates that a period of rapid global cooling followed an era of global warming 8200 years ago. This effect was thought to be due to a disruption in the Gulf Stream caused by changes in ocean currents from melting glacial ice.[17] Rapid global cooling is often seen in the years following major volcanic eruptions, due to the scattering of particles in the atmosphere and the deflection of solar radiation. An average global mean surface temperature decrease of 0.1–0.2°C was seen in the aftermath of several volcanic eruptions over the last 140 years including those in Krakatoa (Indonesia, 1883), El Chichon (Mexico, 1982), and Pinatubo (Philippines, 1991).[18] Mean surface temperature changes following these events were unevenly distributed, with North America and Eurasia seeing temperature increases and Africa and South Asia seeing temperature decreases. The Earth is a complicated system with countless interacting variables, and temperature changes cannot be reliably predicted on a year-to-year basis. Cold related illnesses should therefore be expected to continue to pose a global health issue related to climate change.

FROSTBITE

Frostbite is a peripheral cold injury that occurs primarily in humans as a result of inadequate protection of the extremities in a cold environment. Frostbite has been described for centuries, most notably in military history. Accounts date back to 401 B.C., when over 60% of the army of Athenian commander Xenothon were afflicted while crossing Asia Minor.[19] More recent accounts include the one million cases described over World Wars I and II and the Korean War.[20] Frostbite is also a common hazard for mountain climbers and explorers. Residents or tourists are theoretically at risk for frostbite anywhere temperatures drop below freezing. At-risk areas are found on all seven continents and can be found at any latitude, even equatorial regions depending on the altitude. As mankind pursues more activities in extreme environments such as Antarctica and the Himalayas, frostbite will continue to pose a health risk for selected populations.

PATHOPHYSIOLOGY

Frostbite is caused by the body's efforts to maintain core temperature via peripheral vasoconstriction and shunting, at the expense of extremity perfusion. Below a tissue temperature of 10°C, the *prefreeze* phase begins, characterized by increased viscosity of vascular contents and endothelial plasma leakage. When tissue temperature drops below 0°C, the *freeze-thaw* phase begins. Ice crystals form extracellularly, increasing tissue pressure. Water then exits cells to maintain osmotic equilibrium. The next phase, *progressive vascular collapse,* is characterized by RBC sludging and microthrombi formation that lead to anaerobic metabolism and ultimately ischemia and necrosis.

Impaired local circulation is the primary contributor to frostbite. In addition to the primary cold insult, local circulation is further impaired by factors such as dehydration, wet or tight clothes, ethanol or tobacco consumption, and cardiovascular disease.

SIGNS AND SYMPTOMS

The most common presenting symptom is numbness, present in 75% of cases.[21] Extremities are most commonly affected (lower > upper), as well as the ears, nose, and penis/scrotum. Patients may report a clumsy sensation of the affected extremity. Pain will usually be present if thawing has occurred. Early appearances can be deceiving, as the affected extremity often appears normal even in severe cases. If the extremity is still frozen, it may appear yellowish white or mottled blue.

DIAGNOSIS

It is difficult to assess the extent of injury until the extremity has been rewarmed. Rewarming causes rapid hyperemia, and usually significant pain that can persist for days to weeks. Initial symptoms favoring a good outcome include normal sensation, warmth, and color. A residual blue or purple hue after rewarming predicts a poor outcome. Early formation of large, clear blebs extending to the tips of digits is more favorable than delayed small, hemorrhagic blebs. Edema usually develops within 3 hours post thaw, with a lack thereof suggestive of severe tissue damage.

DIFFERENTIAL CONSIDERATIONS

■ Frostnip
Frostnip is a superficial cold injury with transient parasthesias that resolve after rewarming. It differs from frostbite in that no tissue destruction occurs.

■ Chilblains (pernio)
Chilblains are a mild dry-cold injury, often from repetitive exposure. Sores appear usually on the face, dorsa of hands and/or feet, and the pretibial area.

■ Trench Foot
Trench foot is a nonfreezing cold injury resulting from prolonged exposure to wet cold at above-freezing temperatures. It develops gradually over days and is manifested by cool, pale feet with numbness and/or tingling. After rewarming, the skin remains erythematous, dry, and painful to touch. There may be bullae similar to those found in frostbite. Dry socks can prevent trench foot.

TREATMENT

Pre-thaw: Remove constrictive or wet clothing, and replace with dry loose wraps. Immobilize, elevate, insulate, and keep affected areas dry. Avoid rewarming in the field, during transport, or if a chance of refreezing exists, as refreezing a frostbitten extremity can cause further tissue damage. Friction massage is never indicated. Stabilize core temperature (see the hypothermia section).

Thaw: When a stable location is reached, begin rapid rewarming when core temperature is > 34°C. Rewarming should be achieved by immersion in gently circulating water maintained at temperature of 40–42°C. Continue rewarming until distal erythema is present and tissue feels pliable. Avoid radiant heat sources (campfires, heaters). Administer parenteral analgesia when possible.

Post-thaw: Keep elevated. Apply sterile dressings. Monitor tissue pressures frequently. Aspirate clear vesicles; leave hemorrhagic vesicles intact. Debride broken vesicles, applying topical antibiotics. Tetanus and bacterial prophylaxis (strep, staph, pseudomonas) is indicated, especially in severe cases. NSAIDs are recommended due to their fibrinolytic properties.[5]

PREVENTION

Adequate preparation, education, and health maintenance are effective in the prevention of frostbite. Proper shelter, equipment, and clothing with particular attention paid to the head and neck region maintain core temperature and insulate extremities, delaying the onset of frostbite. Avoid tight-fitting clothing, maintain dry extremities and maintain adequate dietary intake.

HYPOTHERMIA

Unlike frostbite, hypothermia can occur at temperatures above freezing, in any location, and in any season. Hypothermia occurs most frequently in urban settings in industrialized nations.[22] The relationship between mortality and cold temperatures is more complex than that seen with high temperatures, and studies have shown increased mortality in countries with temperate climates (United Kingdom, Western Europe) compared with much harsher climates such as Siberia. This discrepancy may be related to factors such as inadequate housing and clothing as well as fuel poverty.[23,24]

At-risk populations include military personnel, hunters, the homeless, sailors, skiers, climbers, hikers, swimmers, or participants in other outdoor activities. Risk is increased at the extremes of age and in people with chronic medical problems.

PATHOPHYSIOLOGY

Hypothermia is classically defined as a core body temperature below 35°C. At core temperatures below 30°C, humans become poikilothermic, cooling to the ambient temperature.

Table 11-1 Hypothermia

Severity	Temp. F (C)	Features
Mild	> 93.2 (>34)	Maximal shivering + slurred speech at 95F
Moderate	86–93 (30–34)	At 89—altered mental status, mydriasis, shivering ceases, muscles are rigid, incoordination, bradypnea
Severe	< 86 (< 30)	Bradycardia, Osborne waves on ECG, voluntary motion stops, pupils become fixed dilated
	79 (26)	Loss of consciousness, areflexia, no pain response
	77 (25)	No respirations, appear dead, pulmonary edema
	68 (20)	Asystole

Management of Hypothermia

- Evaluate for cause (e.g. sepsis, hypoglycemia, CNS disease, adrenal crisis). Avoid vigorous manipulation (can precipitate ventricular fibrillation).
- **Mild hypothermia** (> 34C): <u>Passive external rewarming</u>, treatment underlying disease only treatment needed. Standard BLS/ACLS if cardiac arrest.
- **Moderate hypothermia** (30–34C): <u>Active external rewarming</u>. Warm humidified O$_2$, warmed fluids. CPR, & advanced life support prn. *If cardiac arrest,* active internal rewarming, standard ACLS with medications spaced at longer intervals.
- **Severe hypothermia** (< 30 C): <u>Active internal warming</u>. Warm humidified O$_2$, warm IV fluids. If nonarrested, consider warm peritoneal dialysis (41C dialysate), or pleural irrigation (41C), cardiopulmonary bypass, or extracorporeal membrane oxygenation (ECMO). If signs of life, and nonarrested, avoid CPR, and ACLS. Do not treat atrial arrhythmias. Treat ↓BP with NS 1st. Use pressors cautiously. Consider underlying cause: empiric D$_{50}$, thiamine 100 mg IV, naloxone 2 mg IV, + hydrocortisone 100 mg IV, sepsis treatment. *If cardiac arrest,* perform standard BLS, intubate and attempt defibrillation for shockable rhythm × 1. If no response, defer defibrillation until rewarmed to 30–32C. Withhold drugs until core temperature > 30C. Consider peritoneal/pleural lavage, ECMO, cardiopulmonary bypass.

Circulation 2005; 112: IV136.

The body's physiological response to hypothermia is variable, depending on the rate of cooling, the patient's fitness, and many other factors. Sometimes a certain response occurs initially, with the opposite response prevailing as the core temperature continues to drop.

■ Central Nervous System
Shivering is triggered at 35°C in an effort to generate heat, and ceases below 31°C. Impaired memory and judgment, and slurred speech develop at 34°C. Most patients become comatose at 30°C.[25]

■ Cardiovascular
Initial response is mediated by catecholamine response including tachycardia, vasoconstriction, and increased blood pressure. As the temperature drops, bradycardia prevails and blood pressure drops. Any atrial or ventricular

dysrythmias are possible below 32°C. Atrial fibrillation is common below a core temperature of 32°C. Asystole and VFib can develop below core temperatures of 25°C. Electrolyte and pH abnormalities can potentiate arrythmias.

■ Renal

Cold exposure induces diuresis, termed *cold diuresis*. Ensuing hypovolemia complicates hypothermia as it progresses.

■ Respiratory

Hypothermia initially stimulates respiratory drive, followed by a progressive decrease in minute ventilation as cellular metabolism diminishes and less CO_2 is produced. Eventually the brain's ventilatory drive ceases.

■ Hematologic

Increased blood viscosity and inhibition of clotting enzymes are seen, as well as platelet alteration and thrombocytopenia. A DIC-type picture may be seen.

Precipitating factors are divided into four categories: 1) decreased heat production such as endocrine failure, insufficient fuel, and neuromuscular inefficiency; 2) increased heat loss from environmental factors, vasodilation, skin losses, and iatrogenic causes; 3) impaired thermoregulation; and 4) miscellaneous causes (e.g., sepsis).

SIGNS AND SYMPTOMS

History usually suggests diagnosis, and severe hypothermia is often obvious. Subtle presentations predominate in urban settings, and vague symptoms are present in mild cases (i.e., hunger, nausea, fatigue, dizziness). Specific signs and symptoms include tachycardia (early finding), bradycardia (late finding), other arrythmias, hypotension, tachypnea (early finding), apnea (late finding), constipation, nausea/vomiting, decreased level of consciousness, ataxia, dysarthria, impaired judgment, apathy, psychoses, increased muscle tone, shivering, rigidity, erythema, pallor, cyanosis, edema, frostbite, and pernio.

DIAGNOSIS

Temperature can be measured via several routes including rectal (most practical for mild cases), esophageal probe (preferable in severe cases or in intubated patients), tympanic, or bladder.

Laboratory studies should include ABG (uncorrected for temperature), CBC, comprehensive metabolic panel with Mg, Ca, amylase/lipase, PT/PTT, and creatinine kinase.

Electrolytes must be continuously monitored during rewarming, as fluctuations can occur. Free water depletion from cold diuresis frequently leads to hypernatremia and increased serum osmolality. Hypokalemia is more common in prolonged hypothermia due to intracellular shifts. K+ supplementation can lead to toxicity as temperature normalizes and the electrolyte reenters circulation, so caution is advised when treating this disorder. Hypothermia enhances cardiac toxicity of K+, so VF can be precipitated at normal or borderline K levels. Rhabdomyolysis is often present. Hyperglycemia is seen initially but hypoglycemia prevails as glycogen stores are depleted.

TREATMENT

"No one is dead until they are warm and dead." The lowest known core temperature in accidental hypothermia in which the patient survived is 13.7°C.[26] Even if a patient appears dead (cold, stiff, unreactive pupils), a chance of successful resuscitation exists unless obvious lethal injuries are present.

Initial stabilization follows the ABCs: airway, breathing, and circulation. An IV should be established while the patient is placed on a cardiac monitor. Core temperature should be obtained and continuously monitored. Remove all clothing, insulate with dry blankets and/or wraps. Comatose patients should be handled delicately, as minimal movement can induce VFib or asystole. Patients are usually dehydrated and aggressive fluid resuscitation is required.

Asystole and VF are common in cases of severe hypothermia. CPR should be initiated and continued until successful resuscitation or death is pronounced after rewarming. ACLS protocols differ in hypothermia. Bradyarrythmias are not responsive to atropine in hypothermia. Vasopressors, epinephrine, and anti-arrhythmics should be avoided when possible as they can be arrhythmogenic. Defibrillation is usually ineffective until a core temperature of 28°–30°C is reached, but three attempts should be made in lower temperatures nevertheless.[9]

As sole treatment, passive external rewarming is generally indicated in mild cases of hypothermia (32.2°–35°C). Treatment consists of removing wet clothing, applying dry clothing and/or wraps, and transferring the patient to a warm environment. It is required that the patient's thermogenesis is still intact.

Active rewarming is the direct transfer of endogenous heat to patient. It is classified as either external or internal (core) active rewarming. Indications for active rewarming include moderate to severe (< 32.2°C) hypothermia and cardiovascular instability. Active external rewarming methods include: forced air surface rewarming, immersion, and arteriovenous anastomoses rewarming. Active core rewarming methods include airway rewarming, heated IV infusion, heated irrigation, and extracorporeal blood rewarming. Patients receiving active external rewarming are susceptible to *core temperature afterdrop*. This phenomenon occurs when rewarming initiates peripheral vasodilation of previously vasoconstricted extremities. Cold blood that was previously confined to the extremities quickly returns to the core circulation, resulting in a precipitous drop in temperature.

PREVENTION

Physical conditioning, adequate rest, and nutrition are paramount. Appropriate garments and shelter should be provided for expeditions where cold conditions are anticipated. Wet garments should be changed immediately. The mnemonic COLD applies to appropriate clothing: *Clean, Open* during exercise to avoid sweating, *Loose* layers to retain heat, and *Dry* to limit conductive heat loss.[9] Maintain hydration, but avoid eating snow, as significant body heat is required to convert ice to water. To prevent urban hypothermia, public services and education are necessary. An adequately warm interior environment (> 21°C) should be maintained.

POLAR MEDICINE

Medicine is increasingly being practiced in the harsh polar regions of both the Arctic Ocean and Antarctica. These polar regions share similar harsh environments, isolation, and darkness. Isolation is particularly a problem during the winter when total darkness and harsh weather conditions can make medical transport difficult or impossible.

The Arctic is generally warmer than Antarctica due to the moderating effects of Arctic waters and the lower elevations than that of Antarctica. The Arctic zone has indigenous populations in eight countries (Canada, Finland, Greenland (Denmark), Iceland, Norway, Russia, Sweden, and the United States) with a permanent population of approximately 4 million people.[27] These populations exhibit similar health problems as those in nonpolar regions of the world, with the addition of psychosocial, environmental, and occupational health problems unique to their harsh climate.[28]

In contrast, the Antarctic has no indigenous population and is governed by 46 nation signatories to the Antarctic Treaty.[29] Seasonal Antarctic populations range from 4000 in summer to 1000 in winter.[30] Antarctic populations are small and tend to be younger and healthier research personnel. Consequently, health problems in the Antarctic are more frequently related to trauma or exposure.

In addition to "regular" health problems experienced at any latitude, visitors and workers in polar regions are particularly susceptible to trauma, hypothermia, frostbite, altitude related illnesses, UV exposure (associated with holes in ozone layer), vitamin D deficiency (underexposure to sunlight), circadian rhythm disturbances, and psychiatric illnesses. Limited resources and transport challenges can make medical problems that would be routine in other environments catastrophic in polar regions. Advances in communication, telemedicine, and the Internet have helped to improve medical care. Travelers to polar regions are encouraged to purchase insurance covering air transport and evacuation for medical reasons.

HIGH ALTITUDE MEDICINE

While high altitude illness is a distinct clinical entity from the illnesses described previously (frostbite and hypothermia), they are often intertwined since high altitude environments are typically cold environments as well.

Worldwide, approximately 40 million people live above 2500 m, and 25 million people live above 3000 m. The highest human habitation is approximately 5100 m at La Rinconada, Peru.[31] Above 5500 m, physiologic deterioration outpaces acclimatization.[32] Visitors to high altitude regions worldwide number in the millions, especially in places such as the American West, the Alps, the Pyrenees and Dolomites in Europe, the Andes in South America, and the Himalayas in Asia.

High altitude illnesses comprise a spectrum ranging from acute mountain sickness (AMS), which is relatively benign, to high altitude pulmonary edema

(HAPE) and cerebral edema (HACE), which are life-threatening. The incidence of altitude illness depends on many variables, including the rate of ascent, sleeping altitude, final peak altitude, duration of stay at the altitude, individual susceptibility, and underlying medical conditions. Most sufferers of high altitude illness are lowland dwelling visitors to high altitude regions. They include regular tourists to the aforementioned regions, mountain climbers, and skiers. Altitude illness is also seen in soldiers stationed at high altitudes, such as the Indian and Pakistani soldiers stationed on the Siachen glacier in the Himalayas—the world's highest battleground—who are often required to ascend quickly with little time for acclimatization.[33] Altitude illness is rarely seen in those who reside at high altitude unless they climb to a significantly higher altitude or in the case of re-entry HAPE when they descend for a brief period and then return to a high altitude.

Clinically significant altitude ranges can be divided into high altitude (1500 m–3500 m), very high altitude (3500 m–5500 m) and extreme altitude (> 5500 m). Physiologic effects of altitude begin in the high altitude range, and incidence of altitude illness is highest here due to the large number of unacclimated individuals ascending to these ranges. The highest incidence of severe altitude illness is seen at the very high altitude range, while at extreme altitude, acclimatization is no longer possible and abrupt ascent can be fatal.[34]

PATHOPHYSIOLOGY

The physiologic effects of high altitude are due to decreased barometric pressure and subsequent hypoxemia. Acclimatization refers to the adaptations the body makes to restore PaO_2 to near sea level values. Acclimatization begins when SaO_2 falls below sea level values. Most healthy, unacclimated persons will not significantly desaturate (< 90% SaO_2) below 2500 m.[16]

Physiologic adaptations to altitude include the following:

■ Increased Ventilation
Above 1500 m, central respiratory centers mediate the hypoxic ventilatory response (HVR), hyperventilation, and ensuing respiratory alkalosis seen at high altitude.

■ Bicarbonate Diuresis
Within 1–2 days of continued respiratory alkalosis, the kidneys respond by excreting bicarbonate, which brings pH to near normal values.

■ Systemic Circulation
Increased sympathetic activity leads to increases in blood pressure, heart rate, cardiac output, and venous tone.

■ Pulmonary Circulation
Hypoxia leads to pulmonary vasoconstriction in an effort to match ventilation and perfusion.

■ Cerebral Circulation
Hypoxemia-induced vasodilation and hypocapnia-induced vasoconstriction compete to increase and decrease cerebral blood flow (CBF), respectively.

Below a PaO$_2$ of 60 mmHg (seen at altitude > 2800 m), the hypoxic response predominates, leading to a net increase in CBF.

■ Hematologic

Erythropoietin secretion is stimulated by hypoxemia, which stimulates bone marrow production of red blood cells (RBCs). New RBCs enter circulation within 4–5 days enabling a greater oxygen-carrying capacity of circulating blood. SaO$_2$ is well maintained (> 90%) until an altitude of approximately 3000 m is reached. At this altitude, PaO$_2$ is approximately 60 mmHg. Excursion above 3000 m causes a precipitous drop in SaO$_2$.

ALTITUDE RELATED ILLNESSES

The most effective treatment of all forms of altitude illness is descent, although pharmaceutical adjuncts exist.

■ High Altitude Headache (HAH)

Headache is generally the first symptom of hypobaric hypoxia. High altitude headache (HAH) is typically a generalized, dull headache exacerbated by movement. It is important to note that HAH never has neurological symptoms, and a headache with neurological symptoms is typically indicative of HACE, a more serious ailment. Pharmacologic treatment of HAH is similar to treatment of other headache syndromes—NSAIDs or Acetaminophen are effective.

■ Acute Mountain Sickness (AMS)

Diagnosis of acute mountain sickness (AMS) is based on setting, history, and symptoms. It is most commonly seen in rapid ascent of unacclimatized persons to altitudes > 2500 m. The initial symptom of AMS is headache, followed by fatigue, nausea, dizziness, and anorexia. AMS symptoms resemble an alcohol hangover. AMS sufferers may also experience disabling apathy, complicating their efforts to descend. Neurological symptoms indicate progression to HACE.

There are no reliable physical findings of AMS. AMS is usually self-limited. For mild cases, halting ascent, rest, and treating symptoms is usually sufficient. Acclimatization will generally occur if ascent is halted. Supplemental oxygen should be provided if available. Portable hyperbaric treatment via inflatable fabric bags is an effective field treatment. For moderate–severe cases descent by 500–1000 m is indicated and usually sufficient.

■ High Altitude Cerebral Edema (HACE)

High altitude cerebral edema (HACE) is an encephalopathy characterized by ataxic gait, listlessness, altered consciousness, drowsiness, stupor, or coma. Focal neurologic deficits have been reported. Headache, nausea, and vomiting are often present. HACE is most common above 3000 m, but has been seen as low as 2100 m.[35] Vasodilation causes increased CBF, cerebral spinal fluid (CSF), and intracranial pressure (ICP), leading to ischemia and cytotoxic edema.

HACE can be fatal. At the first sign of ataxia, immediate descent and parenteral dexamethasone are indicated. Supplemental oxygen or hyperbaric therapy should be administered if available. Loop diuretics (furosemide) or osmotic diuretics (mannitol) will help decrease ICP, but adequate intravascular volume is necessary prior to initiating these therapies. Signs that persist despite adequate treatment for HACE should prompt a search for other causes.

■ High Altitude Pulmonary Edema (HAPE)

High altitude pulmonary edema (HAPE) is the most common cause of death among altitude related illnesses, but is easily reversed if recognized and treated early.[36] HAPE is uncommon below 3000 m, but has been reported to occur at altitudes as low as 1400 m.[37] Victims are typically, but not always, young fit men who ascend rapidly. It usually occurs within 2–4 days of ascent, most commonly on the second night. HAPE occurs as a direct result of pulmonary hypertension leading to noncardiogenic pulmonary edema. Early symptoms include dyspnea on exertion, fatigue, and a dry cough. Progression to dyspnea at rest and copious clear or frothy sputum production mark a serious illness. The condition typically worsens at night. Acute mountain sickness symptoms are present about 50% of the time.[16]

As with other altitude illnesses, descent is the only definitive treatment, and can prevent death in the case of HAPE. 500–1000 m descent is usually sufficient. Bed rest and supplemental oxygen or hyperbaric therapy should be implemented. As with other types of pulmonary edema, furosemide is effective. Nifedipine has pulmonary vasodilating effects and has been shown to be useful in the treatment of HAPE.[38]

PREVENTION

Prevention of altitude illness can be achieved with gradual ascent to permit acclimatization, a high carbohydrate diet, and avoiding alcohol and smoking. If a rapid ascent is attempted, maintaining a lower sleep altitude than peak daytime altitude is advised. The first night should be spent below 2500 m. Subsequent nights should involve ascent of no more than 600 m. Three nights of acclimatization should pass before any increase above 3000 m. One extra night of acclimatization should be added for every 1000 m of the target altitude above 3000 m.[16] Acetazolamide has been shown effective in prevention of AMS and HACE[39], while nifedipine is indicated as HAPE prophylaxis in those who have previously been afflicted.[40]

FURTHER READING

Marx JA, Hockberger RS, Walls RM. *Rosen's Emergency Medicine: Clinical Concepts and Practice.* 6th ed. Philadelphia: Mosby Elsevier; 2006.
Auerbach PS, ed. *Wilderness Medicine.* Philadelphia: Mosby Elsevier; 2007.
Scientific Committee on Antarctic Research Web site: http://www.scar.org

REFERENCES

1. World Health Organization. Climate Change and Human Health—Risks and Responses. Summary. Geneva, Switzerland: World Health Organization; 2003.

2. Intergovernmental Panel on Climate Change. Climate Change 2001: Synthesis Report. Cambridge, MA: World Meteorologic Organization/ United Nations Environment Programme (WMO/UNEP); 2001.

3. Patz JA, et al. Impact of regional climate change on human health. *Nature*. 2005;438:310–317.

4. World Health Organization. Protecting Health from Climate Change— World Health Day 2008. Geneva, Switzerland: World Health Organization; 2008.

5. Kalkstein LS, Greene JS. An evaluation of climate/mortality relationships in large US cities and the possible impacts of climate change. *Env Hlth Pers*. 1997;105(1):84–93.

6. Neira M, Bertollini R, Campbell-Lendrum D, et al. A breakthrough year for health protection from climate change? *Am J Prev Med*. 2008; 35(5):424–425.

7. Millenium Ecosystem Assessment. Ecosystems and Human Well-being: Desertification Synthesis. Washington, D.C.: World Resources Institute. 2005.

8. Campbell-Lendrum D, Corvalan C. Climate Change and Developing-Country Cities: Implications for Environmental Health and Equity. *Journal of Urban Health: Bulletin of the New York Academy of Medicine*: 2007;84(1).

9. Pascoe DD, et al. Clothing and Exercise: Influence of clothing during exercise/work in environmental extremes. *Sports Med*. 1994;18:94.

10. Tek D, Olshaker JS. Heat Illness. *Emergency Medicine Clinics of North America*. 1992;10:299.

11. Bouchama A, Knochel JP. Heat Stroke. *N Engl J Med*. 2002;25(346): 1978–1988.

12. Auerbach PS. Medicine for the Outdoors. 4th ed. Guilford, CT: Globe Pequot Press, 2003.

13. http://www.emedicinehealth.com/heat_exhaustion_and_heat_stroke/ article_em.htm. Accessed April 14, 2009.

14. Simon HB. Hyperthermia. *N Engl J Med*. 1993;329:483.

15. http://www.healthline.com/blogs/outdoor_health/2008_09_01_ outdoor_health_archive.html. Accessed April 10, 2009.

16. http://www.healthline.com/blogs/outdoor_health/2008/10/desert-and-desert-survival-2.html. Accessed April 10, 2009.

17. Barber DC, et al. Forcing of the cold event of 8,200 years ago by catastrophic drainage of Laurentide Lakes. *Nature*. 1999;400:344–348.

18. Robock A, Mao J. The Volcanic Signal in Surface Temperature Observations. *Journal of Climate*. 1995;8:1086–1103.

19. Paton BC. Cold, Casualties, and Conquests: The Effects of Cold on Warfare. In: Pandolf K, Burr R, ed. *Medical Aspects of Harsh Environments*. Vol 1. Washington, D.C.: Office of the Surgeon General; 2001.

20. McCauley R, Killyon G, et al. Frostbite. In: Aurbach PS, ed. *Wilderness Medicine*. Philadelphia: Mosby Elsevier; 2007.

21. Danzl D. Frostbite. In: Marx JA, Hockberger RS, Walls RM, eds. *Rosen's Emergency Medicine: Clinical Concepts and Practice*. 6th ed. Philadelphia: Mosby Elsevier; 2006.

22. Danzl D. Accidental Hypothermia. In: Marx JA, Hockberger RS, Walls RM, eds. *Rosen's Emergency Medicine: Clinical Concepts and Practice*. 6th ed. Philadelphia: Mosby Elsevier; 2006.

23. Curwen M. Excess winter mortality: A British phenomenon? *Health Trends*. 1991;22:169–175.

24. Donaldson GC, Tchernjavskii VE, Ermakov SP, Bucher K, Keatinge WR. Winter mortality and cold stress in Yekaterinburg Russia: interview survey. *Brit Med J*. 1998;316:514–8.

25. Danzl D. Accidental Hypothermia. In: Aurbach PS, ed. *Wilderness Medicine*. Philadelphia: Mosby Elsevier; 2007.

26. Gilbert M, Busund R, et al. Resuscitation from accidental hypothermia of 13.7 degrees C with circulatory arrest. *Lancet*. 2000;355:375–376.

27. http://www.athropolis.com/arctic-facts/fact-arctic-pop.htm

28. Carlisle B, Davis I. "Polar Medicine" Ch 9 in *Wilderness Medicine*, 5th ed., Editor Paul S. Auerbach, Philadelphia: Mosby Elsevier, 2007.

29. http://www.nsf.gov/od/opp/antarct/anttrty.jsp

30. https://www.cia.gov/library/publications/the-world-factbook/geos/ay.html

31. West JB. High Altitude Medicine & Biology. December 2002, 3(4): 401–407.

32. Yaron M and Honigman B. "High Altitude Medicine" Ch 142 in *Rosen's Emergency Medicine: Clinical Concepts and Practice*, 6th edition, ed. Marx, Hockberger, Walls, 2296, Philadelphia: Mosby Elsevier 2006.

33. Anand I. "Letter from the Siachen Glacier", *High Altitude Medicine & Biology*. December 2001, 2(4):553–557.

34. Hackett P, Roach R. "Mountain Medicine", Ch 1 in *Wilderness Medicine*, 5th ed., Editor Paul S. Auerbach, Philadelphia: Mosby Elsevier, 2007.

35. Hackett P, Roach R. "High Altitude Medicine", *High Altitude Medicine & Biology*. May 2004, 5(2):136–146.

36. Hackett P, Roach R. "High Altitude Illness" *New England Journal of Medicine*, 345:107–14, July 12, 2001.

37. Gabry A, Ledoux X. "High Altitude Pulmonary Edema at moderate Altitude (<2,400 m; 7,870 ft)", *Chest*, January 2003 vol. (123)1, 49–53.

38. Oelz O, et al. "Nifedipine for high altitude pulmonary oedema", *The Lancet*, 1989 Nov 25;2(8674):1241–1244.

39. Buddha B, et al., "Efficacy of Low-dose Acetazolamide (125 mg BID) for the Prophylaxis of Acute Mountain Sickness: A Prospective, Double-blind, Randomized, Placebo-controlled Trial." *High Altitude Medicine & Biology*. March 2003;4(1):45–52.

40. Bartsch P, et al. "Prevention of high altitude pulmonary edema by nifedipine", *The New England Journal of Medicine*, Oct 31, 1991, vol 325: 1284–1289.

XII ■ CENTRAL AMERICA AND THE CARIBBEAN

Craig Spencer, MD

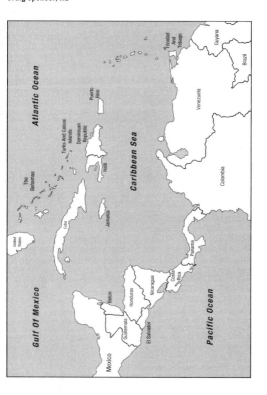

Central America consists of Belize, Costa Rica, El Salvador, Guatemala, Honduras, Nicaragua, and Panama. The Caribbean is made up of many islands across hundreds of miles of water, of which Cuba, Haiti, Dominican Republic, and Jamaica are the largest and most populated.

Human civilizations in the region go back thousands of years, reaching their preconquest pinnacle with the Aztec and Mayan societies that stretched from Mexico to South America. Since Columbus' voyage to the region in the late 15th century, Spanish influence has dominated the area now known as Central America. The British were also influential in the region, particularly in the Caribbean and British Honduras (present-day Belize). In 1821, following periods of war and numerous independence movements, a group of Central American *criollos* declared independence from Spain, and in 1823 finally achieved true independence for Central America. Originally fashioned on the relatively new United States of America, the United Provinces of Central America were not able to keep their union together long—when Honduras left in 1838 it would have been obvious the coalition was falling apart. Although numerous efforts have been made to reorganize the countries into a united force, the only lasting unions have centered on economic issues with minimal political overlap. Since independence, the region has seen many struggles, including the filibuster William Walker, a long civil war in Guatemala, the Contra-Sandinista struggle in Nicaragua, and the Salvadoran civil war. Today the region enjoys relative peace, and there have been significant achievements in bringing the countries together in political, economic, and judicial unions.

In the Caribbean, various European forces wrestled for influence and the region become a hotbed of colonial conflict and rivalries. Although Spain claimed the Caribbean for its own, the Dutch, French, and English also acquired territories. It was only in 1791, when a slave rebellion broke out in Haiti, that a region of the Caribbean gained independence from European oversight. In 1844, the Dominican Republic declared its independence from Haiti. Over the past two centuries, other countries have declared independence or have distanced themselves from their imperial rule. Nevertheless, numerous European dependencies still exist in the region, and the history of colonial intervention is still evident in the language, culture, and politics of the nascent countries.

CLIMATE

Central America and the islands of the Caribbean all enjoy a tropical climate, with little fluctuation between high and low temperatures and only two distinct seasons, characterized by intense rainfall and high humidity. The region suffers annual hurricane and tropical storm activity. Central America itself is an isthmus connecting the much larger landmasses of North and South America, flanked on its sides by both the Pacific and Caribbean and interrupted in the middle by the huge lakes of Nicaragua. It is at the center of four tectonic plates and has both cool, mountainous regions and hotter regions closer to sea level.

HUMAN DIVERSITY AND REGIONAL CULTURAL ISSUES

Indigenous populations lived in the region for thousands of years before the arrival of Europeans in the late 15th century. Since then, mixing of the two groups as well as a dramatic decrease in the indigenous population from war and disease has created a diverse cultural landscape. Indigenous populations are found throughout the region, ranging from 1% in Costa Rica to over 40% in Guatemala, where the vast majority are of Mayan descent. Migration within the region has created diverse and unique groups, such as the Garifuna, also known as "black caribs," who live primarily along the Caribbean seaboard and have a rich linguistic and cultural heritage.

MAJOR HEALTH ISSUES

The most salient health concerns in the region are access to primary care and basic sanitation. Health care differs substantially from the advanced clinics of Costa Rica to the resource-poor facilities in Haiti. Allopathic medications are difficult to obtain, particularly in rural areas, where they are in short supply and expensive to patients.

The region's climate and geography support the numerous tropical diseases whose burden disproportionately affects the poorest people in the region, especially the indigenous populations and people of African descent. Hookworm, helminth infections, and Chagas disease are the most prevalent followed by dengue, schistosomiasis, leishmaniasis, trachoma, leprosy, and lymphatic filariasis.[1]

Over recent years, the region has witnessed a dramatic increase in conditions traditionally associated with wealthier industrialized nations. Ischemic heart disease and cerebrovascular disease are among the leading causes of mortality, and chronic health conditions such as hypertension and diabetes are on the rise.

COUNTRY PROFILES OF CENTRAL AMERICA AND THE CARIBBEAN

BELIZE

Population: 308,000

Religion: Catholic (50%), Protestant (25%)

Languages: English, Creole, Spanish, Mayan

Ethnic Groups: Mestizo, Creole, Maya, Garifuna

Colonial history: 1981 Independence from Britain

Politics: Parliamentary democracy with a Prime Minister and National Assembly.

■ Healthcare System[2]

The Government of Belize is the main provider of health services via the Ministry of Health. This agency is responsible for regulation, financing, health service delivery, sectorial management, and exercise of sanitary authority. Total health expenditure is 5.3% of the gross domestic product (GDP). The funds for health care come from a combination of domestic taxes and international aid. The overwhelming majority of healthcare services in the country are provided free or at low cost. This includes visits to a primary physician, dental care, vaccinations, and access to common prescription medications. Other services, including radiography, hospitalization, and surgery are heavily subsidized but patients are expected to contribute to the costs.

■ Medications and Vaccinations

Immunization coverage has remained stable above 95%, with 100% of vaccination funding supplied by the government.

■ HIV/AIDS[3]

First documented in Belize in 1986, prevalence has been increasing significantly with HIV/AIDS becoming the fourth leading cause of death in 2003. The current estimated prevalence rate is 2.1%, which ranks first in Central America and fourth in the Caribbean for rate of infection per capita. Unfortunately, although Belize initiated a nationwide campaign to "Know Your HIV Status, Get Tested Today" including free antiretroviral (ARV) therapy, stigma and discrimination associated with HIV/AIDS, even in the health sector, remain a barrier to seeking treatment. As a result, most HIV+ people in Belize are not receiving adequate ARV treatment.

■ Tuberculosis[4]

The number of tuberculosis cases has leveled recently after a period of increasing incidence. Directly Observed Treatment, Short-course (DOTS) population coverage and detection rate are 100%, with 75% DOTS treatment success in 2006. HIV/TB co-infection is of particular concern, showing a slight increase over recent years. MDR-TB is only a very small percentage (1.5%) of new TB cases, but represents up to 10% of previously treated patients.

■ Malaria[5]

Most new malaria cases emerge from the northern and southern parts of the country, with no known risk in Belize City and the mangrove isles known as the cayes. According to the World Health Organization (WHO), almost all cases are due to *P. vivax*, and there are no known cases of resistant *P. falciparum*.

■ Leading Causes of Death

In children, the leading causes of death are fetal malnutrition and immaturity, followed by communicable disease, most commonly acute respiratory infections. In schoolchildren and adolescents, transport accidents were the most significant causes of mortality. In adults, external injuries, cardiovascular disease and HIV-related mortality were significant. The infant mortality rate in Belize is 23 deaths per 1000 live births and the life expectancy is 68 years of age.

■ **Special Considerations**

Dengue fever and cholera have been reported in recent years. In the Mayan areas of Belize, traditional medicine is still widely practiced.

EL SALVADOR

Population: 7.2 million

Religion: Catholic (60%), Protestant (20%)

Languages: Spanish

Ethnic Groups: Mestizo, caucasian, Amerindian

Colonial history: Independence from Spain in 1821

Politics: Presidential Republic

■ **Healthcare System[6]**

Health care in El Salvador is provided by three sectors: the public Ministry of Public Health and Social Welfare (MSPAS), social security via the Salvadorian Institute of Social Security (ISSR), and the private sector. The MSPAS covers 80%, the ISSR covers 15%, and the private sector covers the remaining 5% of the population. In theory, there is free access by the entire population to a basic package of prevention-oriented health services and access to essential clinical services, including second-level care such as delivery care, general surgery, outpatient treatment, and hospitalization. The indigent population is subsidized by the State and the rest of the population has access to these services based on a formula that combines direct installment payments and a compulsory minimum health insurance program.

■ **Medications and Vaccinations**

Medications are provided by the government; however, there is a shortage of essential medications in primary care facilities and hospitals. Vaccinations are provided in adequate amounts and the population enjoys high levels of free vaccinations. According to UNICEF, 2007 levels of routine immunizations were all above 93%.[7]

■ **HIV/AIDS[8]**

HIV prevalence is 0.9% with an estimated 36,000 people living with HIV. High-risk communities include sex workers and men who have sex with men, with most transmission in urban areas. It is estimated that 50% of individuals in need of treatment are receiving ART, largely through the MSPAS and ISSR.

■ **Tuberculosis[9]**

There are approximately 2700 new cases of TB every year, with a gradual decrease in recent years. DOTS coverage is 100% and MDR-TB has thus far been minimal. However, as in other parts of Central America, HIV/TB co-infection is on the rise.

■ **Malaria**

There is little to no risk of malaria in most of El Salvador, especially around large urban centers. The Global Fund reports 44 cases of malaria in the country, most arising from migrants.[10]

■ Leading Causes of Death

Cardiovascular disease, lower respiratory infections, trauma, and HIV are the leading causes of death in El Salvador. In children under 5, neonatal infections and diarrheal diseases are the largest causes of death. The infant mortality rate is 21 deaths per 1000 live births and the life expectancy is 72 years of age.

■ Special Considerations

Special attention should be given to Dengue fever and leptospirosis.

GUATEMALA

Population: 13.2 million

Religion: Catholicism and Protestant, indigenous Mayan beliefs

Languages: Spanish, Amerindian languages (23 officially recognized native languages)

Ethnic Groups: Mestizo, K'iche, Kaqchikel

Colonial history: Independence from Spain in 1821; 1960–1996 Civil War

Politics: Presidential Republic

■ Healthcare System[11]

Guatemala's public health expenditure is among the lowest in the Americas (around 1% of the GDP), 20% of its population lacks regular access to health services, and the quality and effectiveness of public services are limited. Although medical care is considered a fundamental right, many people do not have access to affordable health care.

There are three sectors of the healthcare system in Guatemala, the largest of which is the government-run MSPAS. MSPAS is in charge of 1244 primary care centers, 926 health posts, and 300 basic units located in rural areas, as well as 12,000 hospital beds. Health financing comes mainly from out-of-pocket household payments, the central government, companies, and international cooperation.

■ Medications and Vaccinations

The Drug Access Program (PROAM), created in 1997, works to ensure equal access for all Guatemalans to quality, affordable drugs placed in state and municipal pharmacies, hospitals, clinics, and rural infirmaries for the general welfare of all. Over 92% of infants are covered by the immunization program, which includes 10 vaccines. No cases of polio since 1990 or measles since 1997 have been reported.

■ HIV/AIDS[12]

Although HIV prevalence is only 0.9%, the total number of infections in Guatemala represents one-sixth the total of all reported HIV cases in Central America. In all, UNAIDS estimates there are 61,000 people living with HIV in Central America, and 2700 deaths have occurred because of AIDS. The majority of new cases are reported in urban districts and affect young adults, with high rates of infection in sex workers and men who have sex with men.

Seventy-six percent of identified HIV-infected men and women who need treatment receive ART.

■ **Tuberculosis**

The estimated incidence of TB is 8.5 per 100,000 people with an estimated mortality rate of 14 per 100,000. DOTS coverage is only 70%. Although TB incidence is decreasing in the general population, there has been an increase in HIV/TB co-infection. The number of MDR-TB cases has been stable the past few years.[13]

■ **Malaria**

Malaria is a significant health threat in Guatemala, which accounts for 60% of all malaria cases in Central America. Chloroquine prophylaxis is recommended for individuals spending time in low-altitude rural areas (< 1500 m).[14]

■ **Leading Causes of Death**

Infectious diseases and nutritional deficiencies occur mainly in children under 5 years of age. In adults, the leading causes of death are communicable disease, external causes, and circulatory events. The infant mortality rate is 39 deaths per 1000 live births and the life expectancy is 70 years of age.

■ **Special Considerations**

Violence against women has been of particular concern in Guatemala, with a very high level of disappearances and violent deaths among females. Chronic malnutrition affects 50% of Guatemalan children.

HONDURAS

Population: 7.8 million

Religion: Roman Catholic

Languages: Spanish

Ethnic Groups: Mestizo, indigenous

Colonial history: Independence from Spain in 1821

Politics: Presidential representative democratic republic

■ **Healthcare System**[15]

Health care in Honduras is fragmented, with numerous entities in charge of healthcare delivery. The Secretariat of Health (SS) and the Honduran Social Security Institute (IHSS) are responsible for the public sector, and roughly 10% of wealthy Hondurans receive treatment in the private sector. Unfortunately, most Hondurans (83%) are uninsured and roughly 30% of the population receives no health care at all. These disparities are most pronounced in rural and indigenous communities. Health expenditure in Honduras is among the lowest in the region.

■ **Medications and Vaccinations**

The WHO reports that 100% of funding for routine vaccinations is provided by the government, although there is much room for improvement. In 2007, rates for all but two vaccinations were in the 80th percentile, representing a decline over previous years.[16]

■ HIV/AIDS

HIV/AIDS cases in Honduras represents 60% of all cases in Central America. Adult HIV prevalence is 0.7% with an estimated 28,000 adults living with HIV. Each year, approximately 2000 people die of AIDS related deaths, and coverage with ART is at 50%.[17] Particularly vulnerable are sex workers, men who have sex with men, and the Garifuna population. Recent advances have made treatment more accessible to those that need it, largely provided by the public sector with minimal cost to the patient.

■ Tuberculosis[18]

Honduras has the eighth highest TB burden among all countries in the Western Hemisphere. Since the introduction of DOTS programs, new cases have fallen gradually. MDR-TB has remained stable.

■ Malaria[19]

Malaria is endemic in Honduras, with 11,000 new cases annually. Risk of infection is greatest along the eastern coast, on the Bay Islands, and Roatan. Chloroquine is strongly recommended when visiting lowland rural areas and in the departments of Gracias a Dios, Colón, Olancho, Yoro, Alántida, Cortés, and the Bay Islands.

■ Leading Causes of Death

Ischemic heart disease, HIV/AIDS, and perinatal conditions are the leading causes of death in Honduras. The infant mortality rate is 24 deaths per 1000 live births and the life expectancy is 67 years of age.

■ Special Considerations

Dengue fever is endemic in Honduras, and leishmaniasis and Chagas are present, although rare.

NICARAGUA

Population: 5.9 million

Religion: Catholic, Evangelical

Language: Spanish

Ethnic Groups: Mestizo, Caucasian, Black, Amerindian

Colonized: Independence from Spain in 1821, British on Caribbean coast in 19th century.

Politics: Democratic republic with president and National Assembly.

■ Healthcare System[20]

The Ministry of Health (MOH) and Nicaraguan Social Security Institute (INSS) are public providers that cover most consultations, although only 60% are provided free of charge. Private providers require payment for services. Only 6.3% of the population is insured (INSS). Out-of-pocket expenditures represent a significant barrier to healthcare access, especially for rural and minority populations.

■ Medications and Vaccinations

The majority of medications is purchased by patients and drug shortages are common. Routine immunizations are funded by the government and international organizations. Immunization rates have steadily increased, with coverage rates between 84.7% and 97.6%. There were no reported measles, polio, or diphtheria cases in 2007.[21]

■ HIV/AIDS

With a prevalence rate of 0.3%, Nicaragua has one of the lowest HIV rates in Central America. However, new cases of HIV have increased over recent years, and many people are unaware of their HIV status. There are an estimated 8000 individuals living with HIV. Unfortunately, access to HIV/AIDS services and information is limited and only 30% of HIV+ patients are receiving ART due to an inadequate supply of drugs.[22]

■ Tuberculosis

There are an estimated 2700 new cases of TB annually. Most new cases are in poor, rural areas with little access to health care. DOTS is available throughout the country. New cases of MDR-TB are on the decline.[23]

■ Malaria

Malaria is endemic along the Atlantic coast, with minimal or no risk on the Pacific coast.

■ Leading Causes of Death

In young people, traffic accidents and suicide are the leading causes of death, whereas in adults, cardiovascular diseases and diabetes are the leading causes. The infant mortality rate is 25 deaths per 1000 live births and the life expectancy is 69 years of age.

■ Special Considerations

Dengue fever is endemic. High maternal mortality and chronic malnutrition as well as poor access to health care in rural and minority areas represent the greatest public health obstacles.

COSTA RICA

Population: 4.2 million

Religion: Catholic 76%, Evangelical 13%

Languages: Spanish (official), English

Ethnic Groups: White (including mestizo), Black, Amerindian

Colonial history: Independence from Spain (1821)

Politics: Democratic republic

■ Healthcare System

Health care in Costa Rica is universal and of such high quality that it ranks above the United States.[24] The Ministry of Health monitors public health while the Costa Rican Social Security Fund (CCSS) provides maternity and health insurance for the entire population. Contributions from employers, workers, and the State support the system, as well as the unemployed population. Unlike other countries in Latin America, access to comprehensive health care is nearly equal across the country with a large number of healthcare personnel and a strong emphasis on preventative health. There is also private sector that individuals may pay for if desired.

■ Medications and Vaccinations

The majority of medications are provided free or at low cost, with a large network of licensed pharmacies. In addition, routine vaccinations are provided free of charge by the government, with high levels of childhood vaccination across the country, including poor and rural areas.

■ HIV/AIDS

The prevalence rate is 0.4% and there are an estimated 10,000 people living with HIV. Annual incidence of 400–500 new cases over the past few years indicates a steady-state epidemic. The majority of cases are from sexual transmission, particularly in sexual workers and men who have sex with men. Costa Rica is the only region in Central America with universal access to ART. Anti-retroviral therapy levels have remained high, with estimated coverage above 95%.[25]

■ Tuberculosis

The incidence, prevalence, and mortality rates for TB all remain low with 100% DOTS coverage, 100% DOTS detection rate, 90% treatment success, and low levels of MDR-TB.[26]

■ Malaria

Risk is minimal in most of Costa Rica, although present in parts of Alajuela, Limón, Guanacaste, and Heredia provinces. Chloroquine prophylaxis is recommended in these areas.[27]

■ Leading Causes of Death

Cardiovascular disease is the leading cause of death, followed by cancer and external causes. The infant mortality rate in Costa Rica is 9 deaths per 1000 live births and the life expectancy is 77 years of age.

■ Special Considerations

Sporadic cases of dengue fever have been reported, mainly from the provinces of Guanacaste and Puntarenas, both on the Pacific coast, and the province of Limón on the Caribbean coast. Standard insect precautions with DEET and long pants and long-sleeved shirts are advised.

PANAMA

Population: 3.3 million

Religion: Catholic 85%, Protestant 15%

Languages: Spanish (official), English

Ethnic Groups: Mestizo, West Indian, White, Amerindian

Colonial history: Independence from Spain in 1821; United States-backed secession from Colombia in 1903

Politics: Constitutional democracy

■ Healthcare System[28]

Public health in Panama is administered by two separate entities: the Ministry of Health (MINSA) and the Social Security System (CSS). The hospitals and primary healthcare centers administered by MINSA receive funding from the general budget of the government, and cover approximately 30% of the uninsured population. Those administered by CSS are funded with the money collected from workers' wages, and cover 67% of population. Many people do not have health insurance and lack access to health care. For those that can afford to pay for health care, Panama has a large system of excellent private hospitals.

■ Medications and Vaccinations

Individuals covered by CSS receive medications from clinics and hospitals in the Social Security System. Uninsured individuals must pay for medications, which are relatively cheap and readily available. Vaccinations are provided by the government with rates of routine vaccinations between 88% and 99%.[29]

■ HIV/AIDS

Prevalence is 1% and there are an estimated 20,000 people living with HIV, representing a steady increase in both categories since HIV was first identified in Panama two decades ago. The majority of cases are from sexual transmission. Currently, ART is available only to those covered by health insurance. Estimated ART coverage is 60%.[30]

■ Tuberculosis

There are 1600 new cases annually, with low levels of mortality and MDR-TB. DOTS coverage is 99% and DOTS treatment success is 80%.[31]

■ Malaria

Malaria is present in rural areas of Bocas Del Toro, Darién, San Blas provinces, and San Blas Islands. There is no risk in Panama City or in the former Canal Zone. High chloroquine resistance exists, especially in Darien and San Blas.[32]

■ Leading Causes of Death

Cardiovascular disease is the leading cause of death, followed by diabetes. In children under 5 years of age, neonatal complications, diarrhea, and pneumonia are leading causes of mortality. The infant mortality rate in Panama is 18 deaths per 1000 live births and the life expectancy is 76 years of age.

■ Special Considerations

Cases of dengue fever are reported annually, often in the Panama City metropolitan area. Standard insect precautions with DEET and long pants and long-sleeved shirts are advised. An outbreak of hantavirus, a severe viral infection typically leading to respiratory failure and frequently resulting in death, was reported in the province of Los Santos in 1999 and sporadic cases have occurred since then.

CUBA

Population: 11.4 million

Religion: Officially atheist; Catholic 60%, Protestant 5%, Santería

Languages: Spanish (official)

Ethnic Groups: White, Mulatto/mestizo, Black

Colonial history: Independence from Spain in 1898; Independence from US involvement in 1902

Politics: Communist state

■ Healthcare System

Despite trade embargos and widespread poverty, Cuba's healthcare system has remained remarkably strong and compares well to developed countries. Health care is almost exclusively financed by the state, and preventive medical care and diagnostic tests, as well as medications for hospitalized patients are free. The themes of Cuban health care are universality, equitable access, and government control. Health care is focused on preventative and primary care, and Cuba trains vast numbers of physicians to work both at home and across Latin America. Because of limited resources, traditional and alternate treatments are encouraged and widely utilized.

■ Medications and Vaccinations

Due to trade restrictions, Cuba has difficulty accessing many foreign-produced pharmaceuticals. There are often shortages of certain medications and therapeutics. Domestic pharmaceutical production is expansive and innovative, producing cheap and effective medicines for most conditions. These are provided free of charge during hospitalization and subsidized by the state when given on outpatient basis. Vaccinations are free and mandatory, with high levels of coverage across the country (> 95%).[33]

■ HIV/AIDS[34]

Education, HIV testing, and targeted prevention programs have led to the lowest prevalence of HIV/AIDS in the Americas at 0.1%. In 1985, with the first reported case of HIV, the Cuban government instituted broad control and containment strategies, resulting in low levels of new cases and almost non-existent mother to child and blood product transmission. In the past decade, new cases have been rising, with 99% of transmission via sexual relations. Cuba produces its own supplies of anti-retroviral medications and achieves near universal coverage.

■ Tuberculosis

There were 700 new cases in 2007. There were no reported cases of MDR-TB. DOTS coverage and detection rate is 100% and DOTS treatment success is 93%.[35]

■ Malaria
Malaria is not a health issue in Cuba.

■ Leading Causes of Death
Cuba's disease patterns are similar to highly developed countries with an emphasis on deaths from chronic noncommunicable diseases, such as heart disease and cancer. The infant mortality rate is 6 deaths per 1000 live births and the life expectancy is 77 years of age.

■ Special Considerations
Despite enduring embargos and the drastic decrease in funding after the collapse of the former Soviet Union, health care in Cuba continues to perform well when compared to wealthier nations.

DOMINICAN REPUBLIC

Population: 9.6 million

Religion: Catholic 95%

Languages: Spanish

Ethnic Groups: Mixed, White, Black

Colonial history: Independence from Haiti in 1844; independence from Spain in 1865

Politics: Democratic republic

■ Healthcare System
In early 2001, a series of laws established the National Health System (NHS) and the Dominican Social Security System with the intention of developing universal coverage. To date, most individuals have limited access to quality care and 75% of all health expenditures are out-of-pocket. In addition, there is a private sector with higher quality *clínicas*, but only a small percentage of the population is able to afford health insurance coverage.

■ Medications and Vaccinations
Most medications are imported and purchased by patients as needed. In 2006, only 69% of routine vaccinations were funded by the government. According to UNICEF/WHO, vaccination rates range between 59% (second measles) to 96% (first measles vaccination).[36]

■ HIV/AIDS
The adult prevalence of HIV in the Dominican Republic is 1.1%, and UNAIDS estimates that 66,000 Dominicans are HIV-positive. The majority of cases (81%) are from heterosexual transmission. High-risk groups include sex workers, sugar cane workers, and men having sex with men. Currently, 37% of HIV-infected people that need treatment receive ART, and only 50% of pregnant mothers with HIV receive anti-retrovirals.[37]

■ Tuberculosis
Incidence of TB in the Dominican Republic is among the highest in the Americas, and an estimated 10% percent of TB patients are co-infected with

HIV. Almost 7% of new cases are MDR-TB. DOTS coverage is 85% with 78% treatment success.[38]

■ Malaria
P. falciparum malaria is endemic with the highest risk along the western border with Haiti. More recently, cases of malaria have been reported in tourists returning from eastern resort towns, especially Altagracia and Duarte provinces.[39]

■ Leading Causes of Death
Mortality in children (under 5 years of age) is largely from neonatal causes of death, including preterm labor. HIV/AIDS, pneumonia, and diarrheal diseases are other significant causes. In adults, HIV/AIDS and cardiovascular disease are the most common causes of death. The infant mortality rate is 26 deaths per 1000 live births and the life expectancy is 74 years of age.

■ Special Considerations
A recent outbreak of leptospirosis as well as endemic dengue fever pose considerable health risks to both native inhabitants as well as travelers in the Dominican Republic.

HAITI

Population: 9 million

Religion: Catholic 80%, Protestant 16%, Voodoo

Languages: French (official), Creole (official)

Ethnic Groups: Black, Mulatto, white

Colonial history: Independence from France in 1804

Politics: Republic with president and National Assembly

■ Healthcare System[40]
Economic and political instability have had disastrous effects on virtually every aspect of Haiti, especially the healthcare system. The combination of diffuse poverty, poor sanitation, and inadequate access to health care has pushed Haiti to the bottom of the World Bank's rankings of health indicators. In terms of poverty and spending on health care, Haiti ranks last in the Western hemisphere.

There are four healthcare sectors in Haiti: public, private nonprofit, mixed, and private-for-profit. It is estimated that NGOs and religious missions provide up to 40% of health care in Haiti, with Medecins Sans Frontieres (MSF) responsible for three hospitals in the capital and emergency response programs across the country. Approximately 40% of the population has no access to health care.

■ Medications and Vaccinations
Supply of medications is inconsistent and paid for out-of-pocket. The WHO estimates that only 43% of the target population receives the recommended immunizations.[41]

■ **HIV/AIDS**

Haiti has one of the highest levels of HIV/AIDS outside of Africa, with a prevalence of 2.2% and an estimated 120,000 people living with HIV. Fueled by high poverty, illiteracy, and poor access to health care, HIV has become a significant public health problem. Maternal transmission to offspring is high as is the number of children orphaned by AIDS-related deaths. AIDS is the leading cause of death in the country and stigma and discrimination make treatment particularly difficult. Estimated ART coverage is 40%, with most treatment provided by NGOs. Haiti is one of the 15 countries targeted by the United States to receive funding from the U.S. President's Emergency Plan for AIDS Relief (PEPFAR) program.[42]

■ **Tuberculosis**

Haiti has the highest per capita TB burden in the Latin American and Caribbean regions. After HIV/AIDS, TB is the country's greatest infectious cause of mortality in both youth and adults (5400 deaths in 2006). Although DOTS coverage is only 91% and DOTS detection rate is only 55%, both numbers represent a significant improvement over previous years. MDR-TB has increased slightly over the same period, and there is a high rate of co-infection with TB in HIV+ individuals (20%).[43]

■ **Malaria**

P. falciparum malaria is endemic in Haiti. According to the Global Fund, there were over 32,000 reported cases of malaria last year.[44] Risk of malaria is high throughout the country, and prophylaxis with chloroquine is recommended for all visitors.

Infant Mortality Rate: 60 deaths/1,000 live births

Life Expectancy: 60 years

■ **Leading Causes of Death**

Neonatal death is common. Preterm labor, birth asphyxia, and neonatal infection contribute to a high infant mortality rate. Under-5 mortality stems from diarrheal disease and childhood pneumonia. In adults, HIV/AIDS is responsible for 22% of all deaths. The infant mortality rate is 60 deaths per 1000 live births and the life expectancy is 60 years of age.

■ **Special Considerations**

Dengue fever and leptospirosis are endemic.

JAMAICA

Population: 2.8 million

Religion: Protestant 63%, Catholic 3%, None 20%

Languages: English, English Patois

Ethnic Groups: Black, Mixed

Colonial history: Independence from Britain in 1958

Politics: Constitutional parliamentary democracy

■ **Healthcare System**

There are both public and private healthcare sectors in Jamaica though they often overlap. The Ministry of Health runs the public sector, with the Ministry of Finance and Planning the primary financier of health services. The majority of Jamaicans lack health insurance coverage and rely on government-provided health care. Public facilities are available and accessible to the entire population. Most hospitals and preventative institutions are in the public sector. The private sector in Jamaica is loosely regulated and has its own network of hospitals and specialists. Most institutions offering ambulatory care are in the private sector.

■ **Medications and Vaccinations**

Most medications in Jamaica are imported and paid for mostly out-of pocket. Routine vaccinations are financed by the government and rates of immunizations have varied drastically in recent years, representing a steady decline since 2001. Currently, vaccination rates for most routine immunizations are in the 80th percentile.[45]

■ **HIV/AIDS**

Prevalence of HIV in Jamaica has been constant at 1.5% for almost a decade and has probably reached a steady state. There are an estimated 28,000 people living with HIV and 1500 deaths from AIDS annually. Approximately one-half of HIV-infected individuals that need treatment receive ART.

■ **Tuberculosis**

The incidence of TB is approximately 3 per 100,000 people annually. 26% of new TB cases are HIV-positive.[46] The government recently opened a TB testing center at the National Public Health Laboratory.

■ **Malaria**

An outbreak of *P. falciparum* malaria in Kingston in 2006 came as a surprise given the absence of malaria for almost four decades. Eradication efforts have intensified and only sporadic cases are reported. The CDC lists the risk around Kingston as minimal and does not recommend prophylactic therapy.

■ **Leading Causes of Death**

Neonatal complications, diarrheal diseases, and pneumonia are the most common causes of death in children under 5. In adults, cardiovascular disease, diabetes mellitus, and cancer are the leading causes of death. The infant mortality rate is 15 deaths per 1000 live births and life expectancy is 74 years of age.

■ **Special Considerations**

Dengue has occurred sporadically in Jamaica for many years, but a large outbreak occurred in 2007 and affected many parts of the Caribbean.

REFERENCES

1. Hotez PJ, Bottazzi ME, Franco-Paredes C, Ault SK, Periago MR. The Neglected Tropical Diseases of Latin America and the Caribbean: A Review of Disease Burden and Distribution and a Roadmap for Control and Elimination. *PLoS Negl Trop Dis.* 2008;2(9):e300.

2. Pan-American Health Organization. Belize Basic Health Indicator Data Base. http://www.paho.org/English/DD/AIS/cp_084.htm. Accessed June 3, 2009.

3. World Health Organization. Belize Summary Country Profile for HIV/AIDS Treatment Follow-Up. http://www.who.int/hiv/HIVCP_BLZ.pdf. Accessed June 3, 2009.

4. World Health Organization. Belize Tuberculosis Country Profile. http://apps.who.int/globalatlas/predefinedReports/TB/PDF_Files/blz.pdf. Accessed June 3, 2009.

5. The Global Fund. Belize Country Statistics and Indicators. 2008. http://www.theglobalfund.org/programs/countrystats/?lang=en&countryID=bel. Accessed June 3, 2009.

6. Pan-American Health Organization. El Salvador Basic Health Indicator Data Base. http://www.paho.org/english/sha/prflels.htm. Accessed June 3, 2009.

7. UNICEF. At A Glance: El Salvador. http://www.unicef.org/infobycountry/elsalvador_statistics.html. Accessed June 3, 2009.

8. USAID. USAID HIV/AIDS Health Profile for El Salvador. September 2008. http://www.usaid.gov/our_work/global_health/aids/Countries/lac/elsalvad_profile.pdf. Accessed June 3, 2009.

9. World Health Organization. El Salvador Tuberculosis Country Profile. http://apps.who.int/globalatlas/predefinedReports/TB/PDF_Files/slv.pdf. Accessed June 3, 2009.

10. The Global Fund. El Salvador Country Statistics and Indicators. (http://www.theglobalfund.org/programs/countrystats/?lang=en&countryID=SLV. Accessed June 3, 2009.

11. Pan-American Health Organization. Guatemala Basic Health Indicator Data Base. http://www.paho.org/English/DD/AIS/cp_320.htm. Accessed June 3, 2009.

12. USAID. HIV/AIDS Health Profile for Guatemala. September 2008. http://www.usaid.gov/our_work/global_health/aids/Countries/lac/guatemala_profile.pdf. Accessed June 3, 2009.

13. World Health Organization. Guatemala Tuberculosis Country Profile. http://apps.who.int/globalatlas/predefinedReports/TB/PDF_Files/gtm.pdf. Accessed June 3, 2009.

14. Centers for Disease Control. Health Information for Travelers to Guatemala. http://wwwn.cdc.gov/travel/destinations/guatemala.aspx. Accessed June 3, 2009.

15. Pan-American Health Organization. Honduras Basic Health Indicator Data Base. http://www.paho.org/english/sha/prflhon.htm. Accessed June 3, 2009.

16. World Health Organization. Immunization Profile—Honduras. http://www.who.int/vaccines/globalsummary/immunization/countryprofileresult.cfm?C='hnd'. Accessed June 3, 2009.

17. World Health Organization. Summary Country Profile for HIV/AIDS Treatment Scale-Up. http://www.who.int/hiv/HIVCP_HND.pdf. Accessed June 3, 2009.

18. World Health Organization. Honduras Tuberculosis Country Profile. 2009. http://apps.who.int/globalatlas/predefinedReports/TB/PDF_Files/hnd.pdf. Accessed June 3, 2009.

19. Center for Disease Control. Health Information for Travelers to Honduras. 2009. http://wwwn.cdc.gov/travel/destinations/honduras.aspx. Accessed June 3, 2009.

20. Pan-American Health Organization. Nicaragua Basic Health Indicator Data Base. http://www.paho.org/English/sha/prflnic.htm. Accessed June 3, 2009.

21. World Health Organization. Immunization Profile—Nicaragua. http://www.who.int/vaccines/globalsummary/immunization/countryprofileresult.cfm?C='nic'. Accessed June 3, 2009.

22. USAID. HIV/AIDS Health Profile for Nicaragua. September 2008. http://www.usaid.gov/our_work/global_health/aids/Countries/lac/nicaragua_profile.pdf. Accessed June 3, 2009.

23. World Health Organization. Nicaragua Tuberculosis Country Profile. 2009. http://apps.who.int/globalatlas/predefinedReports/TB/PDF_Files/nic.pdf. Accessed June 3, 2009.

24. World Health Organization. World Health Report 2000. Geneva, Switzerland: World Health Organization; 2000.

25. World Health Organization. Costa Rica Summary Country Profile for HIV/AIDS Treatment Scale-Up. http://www.who.int/hiv/HIVCP_CRI.pdf. Accessed June 3, 2009.

26. World Health Organization. Costa Rica Tuberculosis Country Profile. http://apps.who.int/globalatlas/predefinedReports/TB/PDF_Files/cri.pdf. Accessed June 3, 2009.

27. Centers for Disease Control. Health Information for Travelers to Costa Rica. 2009. http://wwwn.cdc.gov/travel/destinations/costarica.aspx. Accessed June 3, 2009.

28. Pan-American Health Organization. Panama Basic Health Indicator Data Base. http://www.paho.org/english/sha/prflpan.htm. Accessed June 3, 2009.

29. World Health Organization. Immunization Profile—Panama. June 2009. http://www.who.int/vaccines/globalsummary/immunization/countryprofileresult.cfm?C='pan'. Accessed June 3, 2009.

30. World Health Organization. Epidemiological Country Profile on HIV and AIDS. http://apps.who.int/globalatlas/predefinedReports/EFS2008/short/EFSCountryProfiles2008_PA.pdf. Accessed June 3, 2009.

31. World Health Organization. Panama Tuberculosis Country Profile. http://apps.who.int/globalatlas/predefinedReports/TB/PDF_Files/pan.pdf. Accessed June 3, 2009.

32. Centers for Disease Control. Health Information for Travelers to Panama. http://wwwn.cdc.gov/travel/destinations/panama.aspx. Accessed June 3, 2009.

33. World Health Organization. Immunization Profile—Cuba. http://www.who.int/vaccines/globalsummary/immunization/countryprofileresult.cfm?C='cub'. Accessed June 3, 2009.

34. Oxfam. Cuba's HIV/AIDS strategy: A Rights Based Approach. July 2008. http://www.medicc.org/ns/assets/documents/Cuban%20HIV%20Strategy.pdf. Accessed June 3, 2009.

35. World Health International. Panama TB Country Profile. 2008. http://apps.who.int/globalatlas/predefinedReports/TB/PDF_Files/pan.pdf. Accessed June 3, 2009.

36. World Health Organization. Immunization Profile—Dominican Republic. http://www.who.int/vaccines/globalsummary/immunization/countryprofileresult.cfm?C='dom'. Accessed June 3, 2009.

37. USAID. HIV/AIDS Health Profile for Dominican Republic. September 2008. http://www.usaid.gov/our_work/global_health/aids/Countries/lac/domreppub_profile.pdf. Accessed June 3, 2009.

38. World Health Organization. Dominican Republic Tuberculosis Country Profile. http://apps.who.int/globalatlas/predefinedReports/TB/PDF_Files/pan.pdf. Accessed June 3, 2009.

39. Centers for Disease Control. Health Information for Travelers to Dominican Republic. 2009. http://wwwn.cdc.gov/travel/destinations/dominicanrepublic.aspx. Accessed June 3, 2009.

40. Pan-American Health Organization. Haiti Basic Health Indicator Data Base. http://www.paho.org/English/SHA/prflhai.htm. Accessed June 3, 2009.

41. World Health Organization. Immunization Profile—Haiti. June 2009. http://www.who.int/vaccines/globalsummary/immunization/countryprofileresult.cfm?C='hti'. Accessed June 3, 2009.

42. President's Emergency Plan for AIDS Relief. 2008 Country Profile—Haiti. 2008. http://www.pepfar.gov/documents/organization/81663.pdf. Accessed June 3, 2009.

43. USAID. Tuberculosis Profile—Haiti. January 2009. http://www.usaid.gov/our_work/global_health/id/tuberculosis/countries/lac/haiti.pdf. Accessed June 3, 2009.

44. The Global Fund. Haiti Country Statistics and Indicators. 2008. http://www.theglobalfund.org/programs/country/index.aspx?countryid=HTI. Accessed June 3, 2009.

45. World Health Organization. Immunization Profile—Jamaica. June 2009. http://www.who.int/vaccines/globalsummary/immunization/countryprofileresult.cfm?C='jam'. Accessed June 3, 2009.

46. World Health International. Jamaica TB Country Profile. 2008. http://apps.who.int/globalatlas/predefinedReports/TB/PDF_Files/jam.pdf. Accessed June 3, 2009.

XIII ■ SOUTH AMERICA

Matthew Dacso, MD, MSc

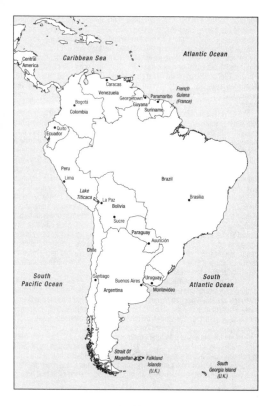

The continent of South America is comprised of fifteen countries: Argentina, Bolivia, Brazil, Chile, Colombia, Ecuador, French Guyana, Guyana, Paraguay, Peru, Suriname, Uruguay, and Venezuela. The Falklands (Malvinas), South Georgia and South Sandwich Islands are British protectorates.

The history of South America is wide, varied, and incredibly region-specific. The initial settlers of the area now called South America are thought to have crossed the Bering Land Bridge around 10,000–25,000 B.C. They gradually settled across the continent and began farming as well as raising livestock. During the pre-Colombian era subsistence farming gradually evolved into commerce. Trade routes were established across South America, connecting civilizations and enabling communication. Cultures such as the Moche (Peru), Aymara (Bolivia/Peru), Nazca (Peru), Cañaris (Ecuador), and Huari (Peru) developed alongside the Inca (Peru), who by the 14–1500s had established themselves as one of the most advanced and developed civilizations in the world.

The arrival of the Spaniards and Portuguese in 1494 heralded an incredible shift in South America's geopolitical and sociocultural landscapes. They brought with them not only technology, weapons, and Catholicism, but also smallpox, influenza, and typhus. Slaves were brought from West Africa to help harvest the land and mine natural resources for use in Europe. Other European colonizers included the Dutch (Guyana, Suriname), French (French Guyana), and British (Guyana, Falklands). French Guyana remains a part of the French Republic. During the 1800s, colonial conflict, slavery, and oppression began to give way to fierce resistance movements and ultimately, independence.

The period of time from independence to the modern era for many South American countries has been defined by massive immigration and emigration, violent border disputes, and frequent shifts in governmental power between military coups and (often) socialist/populist regimes. During the Cold War, the United States supported several military regimes in an attempt to contain the spread of communism and promote neoliberal economic policy on the continent. Meanwhile, urbanization and industrialization created new problems such as rural-urban conflict, governmental corruption, and widening income gaps that resulted in worsening poverty.

Most South American economies were founded upon export-led growth, trading agricultural and mineral goods with Europe and North America. From a marriage of Latin American Marxist political philosophy and economic theory came a school of economic discourse called *dependency theory*. Dependency theorists argued that the center-periphery alignment of global trade would always have poor countries exporting raw materials to rich countries, where they would be processed into final goods and sold back to the poor countries for a profit—in other words, that the terms of trade would always be in favor of rich countries at the expense of the poor. During the latter half of the 20th century several countries such as Argentina, Chile, and Brazil experimented with policies that would internalize all sectors of production such that profits would remain within the region. Such efforts were largely unsuccessful, but the Marxist ideas that informed the politics of the time shaped a very important era in South American history.

Over the past few decades, many parts of South America have been plagued by governmental instability, economic frailty, recession, inflation, and debt. The first decade of the 21st century has been characterized by a relatively stable political economy, with most of the continent adopting free market-friendly economic policies tempered by left-of-center governments.

HEALTH CONCERNS

Health care takes many different forms in South America, ranging from state-sponsored public infrastructure to private pre-paid insurance organizations. In some countries, health care is negotiated by trade unions, in others employers engage in cost sharing with employees. Traditional medicine plays a very important role in the lives of many communities, especially the rural and the underserved. Predominant forms in most countries involve some form of herbalism, bone setting, midwifery, aromatherapy, or shamanism.

COMMUNICABLE DISEASES

In many South American countries communicable diseases are listed as one of the top three causes of mortality. Because of their prevalence, they also account for an even greater proportion of morbidity. Over the past decade, a relative decline in the incidence of malaria has been met with an increased incidence of dengue and dengue hemorrhagic fever. The prevalence of the so-called "neglected" tropical diseases like Chaga's disease, leishmaniasis, schistosomiasis, and trachoma is high, especially in disenfranchised communities.

Lack of formal data collection systems as well as cost issues with tracking diagnoses contribute to general unreliability of epidemiologic data. Many diseases such as dengue, malaria, and tuberculosis (TB) are treated empirically. Diagnosis and treatment of HIV in most countries is state-sponsored and thus better understood. However as the HIV epidemic spreads, the marked increase in morbidity and mortality seen with HIV and TB co-infection is becoming an even more important issue.

CHRONIC DISEASE

The burden of chronic disease is heavy in South America and is often overlooked in the global drive to improve diagnosis and treatment of communicable diseases. Cardiovascular diseases including coronary heart disease and cerebrovascular disease are the leading causes of death in most countries in South America. As the obesity epidemic spreads and ever-growing urban populations become more sedate, increased incidences of type II diabetes, hyperlipidemia, and chronic kidney disease along with alcohol and tobacco abuse are being seen across the continent.

WATER SAFETY AND SANITATION

While the overall trend in South America shows improved access to safe water and sanitation, vast disparities exist between countries and even further between rural and urban populations. Urban rates of sanitation approach 80% across the region, while under 50% of rural communities utilize clean sources of water. This disparity is closely linked to health outcomes, namely diarrhea and malnutrition.

MATERNAL AND CHILD HEALTH

The fifth Millennium Development Goal (MDG) proposes to reduce maternal mortality by three-quarters by 2015. In South America, the lowest income quartiles are disparately affected by low birth weight and in general have less access to health services including having a qualified birth attendant present during delivery. Child survival past the age of 5 depends on numerous factors, including availability of clean drinking water, nutrition, protection from violence and exploitation, adequate vaccination, and safety from vector-borne illness. The AIDS epidemic in South America has also resulted in an increase in the number of orphaned children, encompassing an estimated 6.2% of children under the age of 18.

INSTITUTIONS AND ECONOMIC DEVELOPMENT

Local and international development institutions have played a key role in the unique course of South American social and economic development. Creditors and lending institutions like the International Monetary Fund (IMF) and the Inter-American Development Bank (IADB) have been involved in economic policy in South America since their inception in the 1950s. As a result of the oil crisis of 1973 and the ensuing international debt crisis of the 1980s, South Americans are perhaps more familiar with the concepts of debt, inflation, and structural adjustment programs than anyone else in the world.

The concept of transnational trade agreements has been a prominent feature of South American development over the past three decades. The controversial Free Trade Area of the Americas (FTAA) was proposed in the mid-1990s as a model for transnational trade expanding upon the North American Free Trade Agreement (NAFTA) between the United States, Canada, and Mexico. It has been criticized as neo-colonial or new imperialism of South America by dominant North American economic powers. Mercosur, founded in 1991 as one of South America's answers to the hegemonic World Trade Organization, is a trade agreement between Argentina, Uruguay, Paraguay, and Brazil—it has expanded to include other South American nations in an attempt to regulate trade across the region.

International institutions feature prominently in the healthcare landscape of South America. The Pan American Health Organization (PAHO) is a division of the United Nations (UN) and World Health Organization (WHO) whose mission is to strengthen local health systems, promote primary care and prevention, advocate for reducing health disparities, and better the health of people living in the Americas by working with international, regional, and local health authorities. Both religious and secular medical organizations provide hundreds of medical volunteers to the region every year. Hundreds of nongovernmental organizations (NGOs) operate in South America working on sustainable community-based interventions that range from advocating destigmatization of HIV/AIDS to teaching surgical techniques to promoting primary care and women's health.

COUNTRY PROFILES OF SOUTH AMERICA

ARGENTINA

Population: 39,134,000

Religions: Roman Catholic (~90%), Protestant (2%), Jewish (2%)

Languages: Spanish, Italian, Quechua, Aymara, and Guaraní

Ethnic Makeup: European (86.4%), Mestizo (8%), Asian (4%), Indigenous (1.6%)

Formerly Colonized: Spanish, declared independence July 9th, 1816

Politics/Governance: Federal presidential republic

Type of Health Care System: Three-tiered system: Instituto Nacional de Servicios Sociales para Jubilados y Pensionados (INSSJP, public system) serving ~40% of the population, labor and union-based *Obras Sociales* providing access to ~50% of the population, 10% served by private *prepago* health plans.[1,2]

Life Expectancy (years): 72 (male), 78 (female)[3]

Under 5 Mortality: 16.8/1000 (9.1–26.7)[3]

Vaccinations: > 92% for OPV, DPT, and measles[1]

HIV adult Prevalence: 0.5%[4]

TB: Prevalence 38/100,000, 2.2% of new cases/year are MDR[5]

Malaria: Only 125 cases in 2003, *P. vivax* predominant. Endemic areas are Salta, San Martín, and Orán.[1]

Leading Causes of Death: Cardiovascular disease (~30%), cancer (breast and lung most common), communicable diseases (8.9%), external causes (6.7%)[1]

Key Health Institutions: Ministry of Health, INSSJP (formerly PAMI), *Obras Sociales*

Unusual Pathogens: Chaga's disease, yellow fever, dengue, malaria

Unique Environmental Exposures: Low extreme of temperature in the South (Tierra del Fuego)

Traditional Medicine: 3000 practitioners of homeopathic medicine[6]

BOLIVIA

Population: 9,775,246

Religions: Roman Catholic (~78%), Protestant (16%)

Languages: Spanish (60.7%), Quechua (21.2%), Aymara (14.6%), 34 other native languages

Ethnic Makeup: Quechua (30%), Mestizo (30%), Aymara (25%), European (15%)

Formerly Colonized: Spanish, declared independent August 6th, 1825

Politics/Governance: Federal presidential republic

Type of Health Care System: Basic health insurance plan covers most primary care services, serves ~45% of the population. Social security system provides access to 22%, and private insurance provides 5–10%. 20–25% of the population does not have access to health services. It is estimated that 50% of the population utilizes some form of traditional medicine.[7,8]

Life Expectancy (years): 64 (male), 69 (female)[9]

Under 5 Mortality: 69/1000[9]

Vaccinations: 85% vaccinated against DPT[7]

HIV adult Prevalence: 0.2%[10]

TB: Prevalence 198/100,000, 1.2% of new cases/year are MDR[11]

Malaria: 31,468 cases of *P. vivax* and 2,536 cases of *P. falciparum* in 2000. 75% of the country is at risk for infection. Chloroquine is not effective.[7]

Leading Causes of Death: Organized vital statistics collection not fully developed.

Estimates: Cardiovascular diseases (~40%), communicable diseases (13%), external causes (12%)[7]

Key Health Institutions: National Epidemiological Surveillance and Health Service Analysis System started in 2000 to aid in surveillance/data collection.

Unusual Pathogens: dengue, hepatitis A, typhoid, Chaga's disease, yellow fever, leptospirosis

Unique Environmental Exposures: high altitude exposure in Andes areas, organophosphate pesticides used in some rural areas

Traditional Medicine: Strong preference for traditional medicine in many areas, especially where access to allopathic services is limited. Bolivian Society of Traditional Medicine (SOBOMETRA) present for advocacy and education for traditional healers. 5000 practicing traditional healers, one chiropractor[12]

BRAZIL

Population: 189,323,000

Religions: Roman Catholic (~74%), Protestant (15%), other Christian (1%), Spiritism (1%)

Languages: Portuguese, Spanish (in border areas), 180 other native languages

Ethnic Makeup: European/White (53.7%), Mixed (Pardo) (38.5%), Black (6.2%)

Formerly Colonized: Portugal, declared independence September 7th, 1822

Politics/Governance: Federal presidential republic

Type of Health Care System: A decentralized public system has operated at the municipal level with federal support since the Constitution of 1988. Up to 25% of the population has some form of private insurance.[13,14]

Life Expectancy (years): 68 (male), 75 (female)[15]

Under 5 Mortality: 20/1000 live births[15]

Vaccinations: Comprehensive decentralized vaccination program boasting rates of > 95% in MMR, DPT, OPV, BCG, Hib, and HBV. First country to incorporate rotavirus into scheme.[14]

HIV adult Prevalence: 0.6%[16]

TB: Prevalence 60/100,000, 0.9% of new cases/year are MDR[17]

Malaria: 81,343 cases of *P. falciparum* or mixed, 297,962 of *P. vivax* in 2003. Chloroquine not considered effective prophylaxis[13]

Leading Causes of Death: Cardiovascular diseases (~30%), cancer, external causes (trauma/violence, poisoning), communicable diseases[13]

Key Health Institutions: Unified Health System (SUS)

Unusual Pathogens: leprosy, visceral and cutaneous leishmaniasis, dengue, yellow fever

Unique Environmental Exposures: Some reports of excessive occupational/ environmental lead exposure

Traditional Medicine: Incorporates many South American and African traditions, practiced mainly in the interior and northeast regions by black-native Mestizo populations—draws upon the vast biodiversity of the Amazon.[6]

CHILE

Population: 16,928,873

Religions: Roman Catholic (~70%), Protestant (~15%), Jehovah's Witness (1%), none (8.3%)

Languages: Spanish (majority), Mapudungun, Quechua, Rapa Nui

Ethnic Makeup: White and Mestizo (95%), Mapuche (4%), Other (1%)

Formerly Colonized: Spain, declared independence September 18, 1810

Politics/Governance: Federal presidential republic

Type of Health Care System: public system (FONASA) covers 63% of the population, 23% covered by private insurance (ISAPRES), 14% covered by military or not at all.[18,19]

Life Expectancy (years): 74 (males), 81 (females)[20]

Under 5 Mortality: 9/1000 live births[20]

Vaccinations: 96% vaccinated with measles, polio, BCG, DPT, and Hib in 1999[18]

HIV adult Prevalence: 0.3%[21]

TB: Prevalence 12/100,000, 0.7% of new cases/year are MDR[22]

Malaria: No malaria in Chile[18]

Leading Causes of Death: Cardiovascular diseases, cancer, communicable diseases

Key Health Institutions: FONASA, ISAPRES, and Public Health Institute report to the Ministry of Health[19]

Unusual Pathogens: Chaga's disease prevalent in some areas, no dengue, plague, or schistosomiasis in Chile

Unique Environmental Exposures: Some reports of high levels of arsenic in drinking water.

Traditional Medicine: No official registry, but estimated 2000 practicing healers, including aromatherapy, acupuncture, bone setting, midwifery, and herbalism. Unidad de Medicina Tradicional y Otras Practicas Medicas Alternativas reports to the Ministry of Health.[12]

COLOMBIA

Population: 44,928,970

Religions: ~85% Roman Catholic, ~10% other Christian, 1% Judaism, Islam, Buddhism

Languages: Spanish, Chibchan, Arawak, Cariban, and Quechua

Ethnic Makeup: 58% Mestizo, 20% European, 15% Mulatto, 4% Black, 3% Zambo

Formerly Colonized: Spain, declared independence July 20, 1810

Politics/Governance: Federal presidential republic

Type of Health Care System: 66% of the population covered by either the public system or employer-based plans in which employee and employer contribute to insurance. There is a small percentage of private care. Armed conflict and displacement of communities have contributed to vast health disparities between rural and urban populations.[23,24]

Life Expectancy (years): 71 (male), 78 (female)[25]

Under 5 Mortality: 21/1000[25]

Vaccinations: 92% vaccinated against measles, Hib vaccination and HBV available since late 1990s.[23]

HIV adult Prevalence: 0.6%[26]

TB: Prevalence 43/100,000, 1.5% of new cases/year are MDR[27]

Malaria: 18 million people live in endemic areas, up to 85% of the country endemic (Pacific coast, Amazon areas, and eastern savannahs). *P. vivax* 66% overall, but *P. falciparum* 75% in Pacific coastal area. Chloroquine is not an effective prophylaxis.[24]

Leading Causes of Death: Cardiovascular disease, homicide, COPD, auto accidents, cancer[24]

Key Health Institutions: Law 100 of 1993 saw the creation of General Health and Social Security System (SGSSS), System for the Selection of Beneficiaries of Social Programs (SISBEN), overseen by the Superintendecia de Salud.

Unusual Pathogens: 65% of the urban population is at risk for dengue/dengue hemorrhagic fever. *Aedes aegypti* mosquito present in many municipalities, making yellow fever prevalent in both urban and jungle areas. Leishmaniasis present in lowland/coastal areas.

Unique Environmental Exposures: Cocaine use is estimated at 3.8% of the general population. Domestic violence reported in ~40% of partnered households. Oil infiltration of soil and water has affected large numbers of rural households. Cauca and Magdalena rivers are heavily contaminated with human waste.[24]

Traditional Medicine: Various forms practiced—40% of the population reports using traditional medicine. Only allopathic physicians may practice homeopathy—standardized training in practice of homeopathy since 1914.[6,12]

ECUADOR

Population: 14,573,101

Religions: Roman Catholic (95%), Protestant (4%)

Languages: Spanish, native dialects

Ethnic Makeup: 55% Mestizo, 24% Amerindian, 16% European, 5% Mulatto and Zambo

Formerly Colonized: Spain, achieved independence May 24, 1822

Politics/Governance: Federal presidential republic

Type of Health Care System: Public Health Ministry (MSP) provides services to ~30% of the population. Social Security Institute (IESS) covers 18%, 2% covered by police/military insurance, NGOs provide 5% with coverage, and 20% have private insurance. 25%, mostly rural indigenous communities, have limited or no access to healthcare services.[28,29]

Life Expectancy (years): 70 (male), 76 (female)[30]

Under 5 Mortality: 24/1000 live births[30]

Vaccinations: > 92% vaccinated against measles, DPT, HBV, Hib, polio[28]

HIV adult Prevalence: 0.3%[31]

TB: Prevalence 140/100,000, 4.9% new cases/year are MDR[32]

Malaria: 22.5/1000 annual parasite index, *P. vivax* > *P. falciparum*. Chloroquine is not an effective prophylaxis, although *P. vivax* is 100% susceptible.[29]

Leading Causes of Death: Cardiovascular diseases, cancer, communicable diseases

Key Health Institutions: National Health System (CONASA), National Decentralization Plan[28,29]

Unusual Pathogens: dengue, malaria, leptospirosis

Unique Environmental Exposures: pesticides, volcanic eruptions, floods, only 5% of wastewater treated. Northern border complicated by Colombian armed conflict and displaced refugees.[29]

Traditional Medicine: Widespread use, especially in rural areas. Quichua form commonly found. No registry of practitioners—since 1998 the National Division of Indigenous Health has organized and promoted traditional medicine.[12]

GUYANA

Population: 772,298

Religions: 57% Christian, 23.4% Hindu, 7.3% Muslim. Also, Ba'hai, Judaism, and Rastafarian

Languages: English, Cariban languages, Guyanese Creole

Ethnic Makeup: Indo-Guyanese (43.5%), Afro-Guyanese (30%), Mixed (17%), Amerindian (9%)

Formerly Colonized: United Kingdom, declared independence May 26, 1966

Politics/Governance: Semi-presidential republic

Type of Health Care System: Public decentralized health system with NGO and private actors. Public system built on five levels of care: level 1 = community health workers, level 5 = tertiary care referral hospitals in Georgetown. No national health insurance—mandatory employer-based care for workers between 16 and 60 years of age. Private insurance plans also operate.[33,34]

Life Expectancy (years): 63 (male), 66 (female)[35]

Under 5 Mortality: 62/1000 live births[35]

Vaccinations: > 90% vaccinated with HBV, Hib, DPT, OPV, and BCG. MMR ~88%.[34]

HIV adult Prevalence: 2.5%, responsible for 17.7% of deaths of persons 20–59 yrs old.[36]

TB: Prevalence 136/100,000, 1.7% of new cases/year are MDR[37]

Malaria: 39,000 cases in 2005, 39% *P. falciparum*, 54%. 3% of new cases *P. malariae*. Chloroquine is not considered an effective prophylaxis.[33]

Leading Causes of Death: Cardiovascular disease, HIV/AIDS, and diabetes. Highest suicide rate in South America.[34]

Key Health Institutions: Ministry of Health, Ministry of Local Government, and Regional Development

Unusual Pathogens: leptospirosis, dengue (but no recent DHF), Hansen's disease (leprosy)

Unique Environmental Exposures: floods, pesticides, and mercury exposure in certain areas related to gold mining[34]

Traditional Medicine: Organized resources unavailable

PARAGUAY

Population: 6,831,306

Religions: Roman Catholic (~90%), other Christian (7.3%), indigenous religions (0.6%)

Languages: Spanish (75%), Guaraní understood by ~90%

Ethnic Makeup: Mestizo (95%)

Formerly Colonized: Spain, declared independence May 14th, 1811

Politics/Governance: Constitutional presidential republic

Type of Health Care System: Multi-tiered—services provided through public, private nonprofit, private for-profit, and mixed institutions. 18.4% of the population is insured, while 81.6% is not. Access to resources is extremely limited and traditional medicine is frequently utilized.[38,39]

Life Expectancy (years): 72 (male), 78 (female)[40]

Under 5 Mortality: 22/1000 live births[40]

Vaccinations: 63% of the country's population received measles/rubella vaccine in 2005. DPT/Hib/HBV vaccine introduced in 2002 and administered to 87% of eligible infants.[39]

HIV adult Prevalence: 0.6%[41]

TB: Prevalence 73/100,000, 2.1% of new cases/year are MDR[42]

Malaria: Only 376 cases in 2005 after 1999 epidemic. 99.8% *P. vivax*. 75% of cases found in the east-central zone.[39]

Leading Causes of Death: 79% of deaths without defined causes (data reporting poor).[39]

Key Health Institutions: Ministry of Public Health and Social Welfare (MSPBS) and its various subdepartments

Unusual Pathogens: Dengue, leishmaniasis, hantavirus (both Western and Eastern regions)

Unique Environmental Exposures: drought, pesticides, traffic accidents

Traditional Medicine: Herbalism frequently practiced in rural and underserved areas. Swiss/Paraguayan Red Cross developing 6-year training program in traditional medicine at San Miguel College.[6,12]

PERU

Population: 29,132,013

Religions: Roman Catholic (81%), Evangelical (12.5%)

Languages: Spanish, Quechua (spoken by ~12% of the population)

Ethnic Makeup: Indigenous (45%), Mestizo (37%), European (15%), Black, Asian (3%)

Formerly Colonized: Spain, declared independence July 28th, 1821

Politics/Governance: Federal presidential republic

Type of Health Care System: Ministry of Health (MINSA) regulates the public sector, which operates comprehensive health insurance in conjunction with local communities in a decentralized model (covers ~30% of the population). EsSalud is the social insurance system that covers the majority of the employed population. Private care operates independently and covers ~10%. Between 40–50% of the population has limited or no access to health services.[43,44]

Life Expectancy (years): 71 (male), 75 (female)[45]

Under 5 Mortality: 25/1000 live births[45]

Vaccinations: > 92% coverage for DPT, MR, OPV, BCG[44]

HIV adult Prevalence: 0.5%[46]

TB: Prevalence 136/100,000, 5.3% of new cases/year are MDR[47]

Malaria: 87,699 cases in 2005, 17% *P. falciparum*. Thirteen million people live in at-risk areas. Chloroquine is not considered an effective prophylaxis.[44]

Leading Causes of Death: Cardiovascular diseases, acute pulmonary diseases, TB[44]

Key Health Institutions: MINSA, EsSalud

Unusual Pathogens: Dengue, Chaga's disease, leishmaniasis, brucellosis, yellow fever

Unique Environmental Exposures: River overflows in the north, pesticides, air pollution in city centers[44]

Traditional Medicine: Herbalism, bone setting, and birth attendance are the main specialties. National Institute of Traditional Medicine works under Ministry of Health to help regulate traditional medicine.[6,12]

SURINAME

Population: 494,347

Religions: Roman Catholic and Protestant majority (40%), Hindu (20%), Muslim (14%)

Languages: Dutch (official, first language of 60%), Sranan Tongo, Surinamese Hindi, Javanese, Maroon, and indigenous languages also spoken

Ethnic Makeup: East Indian/Hindoestanen (~30%), Creoles (~20%), Javanese (~15%), Maroons (descendants of West African slaves) ~10%, indigenous groups (~3%)

Formerly Colonized: Netherlands, declared independence November 25th, 1975

Politics/Governance: Constitutional democracy

Type of Health Care System: Public sector consists of regional medical services and Medical Mission (an NGO). Sixty-four percent of the population has health insurance, 36% are uninsured or unsure of coverage. Nineteen percent of costs are out-of-pocket.[48,49]

Life Expectancy (years): 65 (male), 71 (female)[50]

Under 5 Mortality: 39/1000 live births[50]

Vaccinations: 83–86% vaccinated with DPT, OPV, and MMR. Pentavalent vaccine introduced in 2005.[49]

HIV adult Prevalence: 2.4%[51]

TB: Prevalence 155/100,000, incidence of MDR unknown[52]

Malaria: 9000 cases in 2005, highest risk in interior region, highest incidence along Marowijne River near French Guiana border. *P. falciparum* resistant to chloroquine is prevalent.[49]

Leading Causes of Death: Cardiovascular diseases, external causes, HIV/AIDS, cancer[49]

Key Health Institutions: State Health Insurance Fund (SZF), MM, Bureau of Public Health

Unusual Pathogens: yellow fever, leptospirosis (especially in rainy season), HIV/salmonella co-infection

Unique Environmental Exposures: gold mining in the interior with subsequent mercury contamination[49]

Traditional Medicine: Shamans operate in rural indigenous areas with Maroon and Amerindian populations. Kwamalasamutu in the South is an area of research and development of community interventions utilizing traditional medicine in conjunction with the allopathic model.[53]

URUGUAY

Population: 3,241,003

Religions: Roman Catholic (66%), Protestant (~2%), Jewish (~1%)

Languages: Spanish, Portuguese, and Portuñol

Ethnic Makeup: European (88%), Mestizo (6%), West African (4%), Asian (2%)

Formerly Colonized: Brazil, declared independence August 25th, 1825

Politics/Governance: Federal presidential republic

Type of Health Care System: Fragmented with much overlap. Public sector covers ~40%, private sector covers ~40%.[54,55]

Life Expectancy (years): 72 (male), 79 (female)[56]

Under 5 Mortality: 15/1000 live births[56]

Vaccinations: > 95% vaccinated with MMR, DPT, HBV, Hib, OPV, meningitis, BCG.[55]

HIV adult Prevalence: 0.6%[57]

TB: Prevalence 23/100,000 with no new cases/year of MDR[58]

Malaria: No risk of malaria in Uruguay[54]

Leading Causes of Death: cardiovascular disease, cancer, external causes[55]

Key Health Institutions: State Health Services Institution (public sector), Collective Health Care Institutions (private sector)

Unusual Pathogens: leptospirosis, dengue, rare hantavirus, and leprosy

Unique Environmental Exposures: Ninety-eight percent of the country has potable water.[55]

Traditional Medicine: Herbalism is practiced in some rural areas. There is no apparent formal regulatory framework.[6]

VENEZUELA

Population: 26,814,843

Religions: Roman Catholic (92%), Protestant (8%)

Languages: Spanish, 31 indigenous languages

Ethnic Makeup: Mestizo or Mulatto (~70%), European (~20%), Indigenous (~5%)

Formerly Colonized: Spain, declared independence July 5th, 1811

Politics/Governance: Federal presidential republic

Type of Health Care System: Public and private sectors cover ~65% of the population. A large portion of the country has limited or no access.[59,60]

Life Expectancy (years): 71 (male), 78 (female)[61]

Under 5 Mortality: 21/1000 live births[61]

Vaccinations: > 90% vaccinated with BCG and yellow fever. 80–90% vaccinated with OPV, DPT, MMR, Hib, and HBV. Pentavalent vaccine used since 2004.[60]

HIV adult Prevalence: 0.7% (est.)[62]

TB: Prevalence 39/100,000. 0.5% of new cases/year are MDR[63]

Malaria: API 9/1000 in 2004 with *P. vivax* accounting for ~83%[60]

Leading Causes of Death: cardiovascular diseases, cancer, violence/accidents[60]

Key Health Institutions: Venezuelan Social Insurance Administration (IVSS), Health and Social Development Ministry (HSDM), *Misión Barrio Adentro*

Unusual Pathogens: yellow fever, leishmaniasis, Chaga's disease, onchocerciasis

Unique Environmental Exposures: flooding/mudslides, pesticides[60]

Traditional Medicine: Herbalism practiced in the Andes area. 1975 law prohibits practice of medicine unless licensed by ministerial permit.[6,12]

FURTHER READING

Pan-American Health Organization. Health in the Americas Volume I and II. Washington, DC: World Health Organization; 2007.

Pan American Health Organization. Country Profiles. http://www.paho.org/English

World Health Organization. Legal Status of Traditional Medicine and Complementary/Alternative Medicine: A Worldwide Review. Geneva, Switzerland: World Health Organization; 2001.

REFERENCES

1. Pan American Health Organization. Country Profile: Argentina. Health Situation Analysis and Trends Summary. http://www.paho.org/English/DD/AIS/cp_032.htm. Accessed July 19th, 2009.
2. Vasquez E, Castro JL, et al. Argentina. In: Pan American Health Organization, *Health in the Americas Volume II*, Washington, DC, World Health Organization: 2007.
3. World Health Organization. Argentina Country Profile. http://www.who.int/countries/arg/en/. Accessed July 19th, 2009.
4. Central Intelligence Agency. CIA Factbook: Argentina. https://www.cia.gov/library/publications/the-world-factbook/geos/ar.html. Accessed July 19th, 2009.
5. World Health Organization. TB Country Profile: Argentina. http://www.who.int/countries/arg/en/. Accessed July 19th, 2009.
6. Cummings N, Gagne J, et al (eds). *Legal Status of Traditional Medicine and Complementary/Alternative Medicine: A Worldwide Review*, World Health Organization, Geneva: 2001.
7. Pan American Health Organization. Country Profile: Bolivia. Health Situation Analysis and Trends Summary. http://www.paho.org/English/DD/AIS/cp_068.htm. Accessed July 19th, 2009.
8. Ayala C, Caballero D, et al. Bolivia. In: Pan-American Health Organization, *Health in the Americas Volume II*, Washington, DC, World Health Organization: 2007.

9. World Health Organization. Bolivia Country Profile. http://www.who.int/countries/bol/en/. Accessed on July 19th, 2009.
10. Central Intelligence Agency. CIA Factbook: Bolivia. https://www.cia.gov/library/publications/the-world-factbook/geos/bl.html. Accessed on July 19th, 2009.
11. World Health Organization. TB Country Profile: Bolivia. http://www.who.int/countries/bol/en/. Accessed on July 19th, 2009.
12. Pan American Health Organization. Bolivia. In: World Health Organization. *Traditional Health Systems in Latin America and the Carribean: Base Information*. Washington, DC, World Health Organization: 1999.
13. Pan American Health Organization. Country Profile: Brazil. Health Situation Analysis and Trends Summary. http://www.paho.org/English/DD/AIS/cp_076.htm. Accessed on July 20th, 2009.
14. Escamilla JA, Albuquerque Z, et al. Pan-American Health Organization, Brazil. In: *Health in the Americas Volume II*. Washington, D.C., World Health Organization: 2007.
15. World Health Organization. Brazil Country Profile. http://www.who.int/countries/bra/en/. Accessed on July 20th, 2009.
16. Central Intelligence Agency. CIA Factbook: Brazil. https://www.cia.gov/library/publications/the-world-factbook/geos/br.html. Accessed on July 20th, 2009.
17. World Health Organization. TB Country Profile: Brazil. http://www.who.int/countries/bra/en/. Accessed on July 20th, 2009.
18. Pan American Health Organization. Country Profile: Chile. Health Situation Analysis and Trends Summary. http://www.paho.org/English/DD/AIS/cp_152.htm. Accessed on July 20th, 2009.
19. Giusti A, Arteaga O, et al. Pan-American Health Organization, Chile. In: *Health in the Americas Volume II*, Washington, DC. World Health Organization: 2007.
20. World Health Organization. Chile Country Profile. http://www.who.int/countries/chl/en/. Accessed on July 20th, 2009.
21. Central Intelligence Agency. CIA Factbook: Chile. https://www.cia.gov/library/publications/the-world-factbook/geos/ci.html. Accessed on July 20th, 2009.
22. World Health Organization. TB Country Profile: Chile. http://www.who.int/countries/chl/en/. Accessed on July 20th, 2009.
23. Pan American Health Organization. Country Profile: Colombia. Health Situation Analysis and Trends Summary. http://www.paho.org/English/DD/AIS/cp_170.htm. Accessed on July 21st, 2009.
24. Ontaneda RS, Balladelli PP, et al. Pan-American Health Organization, Colombia. In: *Health in the Americas Volume II*. Washington, DC. World Health Organization: 2007.
25. World Health Organization. Colombia Country Profile. http://www.who.int/countries/col/en/. Accessed on July 21st, 2009.
26. Central Intelligence Agency. CIA Factbook: Colombia. https://www.cia.gov/library/publications/the-world-factbook/geos/co.html. Accessed on July 21st, 2009.

27. World Health Organization. TB Country Profile: Colombia. http://www.who.int/countries/col/en/. Accessed on July 21st, 2009.
28. Pan American Health Organization. Country Profile: Ecuador. Health Situation Analysis and Trends Summary. http://www.paho.org/English/DD/AIS/cp_218.htm. Accessed on July 21st, 2009.
29. Machuca M, Aráuz V, et al. Pan-American Health Organization, Ecuador. In: *Health in the Americas Volume II*. Washington, DC. World Health Organization: 2007.
30. World Health Organization. Ecuador Country Profile. http://www.who.int/countries/ecu/en/. Accessed on July 21st, 2009.
31. Central Intelligence Agency. CIA Factbook: Ecuador. https://www.cia.gov/library/publications/the-world-factbook/geos/ec.html. Accessed on July 21st, 2009.
32. World Health Organization. TB Country Profile: Ecuador. http://www.who.int/countries/ecu/en/. Accessed on July 21st, 2009.
33. Pan American Health Organization. Country Profile: Guyana. Health Situation Analysis and Trends Summary. http://www.paho.org/English/DD/AIS/cp_328.htm. Accessed on July 21st, 2009.
34. Griffith T, Baganizi E, et al. Pan-American Health Organization, Guyana. In: Washington, DC. World Health Organization: 2007.
35. World Health Organization. Guyana Country Profile. http://www.who.int/countries/guy/en/. Accessed on July 21st, 2009.
36. Central Intelligence Agency. CIA Factbook: Guyana. https://www.cia.gov/library/publications/the-world-factbook/geos/gy.html. Accessed on July 21st, 2009.
37. World Health Organization. TB Country Profile: Guyana. http://www.who.int/countries/guy/en/ Accessed on July 21st, 2009.
38. Pan American Health Organization. Country Profile: Paraguay. Health Situation Analysis and Trends Summary. http://www.paho.org/English/DD/AIS/cp_600.htm. Accessed on July 22nd, 2009.
39. Moreira M, Almirón M, et al. Pan-American Health Organization, Paraguay. In: *Health in the Americas Volume II*. Washington, DC. World Health Organization: 2007.
40. World Health Organization. Guyana Country Profile. http://www.who.int/countries/pry/en/ Accessed on July 22nd, 2009.
41. Central Intelligence Agency. CIA Factbook: Paraguay. https://www.cia.gov/library/publications/the-world-factbook/geos/pa.html. Accessed on July 22nd, 2009.
42. World Health Organization. TB Country Profile: Paraguay. http://www.who.int/countries/pry/en/. Accessed on July 22nd, 2009.
43. Pan American Health Organization. Country Profile: Peru. Health Situation Analysis and Trends Summary. http://www.paho.org/English/DD/AIS/cp_604.htm. Accessed on July 22nd, 2009.
44. Ramirez FG, Baca ME, et al. Pan-American Health Organization, Peru. In: *Health in the Americas Volume II*. Washington, DC. World Health Organization: 2007.
45. World Health Organization. Peru Country Profile. http://www.who.int/countries/per/en/ Accessed on July 22nd, 2009.

46. Central Intelligence Agency. CIA Factbook: Peru. https://www.cia.gov/library/publications/the-world-factbook/geos/pe.html. Accessed on July 22nd, 2009.

47. World Health Organization. TB Country Profile: Peru. http://www.who.int/countries/per/en/. Accessed on July 22nd, 2009.

48. Pan American Health Organization. Country Profile: Suriname. Health Situation Analysis and Trends Summary. http://www.paho.org/English/DD/AIS/cp_740.htm. Accessed on July 23rd, 2009.

49. VanKanten E, Becker R, et al. Pan-American Health Organization, Suriname. In: Health in the Americas Volume II. Washington, DC. World Health Organization: 2007.

50. World Health Organization. Suriname Country Profile. http://www.who.int/countries/sur/en/. Accessed on July 23rd, 2009.

51. Central Intelligence Agency. CIA Factbook; Suriname. https://www.cia.gov/library/publications/the-world-factbook/geos/ns.html. Accessed on July 23rd, 2009.

52. World Health Organization. TB Country Profile: Suriname. http://www.who.int/countries/sur/en/. Accessed on July 23rd, 2009.

53. Boven K, Morohashi J (eds). Gunther N. Suriname. In: UNESCO. Best Practices on Indigenous Knowledge. The Hague. Nuffic: 2002.

54. Pan American Health Organization. Country Profile: Uruguay. Health Situation Analysis and Trends Summary. http://www.paho.org/English/DD/AIS/cp_858.htm. Accessed on July 23rd, 2009.

55. Gherardi A, Col M, et al. Pan-American Health Organization, Uruguay. In: Health in the Americas Volume II. Washington, DC. World Health Organization: 2007.

56. World Health Organization. Uruguay Country Profile. http://www.who.int/countries/ury/en/. Accessed on July 23rd, 2009.

57. Central Intelligence Agency. CIA Factbook; Uruguay. https://www.cia.gov/library/publications/the-world-factbook/geos/uy.html. Accessed on July 23rd, 2009.

58. World Health Organization. TB Country Profile: Uruguay. http://www.who.int/countries/ury/en/. Accessed on July 23rd, 2009.

59. Pan American Health Organization. Country Profile: Venezuela. Health Situation Analysis and Trends Summary. http://www.paho.org/English/DD/AIS/cp_862.htm. Accessed on July 23rd, 2009.

60. Inzaurralde AL, Cobo OB, et al. Pan-American Health Organization, Venezuela. In: Health in the Americas Volume II. Washington, DC. World Health Organization: 2007.

61. World Health Organization. Venezuela Country Profile. http://www.who.int/countries/ven/en/. Accessed on July 23rd, 2009.

62. Central Intelligence Agency. CIA Factbook: Venezuela. https://www.cia.gov/library/publications/the-world-factbook/geos/ve.html. Accessed on July 23rd, 2009.

63. World Health Organization. TB Country Profile: Venezuela. http://www.who.int/countries/ven/en/. Accessed on July 23rd, 2009.

XIV ■ EASTERN EUROPE

Priya Blazkova-Chandra, MHSA
Amit Chandra, MD, MSc

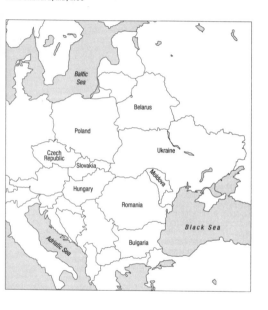

Definitions of Eastern Europe vary, but the UN statistics division includes the following 10 countries in the region: Belarus, Bulgaria, Czech Republic, Hungary, Moldova, Poland, Romania, Russia, Slovakia, and Ukraine.

The region covers an area of over 18 million square kilometers and is home to a population of over 290 million people. It extends from the Ural Mountains in the East to the borders of Western European countries not historically associated with the Warsaw Pact.

The modern history of this region is dominated by the cold war that bound the countries together under the political regime of the Soviet Union. It is one of the only regions of the world experiencing an annual decrease in population, a result of emigration from the region and low fertility rates.

HEALTH CONCERNS

The breakup of the Soviet Union brought enormous changes both politically and socioeconomically to the region. As their systems liberalized and many countries moved toward market-based economies, other challenges emerged. They currently face new crises such as rising unemployment, widening income disparities, and a rise in poverty.

Over the past two decades, most countries of Eastern Europe have progressed in their economic and development indicators across a broad spectrum, although some have fared worse. The Czech Republic, Hungary, Poland, and Slovakia—the first wave of Eastern European countries that acceded to the European Union (EU), have emerged from the transition relatively successfully, with health issues matching those in western European nations. In Bulgaria and Romania, countries in the second wave to join the EU, accessibility to health care is an issue and many inequities exist between rural and urban areas. Belarus, Moldova, Russia, and Ukraine have faced a more difficult transition. By 1999, per capita gross domestic products (GDPs) in Russia and Ukraine had fallen to 57% and 36% respectively, of 1989 levels.[1] Trends in development rankings among these countries have either remained near 1990 levels, as in Belarus, or are significantly lower.

All the countries inherited public health institutions and healthcare infrastructures that were hierarchical, highly centralized, and financed by state revenue sources. Under the state-socialist system, reimbursement for healthcare facilities was fixed based on the number of beds, which led to the establishment of large multibed facilities or megahospitals located in urban centers. These were supported by an integrated network of polyclinics (i.e., outpatient clinics), and other health facilities that brought back basic levels of curative care to a widely dispersed population.[2] Local authorities generally had little input in the mix of services provided or in building greater efficiencies in the system. While this infrastructure was well-suited for large-scale immunization campaigns and for maternal and child health programs, it has struggled to adapt to the changing needs of the people and the increasing complexities of the healthcare environment.

Another legacy of the socialist system was the guarantee of universal healthcare coverage to its citizens and the provision of a broad range of comprehensive services. While the universal entitlement was a key achievement in concept, it hid, in many parts of the region, an informal payment system that was necessary to gain access to the services. The delivery of health care has also been characterized by a wide diversity in clinical practice, driving some to the private sector for comprehensive care.

At the beginning of the 1990s, many governments confronted pressures for cost-containment and the need for sustainability in healthcare spending, and some faced the declining health status of their populations due to ineffective and inefficient healthcare systems. Today the countries in the region are at various stages of reform. Generally, the intent has been to shift away from the centralized state model to a decentralized, contract-based social health insurance structure, one of the key features of the western European model.[3] Nevertheless, some countries in the region have chosen to remain within the old Soviet-style framework. Besides the matter of selected privatization of delivery systems, other common themes have emerged: a new focus on primary care and outpatient services; commitment to reduce the oversupply of hospital beds; and new approaches to public health surveillance and infrastructure.[4] Some have gone as far as recognizing the critical role of individuals—developing patients' rights, and empowering citizens and their communities in improving health.

The leading causes of death among the Eastern European countries are attributed to noninfectious diseases such as cardiovascular disease, respiratory illnesses, cancer, and accidents or injuries.[5] Health systems have also been impacted by the rising threat of HIV/AIDS, resurgence of infectious diseases such as tuberculosis, and chronic diseases of aging populations. These and some additional concerns are further detailed as follows:

■ HIV

Russia, Belarus, and the Ukraine host the majority of new cases of HIV, and unlike other global centers of the epidemic, prevalence in this part of the region has risen at the fastest rate in the world over the past decade.

Insufficient HIV knowledge among a growing number of sex workers and unhygienic needle-sharing practices between illicit drug users are largely to blame for this increase. A shift in cultural values, a widespread sense of uncertainty, and fatalism resulting in increased risk-taking behavior are also factors that have laid the groundwork for the sharp rise.[6]

■ Infectious Diseases

The evidence of the transnational spread of communicable diseases, as in the case of tuberculosis, is well known. As national boundaries fall, population movements will only increase. There is a need for a coordinated regional and global approach to preventing and controlling infectious diseases.[7]

■ Lifestyles

Smoking has traditionally been common in the region among men and a growing number of women. The sustained advertisement campaigns and investments by western tobacco companies in this region ensure that it will be a continued problem.[8]

A diet high in fat content and low in fruits and vegetables, which lead to micronutrient deficiencies, has been recognized as a factor in increasing health risks for chronic diseases. The elimination of borders has had a positive impact on increasing the year-round availability and quality of fruits and vegetables but prices remain high.

Alcoholism is another problem in parts of the region and varies in its severity, contributing to both cardiovascular and liver diseases, as well as death rates from injuries and violence.[9] Falling life expectancies over the past decade in Russia are largely attributed to alcoholism.

■ Chernobyl Fallout

The Chernobyl nuclear disaster occurred in the Ukraine in 1986 and is considered the most devastating accident in the history of nuclear technology. Radioactive contaminants spread throughout Eastern Europe, but particularly affected the Ukraine, Belarus, and Russia. The long-term health effects of this exposure remain unclear and are hotly debated issues. The UN Scientific Committee on the Effects of Atomic Radiation reported an estimated 4000 cases of thyroid cancer over the years following the accident that were directly attributed to Chernobyl material.[10] Several organizations report that this figure is grossly underestimated, and they contend that countries throughout the region suffer from increased rates of leukemia and other malignancies.

REGIONAL ORGANIZATIONS

The Czech Republic, Hungary, Poland, and the Slovak Republic are current members of the Organization for Economic Cooperation and Development (OECD), which has among its goals the mission to support sustainable economic growth in a market-based economy, maintain financial stability, and assist other countries' economic development.

Bulgaria, the Czech Republic, Hungary, Poland, Romania, and Slovakia belong to the North Atlantic Treaty Organization (NATO), the military alliance of democratic states in Europe and North America.

The Czech Republic, Slovakia, Hungary, Poland, Bulgaria, and Romania are the newest members of the European Union (EU).

COUNTRY PROFILES OF EASTERN EUROPE

BELARUS

Population: 9.6 million

Religions: Russian Orthodox, Catholic, Eastern Orthodox, Roman Catholic, Protestant, Jewish, and Muslim

Languages: Belorusian, Russian

Ethnic Makeup: Belorusian, Russian, Polish, Ukrainian

Politics/Governance: Presidential Republic

Type of Healthcare System: Soviet model healthcare system

HIV Prevalence: 0.20%[11]

TB Prevalence: 69 per 100,000 (100% DOTS [Directly Observed Treatment Short-course] coverage)[12]

Percent of Population Vaccinated: 90–99%

Unique Environmental Exposures: Chernobyl-related radiation exposure, high incidence of thyroid cancer in children

Key Health Institutions: The Minsk City Health Administration, Polyclinic #36

BULGARIA

Population: 7.2 million

Religions: Bulgarian Orthodox, Islam, Roman Catholic, Protestant

Languages: Bulgarian

Ethnic Makeup: Bulgarian, Turkish, Roma

Politics/Governance: Parliamentary Democracy

Type of Healthcare System: National Health System with parallel private system, 28 regional health divisions with individual insurance funds.

HIV Prevalence: 0.1%[13]

TB Prevalence: 41 per 100,000 people (100% DOTS coverage)[14]

Percent of Population Vaccinated: 94–99%

Infant Mortality: 11.6 per 1000 live births[15]

Leading Causes of Death: Stroke, heart disease

Key Health Institutions: SAGBAL Eva (Sliven), National Center of Infectious and Parasitic Diseases (Sofia), National Hospital for Cardiology (Sofia), Medical University (Sofia).

CZECH REPUBLIC

Population: 10.2 million

Religions: Agnostic, Roman Catholic, Protestant

Languages: Czech

Politics/Governance: Parliamentary Democracy

Type of Healthcare System: Social Health Insurance (universal coverage), public and private institutional care providers

HIV Prevalence: 1500 people living with HIV[16]

TB Prevalence: 9.3 per 100,000 people (100% DOTS coverage)[17]

Leading Causes of Death: Circulatory system diseases

Key Health Institutions: Charles University Hospital (Pilsen and Prague), The Institute of Clinical and Experimental Medicine (Prague), Motol University Hospital (Prague), Palacky University Faculty of Medicine (Olomouc), Faculty Hospital Brno (Brno), Faculty Hospital Brno at St. Anne (Brno)

HUNGARY

Population: 9.9 million

Religions: Catholic, Protestant, Jewish

Language: Hungarian

Ethnic Groups: Hungarian, Roma

Politics/Governance: Parliamentary Democracy

Type of Healthcare System: Social health insurance, publicly and privately owned care providers

HIV Prevalence: 0.1%[18]

TB Prevalence: 19 per 100,000 people (100% DOTS coverage)[19]

Leading Causes of Death: Cardiovascular disease, cancer

Key Health Institutions: University of Debrecen Medical School, St John's Hospital (Budapest), Vac Municipal Hospital

MOLDOVA

Population: 4.3 million

Religion: Eastern Orthodox

Languages: Moldovan, Russian, Ukrainian, Gagauz

Ethnic Makeup: Moldovan, Russian, Gagauz (turkic)

Politics/Governance: Parliamentary Republic

Type of Healthcare System: Social health insurance, Government-run tertiary care facilities, regional management of primary health care

HIV Prevalence: 0.4%[20]

TB Prevalence: 151 per 100,000 people (100% DOTS coverage)[21]

Leading Causes of Death: Circulatory system diseases

Key Health Institutions: National Center for Preventative Medicine, City Ambulance Hospital xxiii, Republican Clinical Hospital, Medical University of Moldova, The State University of Medicine and Pharmacy "Nicolae Testemitanu" (SMPU)

POLAND

Population: 38.5 million

Religion: Roman Catholic

Language: Polish

Ethnic Makeup: Polish

Politics/Governance: Parliamentary Republic

Type of Healthcare System: Social health insurance, public and private care providers

HIV Prevalence: 0.1%[22]

TB Prevalence: 28 per 100,000 people (100% DOTS coverage)[23]

Leading Causes of Death: Cardiovascular disease, cancer

Key Health Institutions: National Institute of Hygiene and Public Health, Poznan University of Medical Sciences, Medical University of Lodz, University Hospital Krakow

ROMANIA

Population: 22.2 million

Religions: Romanian Orthodox, Roman Catholic, Protestant

Language: Romanian

Ethnic Makeup: Romanian, Hungarian, Roma

Politics/Governance: Presidential Republic

Type of Healthcare System: State owned and operated health system

HIV Prevalence: 0.1%[24]

TB Prevalence: 128 per 100,000 people (100% DOTS coverage)[25]

Leading Causes of Death: Cardiovascular disease, cancer

Key Health Institutions: "Carol Davila" University of Medicine and Pharmacy, Victor Babes University of Medicine and Pharmacy, Coltea Hospital, Pantelimon Hospital, University of Bucharest Hospital, The Institute of Health Services Management (IMSS)

RUSSIA

Population: 140 million

Religions: Russian Orthodox, Catholic, Islam, Jewish

Languages: Russian (27 other regional languages)

Ethnic Makeup: Russian, Tatar, Ukrainian

Politics/Governance: Presidential Republic

Type of Healthcare System: Compulsory health insurance with public and private care providers

HIV Prevalence: 1.1%[26]

TB Prevalence: 115 per 100,000 people (100% DOTS coverage)[27]

Leading Causes of Death: Cardiovascular disease

Key Health Institutions: City Clinical Hospital No. 1 in the name of Pirogov (Moscow), Central Clinical Hospital (CCH) in the Kuntzevo district (Moscow), Savior's Hospital for Peace and Charity (Moscow), Republican Children's Hospital of Moscow, The Institute of Pediatric and Children's Surgery (Moscow), Municipal Hospital No. 13 (Moscow), St. Petersburg State Medical University in the name of Academician Ivan P. Pavlov (SPMU; St. Petersburg), Medical Center of St. Petersburg in the name of Sokolov (formerly Hospital No. 122; St. Petersburg), The Department of Epidemiology of the St. Petersburg Medical Academy in the name of I. I. Mechnikov (St. Petersburg)

SLOVAKIA

Population: 5.5 million

Religions: Roman Catholic, Protestant, Jewish

Language: Slovak

Ethnic Makeup: Slovak, Hungarian, Roma

Politics/Governance: Parliamentary Republic

Type of Healthcare System: Social Health Insurance, most hospitals owned and operated by the Ministry of Health, many private providers.

HIV Prevalence: 185 total cumulative cases as of 2006[28]

TB Prevalence: 20 per 100,000 people (100% DOTS coverage)[29]

Leading Causes of Death: Cardiovascular disease

Key Health Institutions: Ministry of Health, University Teaching Hospital and Polyclinic Bratislava, National Institute of Cardiovascular Diseases, The Faculty Hospital and Polyclinic (Kosice)

UKRAINE

Population: 45.7 million

Religions: Eastern Orthodox, Roman Catholic, Protestant, Islam, Jewish

Language: Ukrainian

Ethnic Makeup: Ukrainians, Russians

Politics/Governance: Presidential Republic

Type of Healthcare System: State-run health system, private facilities available

HIV Prevalence: 1.6%[30]

TB Prevalence: 102 per 100,000 people (100% DOTS coverage)

Leading Causes of Death: Cardiovascular disease, cancer

Key Health Institutions: National Emergency and Trauma Hospital, City Children Clinical Hospital #1, Main Military Clinical Hospital

REFERENCES

1. Coker RJ, Atun RA, McKee M. Health-care system frailties and public health control of communicable disease on the European Union's new eastern border. *Lancet.* 2004;363:1389–1392.

2. Shakarishvili G. *Curing Sick Health Care Systems in Transition Countries.* In Beyond Transition: The Newsletter about Reforming Economies. Washington, DC: The World Bank Group, 2001.

3. Figueras J, McKee M, Cain J, Lessof S. *Health Systems in Transition: Learning from Experience.* Geneva, Switzerland: World Health Organization on behalf of the European Observatory on Health Systems and Policies; 2004.

4. The World Bank Group. *Countries: Europe and Central Asia, Health and Nutrition.* Washington, DC: The World Bank Group; 2009.

5. Health-care system frailties and public health control of communicable disease on the European Union's new eastern border", Richard J. Coker, Rifat A. Atun, Martin McKee. *Lancet.* 2004; Vol 363:1389–1392.

6. Coker RJ, Atun RA, McKee M. Health-care system frailties and public health control of communicable disease on the European Union's new eastern border. *Lancet.* 2004;363:1389–1392.

7. Coker RJ, Atun RA, McKee M. Health-care system frailties and public health control of communicable disease on the European Union's new eastern border. *Lancet.* 2004;363:1389–1392.

8. Figueras J, McKee M, Cain J, Lessof S. *Health Systems in Transition: Learning from Experience.* Geneva, Switzerland: World Health Organization on behalf of the European Observatory on Health Systems and Policies; 2004.

9. Figueras J, McKee M, Cain J, Lessof S. *Health Systems in Transition: Learning from Experience.* Geneva, Switzerland: World Health Organization on behalf of the European Observatory on Health Systems and Policies; 2004.

10. The Chernobyl Forum. Chernobyl's Legacy: Health, Environmental and Socio-Economic Impacts. New York: Council on Foreign Relations; 2006.

11. Kaiser Global Health. Belarus: Statistics on HIV, TB, and Malaria. http://www.globalhealthfacts.org/country.jsp?c=41. Accessed June 12, 2009.

12. Kaiser Global Health. Belarus: Statistics on HIV, TB, and Malaria. http://www.globalhealthfacts.org/country.jsp?c=41. Accessed June 12, 2009.

13. World Health Organization. Epidemiological Fact Sheet on HIV and AIDS: Bulgaria. http://www.who.int/hiv/pub/epidemiology/pubfacts/en/. Update 2008. Accessed June 12, 2009.
14. The World Health Organization. TB Country Profile: Bulgaria. http://apps.who.int/globalatlas/predefinedreports/tb/index.asp. Update 2009. Accessed June 12, 2009.
15. The European Observatory on Health Systems and Policies. Health Systems in Transition: Bulgaria. 2007.
16. World Health Organization. Epidemiological Fact Sheet on HIV and AIDS: Czech Republic. http://www.who.int/hiv/pub/epidemiology/pubfacts/en/. Update 2008. Accessed June 12, 2009.
17. The World Health Organization. TB Country Profile: Czech Republic. http://apps.who.int/globalatlas/predefinedreports/tb/index.asp. Update 2009. Accessed June 12, 2009.
18. World Health Organization. Epidemiological Fact Sheet on HIV and AIDS: Hungary. http://www.who.int/hiv/pub/epidemiology/pubfacts/en/. Update 2008. Accessed June 12, 2009.
19. The World Health Organization. TB Country Profile: Hungary. http://apps.who.int/globalatlas/predefinedreports/tb/index.asp. Update 2009. Accessed June 12, 2009.
20. World Health Organization. Epidemiological Fact Sheet on HIV and AIDS: Moldova. http://www.who.int/hiv/pub/epidemiology/pubfacts/en/. Update 2008. Accessed June 12, 2009.
21. The World Health Organization. TB Country Profile: Moldova. http://apps.who.int/globalatlas/predefinedreports/tb/index.asp. Update 2009. Accessed June 12, 2009.
22. World Health Organization. Epidemiological Fact Sheet on HIV and AIDS: Poland. http://www.who.int/hiv/pub/epidemiology/pubfacts/en/. Update 2008. Accessed June 12, 2009.
23. The World Health Organization. TB Country Profile: Poland. http://apps.who.int/globalatlas/predefinedreports/tb/index.asp. Update 2009. Accessed June 12, 2009.
24. World Health Organization. Epidemiological Fact Sheet on HIV and AIDS: Romania. http://www.who.int/iv/pub/epidemiology/pubfacts/en/. Update 2008. Accessed June 12, 2009.
25. The World Health Organization. TB Country Profile: Romania. http://apps.who.int/globalatlas/predefinedreports/tb/index.asp. Update 2009. Accessed June 12, 2009.
26. World Health Organization. Epidemiological Fact Sheet on HIV and AIDS: Russian Federation. http://www.who.int/hiv/pub/epidemiology/pubfacts/en/. Update 2008. Accessed June 12, 2009.
27. The WHO. The World Health Organization. TB Country Profile: Russian Federation. http://apps.who.int/globalatlas/predefinedreports/tb/index.asp. Update 2009. Accessed June 12, 2009.

28. The World Health Organization Regional Office for Europe. HIV/AIDS in Slovakia. http://www.euro.who.int/aids/ctryinfo/overview/20060118_39. Updated June, 2008. Accessed June 12, 2009.

29. The WHO. The World Health Organization. TB Country Profile: Slovakia. http://apps.who.int/globalatlas/predefinedreports/tb/index.asp. Update 2009. Accessed June 12, 2009.

30. World Health Organization. Epidemiological Fact Sheet on HIV and AIDS: Ukraine. http://www.who.int/hiv/pub/epidemiology/pubfacts/en/. Update 2008. Accessed June 12, 2009.

XV ■ SUB-SAHARAN AFRICA

Nasreen Jessani, MSPH
Matthew Dacso, MD, MSc

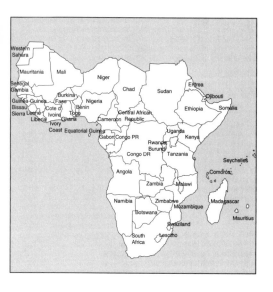

SUB-SAHARAN AFRICA ACCOUNTS FOR 11% OF THE WORLD'S POPULATION AND 24% OF THE GLOBAL DISEASE BURDEN (IFC REPORT, 2007)

The prevailing dominance of colonialism in most of Africa began to wane in the latter part of the 20th century as countries began to gain independence. The desire for democratically elected governments that swept across Africa in the 1980s and 1990s altered political expressions on the continent. By 2002, the number of countries under military rule was only 2% (down from 24% in 1982), the number of one-party states had dropped to 8% (from 54% in 1982) and 81% of countries in Africa could be classified as having some sort of democracy. Recent elections in the region have had mixed results. Violent elections finally settled into the formation of a government of national unity in Zimbabwe, and a Grand Coalition in Kenya. Conversely, recent elections in Ghana and Malawi seem to indicate a positive trend in the improving quality of democracy on the continent. There is no doubt that the quantity of democracies on the continent has dramatically improved, but how does this express itself in the provision of public goods such as health care that impact on all aspects of a country's economy? The statistics vary even within the sub-Saharan African (SSA) region.

The region covers an area of over 25 million square kilometers and is home to a population of over 800 million people—43.3% of which are between the ages of 0 and 14; Uganda has the highest share at this age range (49.3%))[1] Sixty-five percent of SSA's population lives in rural areas.[1] The climate is fairly temperate but varies across the region. Drought and famine are not uncommon. Its geography includes deserts, savannas (tropical grasslands), mountains, and tropical rain forests. The two economic strongholds on the continent are South Africa and Nigeria—comprising 56% of SSA's gross domestic product (GDP)[1]. The region includes 22 million people living with HIV/AIDS.

The Horn of Africa constitutes Djibouti, Somalia, Sudan, and Eritrea—a population of approximately 90 million people. The area exudes a strong Islamic influence as a result of its proximity to the Arabian Peninsula. The landscape is generally mountainous and benefits from arid hot weather in regions close to the Red Sea, as well as monsoon rainfall as a result of its proximity to the equator. The area has suffered numerous bouts of civil conflict and the emergence of local militia-like movements. Traditional medicine is highly valued.

East Africa is comprised of Kenya, Uganda, Tanzania, Rwanda, and Burundi—countries encompassed by a united East African Community (EAC). British, German, French, and Portuguese colonial powers governed parts of the region in the 19th and 20th centuries. The area is relatively dry and cool with unreliable rainy seasons. Cholera, polio, and measles outbreaks have been known to occur. Although HIV/AIDS and malaria continue to be endemic in the region, countries such as Kenya reap the benefits of some of the more advanced healthcare training and treatment institutions.

Southern Africa has borne the brunt of the HIV/AIDS epidemic with national adult HIV prevalence ranging from 11.9% in Malawi to 23.9% in Lesotho. HIV decreases life expectancies and increases the chances of co-morbidities. Infant and child mortality rates are, on average, lower in South West Africa than in South Eastern Africa. Violence-related health emergencies are more prevalent in the area's morbidity and mortality profile. South Africa boasts high-quality private medical facilities and is often frequented by nationals in the region for care and treatment.

West and Central African countries often cite lower respiratory diseases as being the leading cause of death. Civil conflict and displacement has been related to the increase of HIV/AIDS.[2] Torrential rains in the rainy season can result in humanitarian emergencies that have inspired the institution of early warning systems. Deforestation as well as desertification is on the increase. The West African countries have continued to maintain strong ties with their former colonial powers unlike those from East and Southern Africa. They are also united by a common currency, the CFA, which is loosely tied to the Euro.

Throughout the region, the introduction of preventive mechanisms such as insecticide treated bed nets and indoor residual spraying, as well as curative treatment such as artemesinin combination therapy has contributed toward combating the burden of malaria. However, the statistics fail to reflect expected reductions in incidence. This is similar for HIV/AIDS, TB, etc—whereby disease-specific programming, while targeted and well intentioned, have often failed to consider such systemic challenges as true cost, drug storage, health worker retention, environmental challenges, and social determinants.

As in many parts of the developing world, SSA is experiencing a double burden of disease. Better control of infectious disease has aided in the increased life span of the populations. New and emerging contagious diseases, HIV/AIDs, and drug resistance compounded by chronic conditions such as hypertension, diabetes, and heart disease have further strained the health systems and altered the face of health care on the continent.

Political strife and civic displacement has led to habitation in areas with poor water and sanitation. This is particularly noticeable in countries such as Rwanda, the Democratic Republic of Congo, and Zimbabwe. In Eritrea, for instance, 5% of the population has access to improved sanitation facilities in contrast to 94% in Mauritius (MDG7).[1] Continued in-migration of populations to urban centers and constant out-migration of health professionals to regions that provide better opportunities have resulted in a further crippling of healthcare quality. The shortage of human resources for health in the region—the term coined *brain drain*—as a result of poor incentive structures for attraction and retention, amongst others, is creating a new movement of task-shifting whereby countries are exploring means of empowering other cadres of health and community workers to fill in the gaps and alleviate the burden of care.

The inequitable distribution and financing of services tends to mean rural areas are underserved and lower income households in urban areas are also underserved as for-profit outlets and crowded government hospitals are concentrated in the towns. Countries in the region often have three types of health service providers: government, private (for- and not-for-profit), and faith-based. The quality of services varies with type, tier, and location. Funding for health care is often unsubsidized and can lead to catastrophic expenditures for families with health emergencies. In Tanzania, for instance, the government was the principal provider of health services even prior to independence. The private sector—often in the form of traditional healers and birth attendants—existed pre-colonization in much of the continent (Namibia being an exception). The private sector manifests still in response to many governments' compromised ability to provide quality health services due to unfavorable economic conditions. The WHO has encouraged more integration of traditional and alternative medicines due to their continuing importance and popularity.

The statistical summaries outlined reflect the performance of health systems overall and their abilities to react to the health needs of the citizens. From the years 2000–2006, 92% of women in Seychelles were literate; this figure was 13% for Chad and 15% for Niger.[1] The gendered dimensions of a country often reflect in disproportionate access to care. Incidences of corruption, funding shortfalls, and inequitable access for the poor and vulnerable continue to exacerbate the problem.

In 1987, the World Health Organization (WHO)-led Bamako Initiative began the reshaping of health policy in Africa in order to encourage more efficient and equitable provision of services. However, up to and including October 2006, many governments faced difficulties in implementing policies, especially those aimed at mitigating the effects of the AIDS-pandemic. The World Bank, African Development Bank (AfDB), and Agence Française de Développement are among the many institutions that are participating in a project aimed at reshaping the healthcare system in the continent. The plan is to raise at least $15 billion in the next three years to finance the partnerships. Africa endorsed the plan during the African Growth and Opportunity Act (AGOA) conference in Nairobi in August, 2009.

REGIONAL ORGANIZATIONS

The African Union (http://www.africa-union.org) is the principal organization for the promotion of accelerated socioeconomic integration of the entire African continent. The Common Market for Eastern Southern Africa (COMESA; http://www.comesa.int) is a grouping of 21 African states, which have agreed to promote regional integration through trade and development. The Economic Community of West African States (ECOWAS; http://www.ecowas.int) is a regional group of fifteen African countries charged with promoting integration in all fields of economic activity. The East African Community (EAC; http://www.eac.int) is a regional intergovernmental organization comprising Kenya, Uganda, Tanzania, Rwanda and Burundi. The Southern African Development Community (SADC; http://www.sadc.int) is a group of South African states working to achieve economic development, alleviate poverty, and enhance the quality of life of the peoples of Southern Africa. The West African Monetary

Union (UEMOA; http://www.uemoa.int) is an organization of eight states of West Africa established to promote economic integration among countries that share a common currency, the CFA franc. The African Development Bank (AfDB; http://www.afdb.org) aims at assisting African countries in their efforts to achieve sustainable economic development and social progress. The World Health Organization (WHO; http://www.afro.who.int) operates in these countries via their regional office for Africa in the Congo.

COUNTRY PROFILES OF SUB-SAHARAN AFRICA

KENYA

■ Demography[3]

Population: 39,002,772 (2009 national census being conducted at the time of printing)

Religions: Protestant (45%), Roman Catholic (33%), Muslim (10%), indigenous beliefs (10%), other (2%)

Languages: English (official), Kiswahili (official), numerous indigenous languages

Ethnic Makeup: Kikuyu (22%), Luhya (14%), Luo (13%), Kalenjin (12%), Kamba (11%), Kisii (6%), Meru (6%), other African (15%), non-African (Asian, European, and Arab; 1%)

Formerly colonized: British

Politics/governance: Semipresidential/republic—recent elections 2007 were highly contested and resulted in a Grand Coalition constituting a president and prime minister.

HIV Prevalence: Adult—Approximately 8% (2007)[4]

TB Prevalence: Ranks 18th among countries with highest TB burden—24,435 deaths annually. Prevalence: 319/100,000 (2007). DOTS coverage: 100% DOTS rx success: 85%[5]

Malaria: 11,341,750 cases (2006)[6]

Percent of Population Vaccinated: 74–92% depending on the vaccine (2007)[7]

Infant Mortality Rate: 54.7 deaths/1000 live births (2009)[3]

Under-5 Mortality: 121/1000 (2007 estimate)[8]

Leading Causes of Death: HIV/AIDS (38%), lower respiratory infections (10%), diarrheal diseases (7%), TB (5%), and malaria (5%) (2002)[9]

Unusual Pathogens: malaria, Rift Valley Fever, leptospirosis, meningococcal disease, polio[10]

Unique Environmental Exposures: High levels of aflatoxin in homegrown and purchased maize.[11,12] Stagnant water leads to outbreaks of malaria in the rainy seasons. Poor water quality and poor sanitation, particularly during droughts, leads to high incidence of diarrheal and other water-borne diseases.

■ Traditional Medicine

In 1999, Kenya's patent law was revised to include protection for traditional medicine.[13]

■ Healthcare System

Structured in a stepwise manner so that as cases become more complex, they are referred to a higher tier institution. The structure thus consists of dispensaries and private clinics, health centres, subdistrict hospitals and nursing homes, district hospitals and private hospitals, provincial hospitals, and national hospitals. The Ministry of Health (MOH) has been replaced by the Ministry of Medical Services and the Ministry of Public Health (2008).

There are eight provincial hospitals and two national hospitals in the country. Aga Khan University Hospital (Nairobi, Mombasa, and Kisumu); Nairobi Hospital, Kenyatta National Hospital, Karen Hospital, Mariakani Cottage Hospital, Gertrude's Garden Children's Hospital, Moi Teaching and referral Hospital, and Mombasa Hospital.[14]

UGANDA

■ Demography[3]

Population: 32,369,558

Religions: Roman Catholic (41.9%), Protestant (42%: Anglican 35.9%, Pentecostal 4.6%, Seventh Day Adventist 1.5%), Muslim (12.1%), other (3.1%), none (0.9%) (2002 census)

Languages: English (official), Kiswahili, Ganda or Luganda, other Niger-Congo languages, Nilo-Saharan languages, Arabic

Ethnic Makeup: Baganda (16.9%), Banyakole (9.5%), Basoga (8.4%), Bakiga (6.9%), Iteso (6.4%), Langi (6.1%), Acholi (4.7%), Bagisu (4.6%), Lugbara (4.2%), Bunyoro (2.7%), other (29.6%) (2002 census)

Formerly Colonized: British

Politics/Governance: Democratic Republic

HIV Prevalence: Adult—5.4% (2007)[4]

TB: ranks 13th among countries of highest TB burden, with 28,686 deaths annually. Prevalence: 426/100,000 (2007). DOTS coverage: 100%. DOTS rx success: 70%[5]

Malaria: 10,626,930 cases (2006)[6]

Percent of Population Vaccinated: 64–90% depending on the vaccine (2007)[7]

Infant Mortality Rate: 64.82 deaths/1000 live births (2009)[3]

Under-5 mortality: 131/1000 (2007 estimate)[8]

Leading Causes of Death: HIV/AIDS (25%), malaria (11%), lower respiratory infections (11%), diarrheal diseases (8%), TB (5%), and perinatal conditions (4%) (2002)[9]

Unusual Pathogens: malaria, marburg hemorrhagic fever, ebola, cholera[10]

Unique Environmental Exposures: Floods in Eastern and Northern Uganda with a high incidence of water-borne diarrheal illness and cholera. Traditional practices such as bathing in rivers and inadequate hygiene practices exacerbate risk.[15]

■ Traditional Medicine

Practitioners of traditional medicine vastly outnumber allopathic doctors. The government has expressed interest in recognizing traditional health systems. Traditional and Modern Health Practitioners Together against AIDS and other diseases (THETA) organizes training programs for traditional medicine practitioners.[13]

■ Healthcare System

Health provision in Uganda is shared between Government-funded facilities (typically large hospitals—30%); private not-for-profit facilities (45%) that include church-supported hospitals; medium-sized clinics; private for-profit (25%); or commercial health units and self-employed physicians. The MOH presides over allopathic practitioners, while the Ministry of Women in Development, Culture, and Youth presides over traditional medicine practitioners.

There are two national referral hospitals: Butabika Hospital and Mulago Hospital. There are 11 regional referral hospitals, 39 district, 2 other government, 46 NGO, 10 private, 2 military, and 1 prison hospital.[16]

TANZANIA (INCLUDES THE ISLAND OF ZANZIBAR)

■ Demography[3]

Population: 41,048,532

Religions: Mainland: Christian (30%), Muslim (35%), indigenous beliefs (35%); Zanzibar: Muslim

Languages: Kiswahili, English, Arabic (Zanzibar)

Ethnic groups: Mainland: African (99%, of which 95% are Bantu consisting of more than 130 tribes), Asian, European, and Arab (1%); Zanzibar: Arab, African, mixed Arab and African

Formerly Colonized: British

Politics/Governance: Republic

HIV Prevalence: Adult: 6.2% (2007)[4]

TB: ranks 12th among countries of highest TB burden with 31,504 deaths annually. Prevalence: 337/100,000 (2007). DOTS coverage: 100%; DOTS rx success: 85%[5]

Malaria: 11,539,867 cases (2006 estimate)[6]

Percent of Population Vaccinated: 83–90% depending on the vaccine (2007)[7]

Infant Mortality Rate: 59.02 deaths/1000 live births (2009)[3]

Under-5 mortality: 116/1000 (2007 estimate)[8]

Leading Causes of Death: HIV/AIDS (29%), lower respiratory infections (12%), malaria (10%), diarrheal diseases (6%), perinatal conditions (4%), and TB (3%) (2002)[9]

Unusual Pathogens: malaria, Rift Valley Fever, meningococcal disease, cholera[10]

Unique Environmental Exposures: urban area pollution—both air and water—as a result of improper treatment and disposal of solid and liquid wastes contribute to illnesses. In Dar es Salaam, for example, less than 5% of the population is connected to a sewage system.[17] Mining activities are a major cause of environmental degradation by deforestation, destruction of habitat, and loss of biodiversity.

■ Traditional Medicine
Beginning in the 1990s, complementary/alternative systems of health care have emerged in Tanzania. These new medical options include magnetic therapy, homeopathic medicine, massage, and traditional Chinese, Korean, and Indian medicines.[13] Traditional practices play a formidable role in the conservation of medicinal plants.[18]

■ Healthcare System
Health services in Tanzania are provided by the government, parastatal organizations, voluntary organizations, religious organizations, private practitioners (for-profit as well as not-for-profit), and traditional medicine. The referral system (structure) starts from the community level (village) up to treatment abroad. The structure thus consists of village health services, dispensaries, health centers, district hospitals, regional hospitals, and referral/consultant hospitals.[19] The overarching government body is the Ministry of Health and Social Welfare.

The key healthcare institutions are: Muhimbili National Hospital (Dar es Salaam), Aga Khan Hospital (Dar es Salaam, Dodoma, Arusha), and Morogoro regional hospital. There are a total of 126 registered health centers (52% are rural), and 1340 registered private dispensaries. Fifty-six percent of the 121 private hospitals are located in the rural areas. These hospitals are almost all private not-for-profit. The remaining institutions are in urban areas.[19]

RWANDA
■ Demography[3]
Population: 10,473,282

Religions: Roman Catholic (56.5%), Protestant (26%), Adventist (11.1%), Muslim (4.6%), indigenous beliefs (0.1%), none (1.7%) (2001)

Languages: Kinyarwanda (official), English (official), Kiswahili, French, universal Bantu vernacular

Ethnic Makeup: Hutu (Bantu; 84%), Tutsi (Hamitic; 15%), Twa (Pygmy; 1%)

Formerly Colonized: Belgian

Politics/Governance: Republic; presidential, multiparty system

HIV Prevalence: Adult: 2.8% (2007)[4]

TB: Ranks 25th among countries of highest TB burden with 12,403 deaths annually. Prevalence: 590/100,000 (2007). DOTS coverage: 100%; DOTS rx success: 86%[5]

Malaria: 3,251,156 cases (2006 estimate)[6]

Percent of Population Vaccinated: 82–99% depending on the vaccine (2007)[7]

Infant Mortality Rate: 81.61 deaths/1000 live births (2002)[3]

Under-5 mortality: 181/1000 (2007 estimate)[8]

Leading Causes of Death: HIV/AIDS (23%), lower respiratory infections (16%), diarrheal diseases (13%), perinatal conditions (8%), and TB (5%) (2006)[9]

Unusual Pathogens: meningococcal disease.[10]

Unique Environmental Exposures: deforestation due to uncontrolled cutting of trees for fuel, overgrazing, soil exhaustion, soil erosion, widespread poaching, and acid rain

■ Traditional Medicine
Traditional medicine is practiced by five types of people: the umupfumu, the umuhannyi, the umuvuzi, the umurozi, and the magendu—each of them specialized in a particular set of diseases or problems. The most widely used of medicinal plants is *Iboza Riparia*, which is thought to be effective against more than 15 common diseases.

■ Healthcare System
The MOH governs health care in the country with facilities categorized as hospitals, health centers, and health posts/FOSACOMs.[20] The Rwandan government has introduced innovative approaches to increasing the coordination of donors and external aid with government policy, and monitoring the effectiveness of aid; a countrywide independent community health insurance scheme; and the introduction of a performance-based pay initiative.

There are approximately 30 hospitals and 30 health centers including Shyira Hospital, Kibagora Hospital, Gahini Hospital, National University Teaching Hospital, Nyagatare Hospital, Rwamagana district hospital, Ruhengeri district hospital, Polyclinique du Plateau, Bio Medical Center, and Clinique le Bon Samaritain. Referral Hospitals include University Central Hospital of Kigali (CHUK), University Central Hospital of Butare (CHUB), and King Faisal Hospital. There exist a number of traditional medical centers.

BURUNDI
■ Demography[3]
Population: 8,988,091

Religions: Christian (67%: Roman Catholic 62%, Protestant 5%), indigenous beliefs (23%), Muslim (10%)

Languages: Kirundi (official), French (official), Swahili (along Lake Tanganyika and in the Bujumbura area)

Ethnic Makeup: Hutu (Bantu; 85%), Tutsi (Hamitic; 14%), Twa (Pygmy; 1%), Europeans (3000), and South Asians (2000)

Formerly Colonized: Belgian

Politics/Governance: Republic

HIV Prevalence: Adult—2.0% (2007)[4]

TB: Ranks 33rd among countries of highest TB burden with 8685 deaths annually. Prevalence: 647/100,000 (2007). DOTS coverage: 100%; DOTS rx success: 83%[5]

Malaria: 2,270,872 cases (2006 estimate)[6]

Percent of Population Vaccinated: 64–86% depending on the vaccine (2007)[7]

Infant Mortality Rate: 59.64 deaths/1000 live births[3]

Under-5 mortality: 80/1000 (2007 estimate)[8]

Leading Causes of Death: HIV/AIDS (26%), lower respiratory infections (13%), diarrheal diseases (9%), war (8%), and perinatal conditions (7%) (2002)[9]

Unusual Pathogens: meningococcal disease, cholera,[10] trypanosomiasis, schistosomiasis (bilharziasis), malaria.

Unique Environmental Exposures: Deforestation caused by the demands of households and communities for fuel. Overcrowding in refugee camps expose people to unsanitary water and waste disposal.

■ Traditional Medicine
Although widely practiced and sought, there are no procedures for the official approval of traditional medical practices or remedies.[13]

■ Healthcare System
The governing body is the Ministry of Public Health. The key healthcare institutions are the Hospital Prince Regent Charles, Prince Louis Rwagasore Clinic, University hospitals, and military hospitals.

DEMOCRATIC REPUBLIC OF CONGO
■ Demography[3]
Population: 68,692,542 (2009)

Religions: Roman Catholic (50%), Protestant (20%), Kimbanguist (10%), Muslim (10%), other (includes syncretic sects and indigenous beliefs: 10%)

Languages: French (official), Lingala (a lingua franca trade language), Kingwana (a dialect of Kiswahili or Swahili), Kikongo, Tshiluba

Ethnic Makeup: Over 200 African ethnic groups of which the majority are Bantu; the four largest tribes are Mongo, Luba, Kongo (all Bantu), and the Mangbetu-Azande (Hamitic) make up about 45% of the population.

Formerly Colonized: Belgian

Politics/Governance: Republic

HIV Prevalence: Adult—1.2–1.5% (2007)[4]

TB: Ranks 8th among countries of highest TB burden with 51,102 deaths annually. Prevalence: 666/100,000. DOTS coverage: 100%. DOTS rx success: 86%[5]

Malaria: 23,619,960 cases (2006 estimate)[6]

Percent of Population Vaccinated: 79–94% depending on the vaccine (2007)[7]

Infant Mortality Rate: 81.21 deaths/1000 live births (2009)[3]

Under–5 mortality: 161/1000 (2007 estimate)[8]

Leading Causes of Death: Diarrheal diseases (12%), HIV/AIDS (11%), lower respiratory infections (11%), malaria (10%), war (5%), and perinatal conditions (4%) (2002)[9]

Unusual Pathogens: ebola, polio, cholera, typhoid fever, meningococcal disease, sleeping sickness[10]

Unique Environmental Exposures: Wildlife poaching, soil erosion, and increasingly, deforestation are the major environmental threats. Limited access to safe water and sanitation, and waterborne diseases contribute to a low life expectancy in the DRC. The southern region is subject to periodic drought.

■ Traditional Medicine
The government has recognized the role traditional medicine plays as a complement to allopathic medicine and has urged the establishment of a division dedicated to traditional medicine within the Department of Health.[13]

■ Healthcare System
There are 400 hospitals and 5078 health centers in the DRC. The recent commercialization of healthcare delivery is due to weak governance. War and conflict have caused the demolishment of several institutions. Many suffer from stock-outs and low human resources. Trained birth attendants play a large role in safe motherhood initiatives. Several parallel systems have sprung up due to prior donor pressure.[21] The Ministry of Health oversees regulation of the health sector. The key healthcare institutions are the Kindu Hospital, Panzi Hospital, and Kinshasa General Hospital.

ZAMBIA
■ Demography[3]
Population: 11,862,740 (2009)

Religions: Christian (50–75%), Muslim and Hindu (24–49%), indigenous beliefs (1%)

Languages: English (official), major vernaculars: Bemba, Kaonda, Lozi, Lunda, Luvale, Nyanja, Tonga, and about 70 other indigenous languages

Ethnic Makeup: African (99.5%; includes Bemba, Tonga, Chewa, Lozi, Nsenga, Tumbuka, Ngoni, Lala, Kaonde, Lunda, and others), other (0.5%; includes Europeans, Asians, and Americans) (2000 Census)

Formerly Colonized: British

Politics/Governance: Republic

HIV Prevalence: Adult—15.2% (2007)[4]

TB: Ranks 22nd among countries of highest TB burden with 13,661 deaths annually. Prevalence: 387/100,000. DOTS coverage: 100%. DOTS rx success: 85%[5]

Malaria: 3,655,203 cases (2006)[6]

Percent of Population Vaccinated: 77–92% depending on the vaccine (2007)[7]

Infant Mortality Rate: 101.2 deaths/1000 live births[3]

Under-5 Mortality: 170/1000 (2007 estimate)[8]

Leading Causes of Death: HIV/AIDS (43%), lower respiratory infections (12%), malaria (9%), diarrheal diseases (7%), perinatal conditions (4%) (2002)[9]

Unusual Pathogens: cholera, new virus from *Arenaviridae* family (2008)

Unique Environmental Exposures: air pollution and resulting acid rain in the mineral extraction and refining region; chemical runoff into watersheds; poaching; soil erosion; desertification; lack of adequate water treatment presents human health risks[22]

■ Traditional Medicine

At least 70% of Zambians use traditional medicine.[13] Currently, herbal medicine, naturopathy, traditional Chinese medicine, reflexology, spiritualism, and other forms of medicine are practiced in Zambia.

■ Healthcare System

The MOH is the overarching government body. Healthcare facilities run by the Ministry are categorized into hospitals, health centers, or health posts. The hospitals are categorized as primary (district), secondary (provincial), and tertiary (central). The health centers are further divided in urban and rural (or health posts). In addition to the government, there are private and privately funded hospitals (some of which are religiously sponsored), and faith-based hospitals with some governmental funding support.

There are 97 hospitals in Zambia of which 5 are at the tertiary level of care.[23] The major hospitals are the Chipata General Hospital, Kitwe Central Hospital, Ndola Central Hospital, Konkola Mine Hospital, Lubwe Mission Hospital, Maacha Hospital, Mtendere Mission Hospital, Mukinge Mission Hospital, Mwandi Mission Hospital, Nchanga North Hospital, St Francis Hospital, St Luke's Mission Hospital, and the University Teaching Hospital.

ZIMBABWE

■ Demography[3]

Population: 11,392,629 (2009 estimate)

Religions: Syncretic (50%; part Christian, part indigenous beliefs), Christian (25%), indigenous beliefs (24%), Muslim and other (1%)

Languages: English (official), Shona, Sindebele (Ndebele), numerous but minor tribal dialects

Ethnic Makeup: African (98%; Shona 82%, Ndebele 14%, other 2%), mixed and Asian (1%), white (< 1%)

Formerly Colonized: Parliamentary democracy

Politics/Governance: Republic. Coalition government with president and prime minister (August, 2009)

HIV Prevalence: Adult—15.3% (2007)[4]

TB: Ranks 11th among countries of highest TB burden with 35,343 deaths annually. Prevalence: 714/100,000. DOTS coverage: 100%. DOTS rx success: 60%[5]

Malaria: 2,694,304 cases (2006)[6]

Percent of Population Vaccinated: 62–78% depending on the vaccine (2007)[7]

Infant Mortality Rate: 32.31 deaths/1000 live births[3]

Under-5 Mortality: 90/1000 (2007 estimate)[8]

Leading Causes of Death: HIV/AIDS (67%), lower respiratory infections (12%), malaria (4%), TB (3%), diarrheal diseases (2%), cerebrovascular diseases (2%), perinatal conditions (4%) (2002)[9]

Unusual Pathogens: cholera, meningitis[10]

Unique Environmental Exposures: deforestation, soil erosion, land degradation, and air and water pollution; the black rhinoceros herd—once the largest concentration of the species in the world—has been significantly reduced by poaching; poor mining practices have led to toxic waste and heavy metal pollution[3]

■ Traditional Medicine

The Traditional Medical Practitioners Council Act of 1981 is one of the most comprehensive pieces of legislation on the practice of traditional medicine that has been enacted anywhere in the world. There are now over 55,000 traditional medicine practitioners registered with The Zimbabwe National Traditional Healers Association (ZINATHA)[13]

■ Healthcare System

The governing body is the Ministry of Health and Child Welfare. Public primary care is organized at national, district, and municipal hospitals and clinics.

The key healthcare institutions are Ingutsheni Central Hospital, Parirenyatwa Hospital, Central Harare Hospital, Harare Hospital, Sekuru Kaguvi Hospital, The Montague Clinic, The Avenues Clinic, Bulawayo Central Hospital, Masvingo General Hospital, and Kwekwe General Hospital.

MALAWI

■ Demography[3]

Population: 14,268,711 (2009)

Religions: Christian (79.9%), Muslim (12.8%), other (3%), none (4.3%) (1998 census)

Languages: Chichewa (57.2%; official), Chinyanja (12.8%), Chiyao (10.1%), Chitumbuka (9.5%), Chisena (2.7%), Chilomwe (2.4%), Chitonga (1.7%), other (3.6%) (1998 census)

Ethnic Makeup: Chewa, Nyanja, Tumbuka, Yao, Lomwe, Sena, Tonga, Ngoni, Ngonde, Asian, European

Formerly Colonized: British

Politics/Governance: Multiparty Democracy

HIV Prevalence: Adult—11.9% (2007)[4]

TB: Ranks 21st among countries of highest TB burden with 14,167 deaths annually. Prevalence: 305/100,000. DOTS coverage: 100%. DOTS rx success 78%[5]

Malaria: 4,527,651 cases (2006)[6]

Percent of Population Vaccinated: 83–96% depending on the vaccine (2007)[7]

Mortality Rate: 89.05 deaths/1000 live births[3]

Under-5 Mortality: 110/1000 (2007 estimate)[8]

Leading Causes of Death: HIV/AIDS (34%), lower respiratory infections (12%), malaria (8%), diarrheal diseases (8%), cerebrovascular diseases (3%), ischemic heart disease (3%), and perinatal conditions (3%) (2002)[9]

Unusual Pathogens: cholera, plague[10]

Unique Environmental Exposures: deforestation, land degradation, water pollution from agricultural runoff, sewage, and industrial wastes; siltation of spawning grounds endangers fish populations[3]

■ Traditional Medicine

Malawi has a training program in traditional medicine for health workers[13]

■ Healthcare System

Malawi uses a socialized system of health care, with the goal of providing access and basic health services to all Malawians. Traditional medicine also plays a significant role in Malawian health care.[13] The healthcare delivery system consists of private-for-profit providers and government facilities. Malawi has adopted the Integrated Disease Surveillance and Response (IDSR) strategy as a way to strengthen communicable disease surveillance. Health sector reforms are underway as part of the Sector-Wide Approach Program (SWAP). Its main component is the provision of an essential health package.[24] The governing body is the Ministry of Health.

There are 499 government health institutions. Central hospitals are regional referral hospitals while district hospitals are referral facilities for health centers. There are 4 national hospitals, 24 districts hospitals, and 328 health centers. In addition, there are 35 rural hospitals, as well as dispensaries and other types of healthcare institutions.[25] Key institutions include the Blantyre Hospital, Nkhoma Hospital, Lilongwe Central Hospital and Queen Elizabeth Central Hospital (Blantyre), Kamuzu Central Hospital, and Mzuzu Central Hospital.

MOZAMBIQUE

▓ Demography[3]

Population: 21,669,278

Religions: Catholic (23.8%), Muslim (17.8%), Zionist Christian (17.5%), other (17.8%), none (23.1%) (1997 census)

Languages: Emakhuwa (26.1%), Xichangana (11.3%), Portuguese (8.8%; official: spoken by 27% of population as a second language), Elomwe (7.6%), Cisena (6.8%), Echuwabo (5.8%), other Mozambican languages (32%), other foreign languages (0.3%), unspecified (1.3%) (1997 census)

Ethnic Makeup: African (99.66%; Makhuwa, Tsonga, Lomwe, Sena, and others), Europeans (0.06%), Euro-Africans (0.2%), Indians (0.08%)

Formerly Colonized: Portuguese

Politics/Governance: Republic

HIV Prevalence: Adult—12.5% (2007)[4]

TB: Ranks 15th among countries of highest TB burden with 27,200 deaths annually. Prevalence: 504/100,000. DOTS coverage: 100%. DOTS rx success: 83%[5]

Malaria: 7,432,539 cases (2006)[6]

Percent of Population Vaccinated: 70–88% depending on the vaccine (2007)[7]

Infant Mortality Rate: 105.80 deaths/1000 live births[3]

Under-5 Mortality: 168/1000 (2007 estimate)[8]

Leading Causes of Death: HIV/AIDS (28%), malaria (9%), diarrheal diseases (8%), lower respiratory infections (7%), perinatal conditions (5%), measles (3%), and TB (3%) (2002)[9]

Unusual Pathogens: cholera[10]

Unique Environmental Exposures: Long civil war and recurrent drought have resulted in increased migration to urban and coastal areas with adverse environmental consequences; desertification; pollution of surface and coastal waters; and elephant poaching for ivory is a problem[3]

▓ Traditional Medicine

Collaborative programs with traditional medicine practitioners take place under the umbrella of the Department of Health.[13] Traditional healers known as *curandeiros* are highly sought after. Religious healers known as *profetas* (spirit mediums) and *feticeiros* (witch doctors) are also used.

■ Healthcare System

The health system in Mozambique is provided by the Ministério de Saúde (MISAU), through hospitals, health centers, and health posts. There are three levels of organization of health through the government: national, provincial, and district level. The public sector is complemented by services being provided by the private sector (mainly in large cities) and NGOs. Traditional doctors or Curandeiros, are still a popular (and more affordable) source of care for many rural and urban populations.[26] Mozambique adopted a SWAP in 2000.

There are 1277 health institutions including 4 national, 7 provincial, 2 specialist, 8 district, 27 rural, and 6 general hospitals for secondary and tertiary health care. Primary healthcare is served by 104 urban health centers, 755 rural health centers, and 365 health posts.[27] Key health institutions include the Maputo Central Hospital, Nampula Central Hospital Mavalane and Jose Macamo general hospitals, Phoenix Centro Medico, Clinica da Sommerschield, Clinica Especial, Dr Soares UN Dispensary, and the Swedish Medical Clinic.

SOUTH AFRICA

■ Demography[3]

Population: 49,052,489 (2009 estimate)

Religions: Zion Christian (11.1%), Pentecostal/Charismatic (8.2%), Catholic (7.1%), Methodist (6.8%), Dutch Reformed (6.7%), Anglican (3.8%), Muslim (1.5%), other Christian (36%), other (2.3%), unspecified (1.4%), none (15.1%) (2001 census)

Languages: IsiZulu (23.8%), IsiXhosa (17.6%), Afrikaans (13.3%), Sepedi (9.4%), English (8.2%), Setswana (8.2%), Sesotho (7.9%), Xitsonga (4.4%), other (7.2%) (2001 census)

Ethnic Makeup: Black African (79%), White (9.6%), colored (8.9%), Indian/Asian (2.5%) (2001 census)

Formerly Colonized: British

Politics/Governance: Republic

HIV Prevalence: Adult—18.1% (2007)[4]

TB: Ranks 4th among countries of highest TB burden with 111,924 deaths annually. Prevalence: 692/100,000 (2007). DOTS coverage: 100%. DOTS rx success: 74%[5]

Malaria: 32,530 cases (2006 estimate)[6]

Percent of Population Vaccinated: 72–99% depending on the vaccine (2007)[7]

Infant Mortality Rate: 44.42 deaths/1000 live births (2009)[3]

Under-5 Mortality: 59/1000 (2007 estimate)[8]

Leading Causes of Death: HIV/AIDS (52%), cerebrovascular disease (5%), ischemic heart disease (4%), lower respiratory infections (4%), violence (3%), and TB (3%) (2002)[9]

Unusual Pathogens: New virus from *Arenaviridae* family, SARS (2003), cholera[10]

Unique Environmental Exposures: Lack of important arterial rivers or lakes requires extensive water conservation and control measures; growth in water usage outpacing supply; pollution of rivers from agricultural runoff and urban discharge; air pollution resulting in acid rain; soil erosion; and desertification[3]

■ Traditional Medicine

Inyangas, *sangomas*, and witchdoctors have a crucial role in providing health care to the majority of South Africans. The Traditional Healers' Organization was created in 1980 and currently represents more than 180,000 South African traditional healers. They are regulated under the Associated Health Service Professions Act of 1982.[13]

■ Healthcare System

Health care is decentralized to the nine provinces and considered a district health system. The government, private practitioners (for-profit as well as not-for-profit), the mining industry, and traditional healers provide health services in South Africa. With the exception of nurses, most healthcare professionals are associated with private services. Public health consumes 11% of the budget. The state contributes about 40% of all expenditures on health and is responsible for delivering services to about 80% of the population.[28] The overarching government body is the Department of Health.

The number of private hospitals and clinics continues to grow. There are approximately 200 private hospitals with the majority in urban areas. The mining industry also provides its own hospitals, and has 60 hospitals and clinics around the country.[28] Key institutions include the Port Elizabeth Provincial Hospital (Eastern Cape), Rosepark Hospital (Free State), Johannesburg General Hospital (Gauteng), Addington Hospital (KwaZulu-Natal), Mankweng Hospital (Limpopo), Witbank Provincial Hospital (Mpulamanga), Kimberley Medi-Clinic (Northern Cape), Wilmed Private Hospital (North West), and the Alexandra Hospital (Western Cape).

LESOTHO

■ Demography[3]

Population: 2,130,819

Religions: Christian (80%), indigenous beliefs (20%)

Languages: Sesotho (southern Sotho), English (official), Zulu, Xhosa

Ethnic Makeup: Sotho (99.7%), Europeans, Asians, and other (0.3%)

Formerly Colonized: British

Politics/Governance: Parliamentary constitutional monarchy

HIV Prevalence: Adult—23.2% (2007)[4]

TB: Ranks 46th among countries of highest TB burden with 5282 deaths annually. Prevalence: 568/100,000 (2007). DOTS coverage: 100%. DOTS rx success: 66%[5]

Malaria: not endemic (2006 estimate)[6]

Percent of Population Vaccinated: 76–96% depending on the vaccine (2007)[7]

Infant mortality rate: 77.4 deaths/1000 live births (2009)[3]

Under-5 mortality: 84/1000 (2007 estimate)[8]

Leading Causes of Death: HIV/AIDS (63%), lower respiratory infections (4%), diarrheal diseases (3%), cerebrovascular disease (3%), ischemic heart disease (3%), perinatal conditions (3%), and TB (2%) (2002)[9]

Unusual Pathogens: dysentery[10]

Unique Environmental Exposures: population pressure forcing settlement in marginal areas results in overgrazing, severe soil erosion, and soil exhaustion; desertification; Highlands Water Project controls, stores, and redirects water to South Africa[3]

■ Traditional Medicine

The Universal Medicinemen and Herbalists Council was established to promote and control the activities of traditional medicine practitioners, to provide facilities for the improvement of skills of traditional medicine practitioners, and to bring together all traditional medicine practitioners into one associated group. Lesotho has a training program in traditional medicine for health workers.[13]

■ Healthcare System

Divided into four tiers: Primary, which includes health posts that provide basic services and operate at regular intervals rather than daily, and health centers that provide basic preventive, promotive, curative, and rehabilitative services; secondary includes filter clinics and district hospitals that provide services similar to health centers (though at this level services are more comprehensive); tertiary includes hospitals providing specialized referral services for all the district hospitals in the country. For conditions that cannot be managed within the country patients are referred to neighboring South Africa through the national referral hospital.[29] The overarching government body is the Ministry of Health and Social Welfare.

There are 16 district hospitals. The tertiary level is comprised of Queen Elizabeth II Hospital, Mohlomi Mental Hospital, Bots`abelo Leprosy Hospital, and Senakatana AIDS Clinic.[29]

BOTSWANA

■ Demography[3]

Population: 1,990,876

Religions: Christian (71.6%), Badimo (6%), other (1.4%), unspecified (0.4%), none (20.6%) (2001 census)

Languages: Setswana (78.2%), Kalanga (7.9%), Sekgalagadi (2.8%), English (2.1%; official), other (8.6%), unspecified (0.4%) (2001 census)

Ethnic Makeup: Tswana (or Setswana; 79%), Kalanga (11%), Basarwa (3%), other, including Kgalagadi and White (7%)

Formerly Colonized: British

Politics/Governance: Parliamentary republic

HIV Prevalence: Adult—23.9% (2007)[4]

TB: Ranks 54th among countries of highest TB burden with 3649 deaths annually. Prevalence: 622/100,000 (2007). DOTS coverage: 100%. DOTS rx success: 72%[5]

Malaria: 6722 cases (2006 estimate)[6]

Percent of Population Vaccinated: 78–99% depending on the vaccine (2007)[7]

Infant Mortality Rate: 12.59 deaths/1000 live births (2009)[3]

Under-5 Mortality: 40/1000 (2007 estimate)[8]

Leading Causes of Death: HIV/AIDS (80%), ischemic Heart Disease (2%), cerebrovascular disease (2%), perinatal conditions (2%) (2002)[9]

Unusual Pathogens: none[10]

Unique Environmental Exposures: periodic drought; overgrazing; desertification; limited fresh water resources[3]

■ Traditional Medicine

Practitioners of traditional medicine provided the only healthcare services available in most of Botswana until the first part of the decade following independence in 1966.[13] There are about 3100 traditional health practitioners in Botswana, approximately 95% reside in rural areas.[30]

■ Healthcare System

The government, parastatal organizations, voluntary organizations, private practitioners (for-profit as well as not-for-profit) and traditional medicine provide health services in Botswana. The referral system (structure) includes mobile stops, health posts, clinics, primary hospitals, district hospitals, and referral hospitals as national health laboratories. The overarching government body is the Ministry of Health and a department of public health.[31]

There are three referral hospitals: Nyangabgwe Hospital in Francistown, Princess Marina in Gaborone, and Lobatse Mental Hospital.

NAMIBIA

■ Demography[3]

Population: 2,108,665

Religions: Christian (80–90%; Lutheran 50% at least), indigenous beliefs (10–20%)

Languages: English (7%; official), Afrikaans (common language of most of the population and about 60% of the White population), German (32%), indigenous languages (1%; includes Oshivambo, Herero, and Nama)

Ethnic Makeup: Black (87.5%), White (6%), mixed (6.5%)

Formerly Colonized: South African/German

Politics/Governance: Republic

HIV Prevalence: Adult—15.3% (2007)[4]

TB: Ranks 70th among countries of highest TB burden with 2124 deaths annually. Prevalence: 532/100,000 (2007). DOTS coverage: 100%. DOTS rx success: 76%[5]

Malaria: 34,761 cases (2006 estimate)[6]

Percent of Population Vaccinated: 69–95% depending on the vaccine (2007)[7]

Infant Mortality Rate: 45.51 deaths/1000 live births (2009)[3]

Under-5 Mortality: 68/1000 (2007 estimate)[8]

Leading Causes of Death: HIV/AIDS (51%), perinatal conditions (4%), cerebrovascular disease (4%), ischemic heart disease (4%), and TB (4%) (2002)[9]

Unusual Pathogens: polio, plague (1999)[10]

Unique Environmental Exposures: prolonged periods of drought; limited natural fresh water resources; desertification; wildlife poaching; land degradation has led to few conservation areas[3]

■ Traditional Medicine
Before independence, health services were fragmented and traditional medicine was outlawed. After Namibia's independence in 1990, traditional medicine was legalized. Those who practice traditional medicine are classified as herbalists, faith-herbalists, diviner-herbalists, diviners, faith healers, and traditional birth attendants. The Namibia Eagle Traditional Healers Association was created in 1990.[13]

■ Healthcare System
The government, private practitioners (for-profit as well as not-for-profit), and traditional medicine, provide health services in Namibia. Limited private practice for full-time medical specialists may be allowed under strict control. The referral system (structure) starts from the rural health posts to clinics to health centers and, finally, to hospitals. Secondary and tertiary healthcare levels of services are also used for training health and social workers.[32] The overarching government body is the Ministry of Health and Social Services.

The key healthcare institutions are the Katutura State Hospital and the Windhoek Central Hospital.[33]

ANGOLA
■ Demography[3]
Population: 12,799,293 (July, 2009 estimate)

Religions: Indigenous beliefs (47%), Roman Catholic (38%), Protestant (15%) (1998 estimate)

Languages: Portuguese (official), Bantu, and other African languages

Ethnic Makeup: Ovimbundu (37%), Kimbundu (25%), Bakongo (13%), mestico (mixed European and Native African; 2%), European (1%), other (22%)

Formerly Colonized: Portuguese

Politics/Governance: Republic; multiparty presidential regime

HIV Prevalence: Adult—2.1% (2007)[4]

TB: Ranks 43rd among countries of highest TB burden with 5684 deaths annually. Prevalence: 294/100,000 (2007). DOTS coverage: 63%. DOTS rx success: 18%[5]

Malaria: 3,554,908 cases (2006 estimate)[6]

Percent of Population Vaccinated: 81–99% depending on the vaccine (2007)[7]

Infant Mortality Rate: 180.21 deaths/1000 live births (2009)[3]

Under-5 Mortality: 158/1000 (2007 estimate)[8]

Leading Causes of Death: Diarrheal diseases (16%), lower respiratory infections (15%), HIV/AIDS (7%), perinatal conditions (4%), and malaria (6%) (2002)[9]

Unusual Pathogens: Polio, Marburg haemorrhagic fever, meningococcal disease, cholera[10]

Unique Environmental Exposures: Overuse of pastures and subsequent soil erosion attributable to population pressures; desertification; deforestation of tropical rain forest—in response to both international demand for tropical timber and to domestic use as fuel—resulting in loss of biodiversity; soil erosion contributing to water pollution and siltation of rivers and dams; inadequate supplies of potable water[3]

■ **Traditional Medicine**
Though the practice exists, there is no official governance of practitioners[13]

■ **Healthcare System**
Prior to independence, only urban inhabitants, many of whom were Portuguese, had access to health facilities. In 2001, the health system was decentralized. Facilities are run by public and private institutions. The referral system includes health posts, health centers, municipal hospitals, and provincial hospitals.[34] The overarching government body is the Ministry of Health.

The key healthcare institutions are the Cameron Hospital and Land Lakes family health service.

MADAGASCAR
■ **Demography**[3]
Population: 20,653,556 (July 2009 estimate)

Religions: Indigenous beliefs (52%), Christian (41%), Muslim (7%)

Languages: English (official), French (official), Malagasy (official)

Ethnic Makeup: Malayo-Indonesian (Merina and related Betsileo), Cotiers (mixed African, Malayo-Indonesian, and Arab ancestry; Betsimisaraka, Tsimihety, Antaisaka, Sakalava), French, Indian, Creole, Comoran

Formerly Colonized: French

Politics/Governance: Republic

HIV Prevalence: Adult—0.1% (2007)[4]

TB: Ranks 30th among countries of highest TB burden with 9371 deaths annually. Prevalence: 417/100,000 (2007). DOTS coverage: 100%. DOTS rx success: 78%[5]

Malaria: 642,957 cases (2006 estimate)[6]

Percent of Population Vaccinated: 72–94% depending on the vaccine (2007)[7]

Infant Mortality Rate: 54.2 deaths/1000 live births (2009)[3]

Under-5 Mortality: 112/1000 (2007 estimate)[8]

Leading Causes of Death: Lower respiratory infections (14%), malaria (11%), diarrheal diseases (9%), perinatal conditions (7%), measles (5%), cerebrovascular diseases (5%), ischemic heart disease (4%), and TB (4%) (2002)[9]

Unusual Pathogens: Rift Valley Fever, influenza, rabies, acute respiratory syndrome, cholera[10]

Unique Environmental Exposures: Periodic cyclones, drought, and locust infestation; soil erosion results from deforestation and overgrazing; desertification; surface water contaminated with raw sewage and other organic wastes[3]

■ Traditional Medicine

More than 10,000 practitioners are involved in Madagascar's primary healthcare program and regulations for herbal medicines were instituted in 2000.[13]

■ Healthcare System

The government, religious organizations, private practitioners (for-profit as well as not-for-profit), and traditional medicine, provide health services. Each province has a central hospital and local clinics, dispensaries, and maternity-care centers that are supplemented by mobile health units. The overarching government body is the Ministry of Health.[35]

There are 8 hospitals and 14 clinics supported by Malagasy Lutheran Church. Key healthcare institutions include Hopitaly Loterana Antanimalandy in Mahajanga, Hopital Principal de Toamasina, Befeletanana General Hospital in Antananarivo, Centre Hospitalier Regional in Toliara, and Hopitaly Loterana Manambara in Tolanaro. Another commendable hospital is the Fort Dauphin hospital.

ETHIOPIA

■ Demography[3]

Population: 85,237,338 (2009 estimate)

Religions: Christian (60.8%; Orthodox 50.6%, Protestant 10.2%), Muslim (32.8%), traditional (4.6%), other (1.8%) (1994 census)

Languages: Amarigna (32.7%), Oromigna (31.6%), Tigrigna (6.1%), Somaligna (6%), Guaragigna (3.5%), Sidamigna (3.5%), Hadiyigna (1.7%), other (14.8%), English (major foreign language taught in schools) (1994 census)

Ethnic Makeup: Oromo (32.1%), Amara (30.1%), Tigraway (6.2%), Somalie (5.9%), Guragie (4.3%), Sidama (3.5%), Welaita (2.4%), other (15.4%) (1994 census)

Formerly Colonized: Oldest independent country in Africa and one of the oldest in the world (at least 2000 years)

Politics/Governance: Federal Republic

HIV Prevalence: Adult—2.1% (2007)[4]

TB: Ranks 6th among countries of highest TB burden with 76,421 deaths annually. Prevalence: 579/100,000 (2007). DOTS coverage: 95%. DOTS rx success: 84%[5]

Malaria: 12,405,124 cases (2006 estimate)[6]

Percent of Population Vaccinated: 65–85% depending on the vaccine (2007)[7]

Infant Mortality Rate: 80.8 deaths/1000 live births (2009)[3]

Under-5 Mortality: 119/1000 (2007 estimate)[8]

Leading Causes of Death: HIV/AIDS (12%), lower respiratory infections (12%), perinatal conditions (8%), diarrheal diseases (6%), measles (4%), and TB (4%) (2002)[9]

Unusual Pathogens: Diarrheal diseases, polio, meningococcal disease[10]

Unique Environmental Exposures: geologically active Great Rift Valley susceptible to earthquakes and volcanic eruptions; frequent droughts; deforestation; overgrazing; soil erosion; desertification; water shortages in some areas from water-intensive farming and poor management[3]

■ Traditional Medicine

Traditional medicine includes spiritual healing, traditional midwifery, hydrotherapy, massage, cupping, counter-irritation, surgery, and bone-setting.[13] Over 80% of the Ethiopian population relies on traditional medicine.[36]

■ Healthcare System

Healthcare services are provided by the government, religions organizations, private practitioners (for-profit as well as not-for profit), and traditional healers. Western medicine came to Ethiopia during the last quarter of the 19th century with the arrival of missionary doctors, nurses, and midwives. The referral system (structure) includes hospitals, health centers, and outpatient clinics. The Health Extension Program (HEP) is a community-based health-care delivery system aimed at providing essential promotion and preventive healthcare services. It was introduced due to inadequate reach of essential services to communities in remote parts of Ethiopia. The overarching government body is the Federal Ministry of Health.[37]

Key healthcare institutions include Saint Gabriel General Hospital, Tzna General Hospital, Zenbaba General Hospital, and Awassa Referral Hospital.

SOMALIA

■ Demography[3]

Population: 9,832,017 (2009 estimate)

Religions: Sunni Muslim

Languages: Somali (official), Arabic, Italian, English

Ethnic Makeup: Somali (85%), Bantu and other non-Somali (15%; including Arabs 30,000)

Formerly Colonized: British and Italian Somaliland

Politics/Governance: No permanent national government; transitional, parliamentary federal government

HIV Prevalence: Adult—0.5% (2007)[4]

TB: Ranks 44th among countries of highest TB burden: 5,483 deaths annually. Prevalence: 352/100,000 (2007). DOTS coverage: 100%. DOTS rx success: 89%[5]

Malaria: 608,831 cases (2006 estimate)[6]

Percent of Population Vaccinated: 34–68% depending on the vaccine (2007)[7]

Infant Mortality Rate: 109.19 deaths/1000 live births (2009)[3]

Under-5 Mortality: 142/1000 (2007 estimate)[8]

Leading Causes of Death: Lower respiratory infections (11%), perinatal conditions (11%), diarrheal diseases (9%), measles (7%), and TB (6%) (2002)[9]

Unusual Pathogens: Polio, Rift Valley Fever, meningococcal disease, cholera[10]

Unique Environmental Exposures: Recurring droughts; frequent dust storms over the eastern plains in summer; floods during rainy season; famine; use of contaminated water contributes to human health problems; deforestation; overgrazing; soil erosion; desertification; conflict[3]

■ Traditional Medicine

Herbal medicine is among the more popular method of traditional healing in Somalia. Bone setting as well as religious traditions and dances are often exercised as a source of energy for treatment.[38]

■ Healthcare System

The village level usually has one primary healthcare post, staffed by one locally recruited community health worker and one traditional birth attendant. Primary healthcare units serve from 10,000 to 15,000 persons and are staffed by one public health nurse, one nurse midwife, and one sanitarian. The district health center, is responsible for four primary health care units. The regional health center is, in effect, the district health center of the regional capital. Governmental health curative services are offered at district and regional hospitals. Recurrent conflict has rendered the health system ineffective.[39] The overarching government body is the Ministry of Health.

As a result of the 1990–1991 conflict in Somalia, several of the urban hospitals lost function and virtually none of the rural ones are operational. In addition to hospitals, there were 411 primary healthcare posts, 50 primary healthcare units, and 94 maternal and child health centers reported at the end of 1990. East Bardera Mothers and Children's Hospital, Edna Adan Maternity Hospital, and Hargeisa Canadian Medical Center are among the key healthcare institutions.

SUDAN

■ Demography[3]

Population: 41,087,825 (July 2009 estimate)

Religions: Sunni Muslim (70% in north), Christian (5% mostly in south and Khartoum), indigenous beliefs (25%)

Languages: Arabic (official), English (official), Nubian, Ta Bedawie, diverse dialects of Nilotic, Nilo-Hamitic, Sudanic languages. *Note:* program of "Arabization" in process

Ethnic Makeup: Black (52%), Arab (39%), Beja (6%), foreigners (2%), other (1%)

Formerly Colonized: British and Egyptian

Politics/Governance: Power-sharing government under the 2005 Comprehensive Peace Agreement (CPA); the NCP came to power by military coup in 1989 and is a majority partner; elections expected in 2010.

HIV Prevalence: Adult: 1.4% (2007)[4]

TB: Ranks 14th among countries of highest TB burden with 27,450 deaths annually. Prevalence: 402/100,000 (2007). DOTS coverage: 91%. DOTS rx success: 82%[5]

Malaria: 5,022,809 cases (2006 estimate)[6]

Percent of Population Vaccinated: 72–95% depending on the vaccine (2007)[7]

Infant Mortality Rate: 82.43 deaths/1000 live births (2009)[3]

Under-5 Mortality: 109/1000 (2007 estimate)[8]

Leading Causes of Death: Ischemic heart disease (8%), malaria (6%), HIV/AIDS (6%), diarrheal diseases (6%) (2002)[9]

Unusual Pathogens: Polio, Rift Valley Fever, yellow fever, shigellosis, ebola, hepatitis E, meningococcal disease, cholera[10]

Unique Environmental Exposures: Dust storms; inadequate supplies of potable water; wildlife populations threatened by excessive hunting; soil erosion; desertification; periodic drought[3]

■ Traditional Medicine
Traditional medicine is rooted in Islamic and West African practices. People travel to herbalists in rural regions for complicated cases[13]

■ Healthcare System
At the village level, primary healthcare units represent the first level of contact between the community and the health services. Secondary health care is available in small towns through rural hospitals and urban health centers. Tertiary healthcare services are comprised of provincial, regional, university, and specialist hospitals.[40] Service provision is through government as well as NGOs. The overarching government body is the Ministry of Health.

The key healthcare institutions are the Khartoum Hospital, Soba Hospital, Al Baraha Hospital, Bahry (Khartoum North) Hospital, and the Academy University Hospital.

DJIBOUTI
■ Demography[3]
Population: 516,055 (July 2009 estimate)

Religions: Muslim (94%), Christian (6%)

Languages: French (official), Arabic (official), Somali, Afar

Ethnic Makeup: Somali (60%), Afar (35%), other (5%; includes French, Arab, Ethiopian, and Italian)

Formerly Colonized: British and Egyptian

Politics/Governance: Power-sharing government under the 2005 Comprehensive Peace Agreement (CPA); the NCP came to power by military coup in 1989 and is majority partner; elections are expected in 2010.

HIV Prevalence: Adult: 3.1% (2007)[4]

TB: Ranks 82nd among countries of highest TB burden with 1304 deaths annually. Prevalence: 1104/100,000 (2007). DOTS coverage: 100%. DOTS rx success: 78%[5]

Malaria: 38,673 cases (2006 estimate)[6]

Percent of Population Vaccinated: 25–92% depending on the vaccine (2007)[7]

Infant Mortality Rate: 97.51 deaths/1000 live births (2009)[3]

Under-5 Mortality: 127/1000 (2007 estimate)[8]

Leading Causes of Death: Lower respiratory infections (12%), diarrheal diseases (10%), ischemic heart disease (9%), HIV/AIDs (8%), perinatal conditions (8%), and TB (6%) (2002)[9]

Unusual Pathogens: Avian influenza[10]

Unique Environmental Exposures: Earthquakes; droughts; occasional cyclonic disturbances from the Indian Ocean bring heavy rains and flash floods[3]

■ Traditional Medicine

Cheiks are medical providers who use the Quran or other Islamic scriptures to treat patients. Herbalists also provide traditional medicine. Only traditional birth attendants have gained official recognition.[13]

■ Healthcare System

Health care is provided by a tiered system. The primary level consists of small units, providing health care to remote or nomadic communities. The secondary level includes district hospitals that provide nonspecialized inpatient or outpatient care and supervise the activities of the rural health units under their jurisdiction. General hospitals make up the tertiary level.[41] Government, NGOs, and communities play a strong role in healthcare provision. The overarching government body is the Ministry of Public Health and Social Affairs. Urban and rural facilities manage their own budgets. The key healthcare institution is the Hôpital Générale Peltier.

ERITREA

■ Demography[3]

Population: 5,647,168 (July 2009 estimate)

Religions: Muslim, Coptic Christian, Roman Catholic, Protestant

Languages: Afar, Arabic, Tigre and Kunama, Tigrinya, other Cushitic languages

Ethnic Makeup: Tigrinya (50%), Tigre and Kunama (40%), Afar (4%), Saho (Red Sea coast dwellers; 3%), other (3%)

Formerly Colonized: Ethiopian

Politics/Governance: Transitional government

HIV Prevalence: Adult—1.3% (2007)[4]

TB: Ranks 92nd among countries of highest TB burden with 793 deaths annually. Prevalence: 134/100,000 (2007). DOTS coverage: 93%. DOTS rx success: 90%[5]

Malaria: 18,964 cases (2006 estimate)[6]

Percent of Population Vaccinated: 80–99% depending on the vaccine (2007)[7]

Infant Mortality Rate: 43.3 deaths/1000 live births (2009)[3]

Under-5 Mortality: 70/1000 (2007 estimate)[8]

Leading Causes of Death: HIV/AIDS (16%), lower respiratory infections (16%), malaria (6%), diarrheal diseases (6%), perinatal conditions (6%), and TB (5%) (2002)[9]

Unusual Pathogens: None[10]

Unique Environmental Exposures: Frequent droughts; locust swarms; deforestation; desertification; soil erosion; overgrazing; loss of infrastructure from civil warfare[3]

■ Traditional Medicine

Perceived inadequate modern health care leads many Eritreans to frequent traditional healers who prefer an exchange of goods rather than cash payments.[42]

■ Healthcare System

The healthcare system is predominantly public. Few private clinics serve the minority. Catholic missions own about 10% of the facilities. Based on the principle of primary health care. The tiered system includes health stations, health centers (community hospitals), sub-Zoba hospitals (district), Zoba referral hospitals (regional), and National Referral Hospitals. Medical care is improving rapidly in Eritrea with new hospitals and health centers opening every year. The first medical college opened in 2003 to fill the critical health worker gap. Modern facilities may not always be available outside Asmara.[43] The overarching government body is the Ministry of Health.

The key healthcare institutions include the Orota Referral Hospital, Sembel Hospital, Hospitem-Ospedale Italiano Ente Morale, and Edaga Hamus Hospital and Health Center.

GABON

■ Demography[3]

Population: 1,514,993 (2009 estimate)

Religions: Christian (55–75%), animist, Muslim (less than 1%)

Languages: French (official), Fang, Myene, Nzebi, Bapounou/Eschira, Bandjabi

Ethnic Makeup: Bantu tribes, including four major tribal groupings: Fang, Bapounou, Nzebi, Obamba; other Africans and Europeans (154,000, including 10,700 French and 11,000 persons of dual nationality)

Formerly Colonized: French

Politics/Governance: Republic; multiparty presidential regime

HIV Prevalence: Adult: 5.9% (2007)[4]

TB: Ranks 85th among countries of highest TB burden with 1011 deaths annually. Prevalence: 379/100,000 (2007). DOTS coverage: 31%. DOTS rx success: 46%[5]

Malaria: 386,506 cases (2006 estimate)[6]

Percent of Population Vaccinated: 31–89% depending on the vaccine (2007)[7]

Infant Mortality Rate: 51.78 deaths/1000 live births (2009)[3]

Under-5 Mortality: 91/1000 (2007 estimate)[8]

Leading Causes of Death: HIV/AIDS (19%), malaria (8%), ischemic heart disease (7%), cerebrovascular disease (6%), lower respiratory infections (5%), measles (5%), and perinatal conditions (4%) (2002)[9]

Unusual Pathogens: Ebola hemorrhagic fever[10]

Unique Environmental Exposures: Deforestation[3]

■ Traditional Medicine

Traditional medicine is included in the primary healthcare system. There is no oversight or governance mechanism.[13]

■ Healthcare System

Gabon has a public healthcare system with few private institutions. The overarching government body is the Ministry of Health.

Gabon has 27 hospitals and 660 medical centers. The Albert Schweitzer Hospital in Lambarene and the Libreville General Hospital in the capital are the key healthcare institutions.

GAMBIA

■ Demography[3]

Population: 1,782,893 (2009 estimate)

Religions: Muslim (90%), Christian (8%), indigenous beliefs (2%)

Languages: English (official), Mandinka, Wolof, Fula, other indigenous vernaculars

Ethnic Makeup: African (99%: Mandinka 42%, Fula 18%, Wolof 16%, Jola 10%, Serahuli 9%, other 4%), non-African (1%) (2003 census)

Formerly Colonized: British

Politics/Governance: Republic

HIV Prevalence: Adult: 0.9% (2007)[4]

TB: Ranks 87th among countries of highest TB burden with 936 deaths annually. Prevalence: 404/100,000 (2007). DOTS coverage: 100%. DOTS rx success: 58%[5]

Malaria: 469,382 cases (2006 estimate)[6]

Percent of Population Vaccinated: 85–95% depending on the vaccine (2007)[7]

Infant Mortality Rate: 67.33 deaths/1000 live births (2009)[3]

Under-5 Mortality: 109/1000 (2007 estimate)[8]

Leading Causes of Death: Lower respiratory infections (13%), malaria (8%), perinatal conditions (7%), diarrheal diseases (6%), ischemic heart disease (5%), and cerebrovascular disease (5%) (2002)[9]

Unusual Pathogens: Meningococcal disease[10]

Unique Environmental Exposures: Drought; deforestation; desertification; water-borne diseases prevalent[3]

■ **Traditional Medicine**

Legislation and licensing exists for practitioners of traditional medicine in Gambia.[13]

■ **Healthcare System**

The public health service delivery system is three tiers based on the primary healthcare strategy (primary, secondary, and tertiary). It is complemented by numerous private and NGO clinics.[44] The overarching government body is the Department of State for Health.

There are 4 government-run referral hospitals, 8 major health centers, 16 minor health centers, 1 research health center, several NGO and private clinics, and over 200 mobile/trekking clinics.[45] The Royal Victoria Hospital, Bansang Hospital, Sulayman Junkung General Hospital, and AFPRC Farafenni Hospital are among the key healthcare institutions.

CENTRAL AFRICAN REPUBLIC

■ **Demography[3]**

Population: 4,511,488 (July 2009 estimate)

Religions: Indigenous beliefs (35%), Protestant (25%), Roman Catholic (25%), Muslim (15%). *Note:* animistic beliefs and practices strongly influence the Christian majority.

Languages: French (official), Sangho (lingua franca and national language), tribal languages

Ethnic Makeup: Baya (33%), Banda (27%), Mandjia (13%), Sara (10%), Mboum (7%), M'Baka (4%), Yakoma (4%), other (2%)

Formerly Colonized: British

Politics/Governance: Republic

HIV Prevalence: Adult: 6.3% (2007)[4]

TB: Ranks 51st among countries of highest TB burden with 4330 deaths annually. Prevalence: 425/100,000 (2007). DOTS coverage: n/a. DOTS rx success: n/a[5]

Malaria: 1,574,295 cases (2006 estimate)[6]

Percent of Population Vaccinated: 47–65% depending on the vaccine (2007)[7]

Infant Mortality Rate: 80.62 deaths/1000 live births (2009)[3]

Under-5 Mortality: 172/1000 (2007 estimate)[8]

Leading Causes of Death: HIV/AIDS (32%), lower respiratory infections (9%), malaria (8%), diarrheal diseases (6%), measles (5%), perinatal conditions (4%), and cerebrovascular disease (4%) (2002)[9]

Unusual Pathogens: Shigellosis, yellow fever, meningococcal disease[10]

Unique Environmental Exposures: Dusty harmattan winds affect northern areas; floods are common; deforestation; poaching

■ **Traditional Medicine**

There are local intersectoral councils for traditional medicine and a registry of traditional health practitioners but no legislation.[13]

■ **Healthcare System**

Public and private practitioners (for-profit as well as not-for-profit) provide health services in CAR. The overarching government body is the Ministry of Health.

The key healthcare institutions are the Vakaga Prefectural Hospital and the Kaga-Bandoro District Hospital.

EQUATORIAL GUINEA

■ **Demography[3]**

Population: 633,441 (July 2009 estimate)

Religions: Nominally Christian and predominantly Roman Catholic, pagan practices

Languages: Spanish 67.6% (official), other 32.4% (includes French, which is official, Fang, and Bubi) (1994 census)

Ethnic Makeup: Fang (85.7%), Bubi (6.5%), Mdowe (3.6%), Annobon (1.6%), Bujeba (1.1%), other (1.4%) (1994 census)

Formerly Colonized: Spanish

Politics/Governance: Republic

HIV Prevalence: Adult: 3.4% (2007)[4]

TB: Ranks 105th among countries of highest TB burden with 442 deaths annually. Prevalence: 469/100,000 (2007). DOTS coverage: n/a. DOTS rx success: n/a[5]

Malaria: 193,341 cases (2006 estimate)[6]

Percent of Population Vaccinated: 33–73% depending on the vaccine (2007)[7]

Infant Mortality Rate: 81.58 deaths/1000 live births (2009)[3]

Under-5 Mortality: 150/1000 (2007 estimate)[8]

Leading Causes of Death: HIV/AIDS (17%), malaria (11%), diarrheal diseases (6%), lower respiratory infections (6%), perinatal conditions (5%), and measles (5%) (2002)[9]

Unusual Pathogens: None[10]

Unique Environmental Exposures: Deforestation, violent windstorms; flash floods[3]

■ **Traditional Medicine**

Legislation and licensing exists but traditional medicine practitioners are not involved in Equatorial Guinea's primary healthcare program.[13]

■ **Healthcare System**

The government, religious organizations, and private practitioners (for-profit as well as not-for-profit) offer four levels of health care: health posts in each village of 600 people, dispensaries in health centers with a qualified nurse at the intermediate level, district level hospitals, and two referral hospitals at the most centralized level. The overarching government body is the Ministry of Health and Social Well-being.[46]

The key healthcare institution is the Bata Hospital.

SWAZILAND

■ Demography[3]

Population: 1,123,913 (July 2009 estimate)

Religions: Zionist (a blend of Christianity and indigenous ancestral worship; 40%), Roman Catholic (20%), Muslim (10%), other (includes Anglican, Bahai, Methodist, Mormon, Jewish; 30%)

Language: English (official, government business conducted in English), siSwati (official)

Ethnic Makeup: African (97%), European (3%)

Formerly Colonized: British

Politics/Governance: Monarchy

HIV Prevalence: Adult—26.1% (2007)[4]

TB: Ranks 55th among countries of highest TB burden with 3619 deaths annually. Prevalence: 812/100,000 (2007). DOTS coverage: 100%. DOTS rx success: 43%[5]

Malaria: 198 cases (2006 estimate)[6]

Percent of Population Vaccinated: 86–99% depending on the vaccine (2007)[7]

Infant Mortality Rate: 68.63 deaths/1000 live births (2009)[3]

Under-5 mortality: 91/1000 (2007 estimate)[8]

Leading Causes of Death: HIV/AIDS (64%), lower respiratory infections (5%), and TB (4%) (2002)[9]

Unusual Pathogens: None[10]

Unique Environmental Exposures: Drought; limited supplies of potable water; wildlife populations being depleted because of excessive hunting; overgrazing; soil degradation; soil erosion[3]

■ Traditional Medicine
There are no official training facilities or programs offered in traditional medicine[13]

■ Healthcare System
The healthcare system consists of public, private not-for-profit, private for-profit, and industry-owned facilities. The majority of the private not-for-profit facilities are owned by missions but receive most of their subsidies from the Swazi government. Community-based care is prevalent. The overarching government body is the Ministry of Health and Social Welfare.

There are 7 hospitals, 12 health centers, 162 clinics, 8 public health units, and 187 outreach sites.[47] Mankayane, Mbabane General, Piggs Peak, Raleigh Fitkin, Good Shepherd, Hlatikulu, and National Psychiatric are the key health-care institutions.

CAMEROON

■ Demography[3]

Population: 18,879,301 (2009 estimate)

Religions: Indigenous beliefs (40%), Christian (40%), Muslim (20%)

Languages: 24 major African language groups, English (official), French (official)

Ethnic Makeup: Cameroon Highlanders (31%), Equatorial Bantu (19%), Kirdi (11%), Fulani (10%), Northwestern Bantu (8%), Eastern Nigritic (7%), other African (13%), non-African (less than 1%)

Formerly Colonized: French administered UN trusteeship

Politics/Governance: Republic; multiparty presidential regime

HIV Prevalence: Adult: 5.1% (2007)[4]

TB: Ranks 37th among countries of highest TB burden with 7159 deaths annually. Prevalence: 195/100,000 (2007). DOTS coverage: 100%. DOTS rx success: 74%[5]

Malaria: 5,091,300 cases (2006 estimate)[6]

Percent of Population Vaccinated: 74–90% depending on the vaccine (2007)[7]

Infant Mortality Rate: 63.34 deaths/1000 live births (2009)[3]

Under-5 mortality: 148/1000 (2007 estimate)[8]

Leading Causes of Death: HIV/AIDS (21%), lower respiratory infections (14%), malaria (8%), diarrheal diseases (6%), perinatal conditions (5%), cerebro-vascular disease (4%), ischemic heart disease (4%)[9]

Unusual Pathogens: Cholera, meningococcal disease[10]

Unique Environmental Exposures: Waterborne diseases are prevalent; defor-estation; overgrazing; desertification; poaching; overfishing[3]

■ Traditional Medicine

Traditional medicine is governed in part by the Office of Traditional Medicine in the Ministry of Public Health.[13]

■ Healthcare System

Health facilities in Cameroon consist of government services or private ser-vices managed by the various churches and other private individuals. It is a decentralized system. The overarching government body is the Ministry of Public Health.

The key healthcare institutions are the Limbe Provincial Hospital, Bamenda Regional Hospital, Hôpital Général de Yaoundé, Hôpital Général de Dla, Hôpital Laquintinie, Hôpital Central de Yaoundé, Hopital Gyneco-Obstetrique de Yaoundé, Hopital Jamot de Yaoundé (HJY), and the Centre Hospitalier et Universitaire de Yaoundé.[48]

NIGERIA

■ Demography[3]

Population: 149,229,090 (2009 estimate)

Religions: Muslim (50%), Christian (40%), indigenous beliefs (10%)

Languages: English (official), Hausa, Yoruba, Igbo (Ibo), Fulani

Ethnic Makeup: Nigeria, Africa's most populous country, is composed of more than 250 ethnic groups; the following are the most populous and politically influential: Hausa and Fulani (29%), Yoruba (21%), Igbo (Ibo; 18%), Ijaw (10%), Kanuri (4%), Ibibio (3.5%), Tiv (2.5%)

Formerly Colonized: British

Politics/Governance: Federal Republic

HIV Prevalence: Adult: 3.1% (2007)[4]

TB: Ranks 3rd among countries of highest TB burden with 137,845 deaths annually. Prevalence: 521/100,000 (2007). DOTS coverage: 91%. DOTS rx success: 76%[5]

Malaria: 57,506,430 cases (2006 estimate)[6]

Percent of Population Vaccinated: 41–72% depending on the vaccine (2007)[7]

Infant Mortality Rate: 94.35 deaths/1000 live births (2009)[3]

Under-5 mortality: 189/1000 (2007 estimate)[8]

Leading Causes of Death: HIV/AIDS (16%), lower respiratory infections (11%), malaria (11%), diarrheal diseases (7%), measles (6%), perinatal conditions (5%), and TB (4%) (2002)[9]

Unusual Pathogens: Polio, avian influenza, meningococcal disease, cholera[10]

Unique Environmental Exposures: Soil degradation; rapid deforestation; urban air and water pollution; desertification; oil pollution—water, air, and soil; serious damage from oil spills; loss of arable land; rapid urbanization[3]

■ Traditional Medicine
Traditional medicine is accessed by the majority of Nigerians. The Traditional Medicine Council of Nigeria Act facilitates the practice and development of traditional medicine; establishing model traditional medicine clinics, herbal farms, botanical gardens etc.[13]

■ Healthcare System
The federal government coordinates the university teaching hospitals, while the state government manages the various general hospitals. The local

governments focus on dispensaries. The overarching government body is the Ministry of Health.

The key healthcare institutions are National Hospital-Abuja, Asokoro General Hospital, University of Abuja Teaching Hospital, Badagari General Hospital, and Lagos General Hospital.

NIGER

■ Demography[3]

Population: 15,306,252 (July 2009 estimate)

Religions: Muslim (80%), other (includes indigenous beliefs and Christian; 20%)

Languages: French (official), Hausa, Djerma

Ethnic Makeup: Haoussa (55.4%), Djerma Sonrai (21%), Tuareg (9.3%), Peuhl (8.5%), Kanouri Manga (4.7%), other (1.2%) (2001 census)

Formerly Colonized: French

Politics/Governance: Republic

HIV Prevalence: Adult—0.8% (2007)[4]

TB: Ranks 45th among countries of highest TB burden with 5443 deaths annually. Prevalence: 292/100,000 (2007). DOTS coverage: 100%. DOTS rx success: 77%[5]

Malaria: 5,759,935 cases (2006 estimate)[6]

Percent of Population Vaccinated: 47–72% depending on the vaccine (2007)[7]

Infant Mortality Rate: 116.66 deaths/1000 live births (2009)[3]

Under-5 Mortality: 176/1000 (2007 estimate)[8]

Leading Causes of Death: Lower respiratory infections (14%), perinatal conditions (11%), diarrheal diseases (10%), malaria (10%), and measles (6%) (2002)[9]

Unusual Pathogens: Avian influenza, meningococcal disease, cholera[10]

Unique Environmental Exposures: Droughts; overgrazing; soil erosion; deforestation; desertification; wildlife populations threatened because of poaching and habitat destruction[3]

■ Traditional Medicine

Legislation and licensing exists for the practitioners of traditional medicine.[13]

■ Healthcare System

The government, religious organizations, private practitioners (for-profit as well as not-for-profit), and traditional medicine provide health services in Niger. The overarching government body is the Ministry of Health.

The key healthcare institutions are the Hôpital National de Niamey and the Hôpital National De Lamordé, Dosso Regional Hospital, and Mayahi District Hospital.

CONGO

■ Demography[3]

Population: 4,012,809 (July 2009 estimate)

Religions: Christian (50%), animist (48%), Muslim (2%)

Languages: French (official), Lingala and Monokutuba (lingua franca trade languages), many local languages and dialects (of which Kikongo is the most widespread)

Ethnic Makeup: Kongo (48%), Sangha (20%), M'Bochi (12%), Teke (17%), Europeans and other (3%)

Formerly Colonized: British

Politics/Governance: Republic

HIV Prevalence: Adult—3.5% (2007)[4]

TB: Ranks 57th among countries of highest TB burden with 3405 deaths annually. Prevalence: 485/100,000 (2007). DOTS coverage: 60%. DOTS rx success: 53%[5]

Malaria: 1,331,668 cases (2006 estimate)[6]

Percent of Population Vaccinated: 67–90% depending on the vaccine (2007)[7]

Infant Mortality Rate: 79.78 deaths/1000 live births (2009)[3]

Under-5 Mortality: 125/1000 (2007 estimate)[8]

Leading Causes of Death: HIV/AIDS (25%), malaria (12%), measles (7%), perinatal conditions (5%), and TB (4%) (2002)[9]

Unusual Pathogens: Yellow fever, ebola[10]

Unique Environmental Exposures: Seasonal flooding; air pollution from vehicle emissions; water pollution from the dumping of raw sewage; tap water is not potable; deforestation[3]

■ Traditional Medicine

Herbalists and spiritualists are common in rural areas. Acupuncturists and natural medicine providers are more common in urban centers. Congolese traditional medical products include manadiar, antougine, meyamium, and diazostimul. Legislation and licensing exists.[13]

■ Healthcare System

The overarching government body is the Ministry of Health and Population. The University Hospital of Brazzaville is the key healthcare institution.

CHAD

■ Demography[3]

Population: 10,329,208 (July 2009 estimate)

Religions: Mainland—Muslim (53.1%), Catholic (20.1%), Protestant (14.2%), animist (7.3%), other (0.5%), unknown (1.7%), atheist (3.1%) (1993 census)

Languages: French (official), Arabic (official), Sara (in south), more than 120 different languages and dialects

Ethnic Makeup: Sara (27.7%), Arab (12.3%), Mayo-Kebbi (11.5%), Kanem-Bornou (9%), Ouaddai (8.7%), Hadjarai (6.7%), Tandjile (6.5%), Gorane (6.3%), Fitri-Batha (4.7%), other (6.4%), unknown (0.3%) (1993 census)

Formerly Colonized: French

Politics/Governance: Republic

HIV Prevalence: Adult—3.5% (2007)[4]

TB: Ranks 29th among countries of highest TB burden with 9690 deaths annually. Prevalence: 497/100,000 (2007). DOTS coverage: 33%. DOTS rx success: 54%[5]

Malaria: 4,178,935 cases (2006 estimate)[6]

Percent of Population Vaccinated: 23–60% depending on the vaccine (2007)[7]

Infant Mortality Rate: 98.69 deaths/1000 live births (2009)[3]

Under-5 Mortality: 209/1000 (2007 estimate)[8]

Leading Causes of Death: Lower respiratory infections (14%), HIV/AIDS (12%), malaria (11%), diarrheal diseases (8%), perinatal conditions (6%), measles (5%) (2002)[9]

Unusual Pathogens: Hepatitis E, meningococcal disease[10]

Unique Environmental Exposures: Dusty harmattan winds occur in north; periodic droughts; locust plagues; inadequate supplies of potable water; improper waste disposal in rural areas contributes to soil and water pollution; desertification[3]

■ **Traditional Medicine**
No legislation or licensing exists in Chad, but practitioners are part of the primary healthcare program.[13]

■ **Healthcare System**
The overarching government body is the Ministry of Health and the key health-care institution is the Abeche Regional Hospital.

BENIN
■ **Demography**[3]
Population: 8,760,000

Religions: Christian (43%), Muslim (24%), Vodun (17%), other (6%)

Languages: Beninese (e.g., Yoruba, Yon), French (official)

Ethnic Makeup: Fon (39.2%), Adja (15.2%), Yoruba (12.3%), Bariba (9.2%), Peulh (7%), Ottamari (6.1%), Yoa-Lokpa (4%), Dendi and other (4.1%)

Formerly Colonized: France

Politics/Governance: Multiparty democracy

HIV Prevalence: Adult—1.9%

TB: 1,600 deaths annually. Prevalence: 135/100,000 (2007). DOTS coverage: 100%; DOTS rx success: 87%[5]

Malaria: 3,238,973 cases (2006 estimate)[6]

Percent of Population Vaccinated: 83–89% vaccinated with DPT, measles, and HBV

Infant Mortality Rate: 64.64 deaths/1000 live births (2009)[3]

Under-5 mortality: 148/1000 live births[8]

Leading Causes of Death: Lower respiratory infections (17%), malaria (14%), diarrheal diseases (8%), and HIV/AIDS (7%) (2006)[9]

Unusual Pathogens: Yellow fever, typhoid fever, meningococcal meningitis, rabies.

Unique Environmental Exposures: potable water supplies are insufficient, poaching, deforestation, and desertification.

■ **Traditional Medicine**
Eighty percent of the country relies on traditional Beninese "voodoo" medicine. The government registers and licenses practitioners.

■ **Healthcare System**
The healthcare system is decentralized, and comprised of public and private elements. Rural penetration is low. The Bamako Initiative in the 1990s resulted in improved access to necessary medications and collaboration between government, communities, and donors.[49] The overarching government body is the Ministry of Health.

BURKINA FASO
■ **Demography**
Population: 14,359,000

Religions: Muslim (~60%), local religions (~24%), Catholic (17%)

Languages: French (official), Mòoré, Dioula, other native African languages spoken by 90% of the population

Ethnic Makeup: Mossa (over 40%), Gurunsi, Mande, Lobi, Bobo, Senufo, and Fulani compose other 60%

Formerly Colonized: France

Politics/Governance: Parliamentary republic

HIV Prevalence: Adult—1.6%

TB: 10,000 deaths annually. Prevalence: 403/100,000 (2007). DOTS coverage: 100%; DOTS rx success: 73%[5]

Malaria: 6,226,667 cases (2006 estimate)[6]

Percent of Population Vaccinated: 78% with measles, 88% with DPT

Infant Mortality Rate: 84.49 deaths/1000 live births (2009)[3]

Under-5 mortality: 204/1000 live births [8]

Leading Causes of Death: Lower respiratory infections (20%), HIV/AIDS (13%), malaria (10%), and diarrheal diseases (9%) (2006)[9]

Unusual Pathogens: Yellow fever, meningococcal meningitis, schistosomiasis, rabies, H5N1 (avian) influenza, onchocerciasis (river blindness)

Unique Environmental Exposures: Agricultural activity affected by drought and desertification; overgrazing has caused soil degradation; deforestation.

■ **Traditional Medicine**
More than eighty percent of the population uses traditional medicine. Female genital mutilation is commonly practiced in Burkina Faso. The Ministry of Health recognizes and regulates traditional medicines and its practitioners.

■ **Healthcare System**
The healthcare system is a decentralized public system with some private care, mostly in the capital Ouagadougou. Rural penetration is limited.

The key healthcare institution is the Hospital Ouagadougou, where tertiary and specialty care is available. The overarching government body is the Ministry of Health.

COTE D'IVOIRE
■ **Demography**
Population: 18,914,000

Religions: Islam (39%), Christian (33%), local beliefs (12%)

Languages: French (official), estimated 65 other languages spoken, Dioula most common

Ethnic Makeup: Akan (42.1%), Gur (17.6%), Northern and Southern Mandes (26.5%), Krous (11%), other, including Lebanese and French (2.8%)

Formerly Colonized: France

Politics/Governance: Multiparty presidential republic (currently operating under a power-sharing agreement)

HIV Prevalence: Adult—3.9%

TB: 25,000 deaths annually. Prevalence: 582/100,000 (2007). DOTS coverage: 100%; DOTS rx success: 73%[5]

Malaria: 7,028,990 cases (2006 estimate)[6]

Percent of Population Vaccinated: 49–50% vaccinated with measles, DPT, and HBV

Infant Mortality Rate: 68.06 deaths/1000 live births (2009)[3]

Under-5 mortality: 127/1000 live births [8]

Leading Causes of Death: HIV/AIDS (19%), malaria (10%), lower respiratory infections (8%), and diarrheal diseases (7%) (2006)[9]

Unusual Pathogens: Typhoid, yellow fever, schistosomiasis, H5N1 (avian) influenza.

Unique Environmental Exposures: Seforestation; water pollution from sewage

■ **Traditional Medicine**
Medicinal plants used in rural areas. No formal recognition or regulation by government.

■ **Healthcare System**
Strong community-based public health system until 2002—civil war has disrupted healthcare delivery in most of the country, especially the north. Private facilities are available mostly in urban centers.
   The key healthcare institutions are the Hopital de Port Bouet and the Polyclinique Internationale Sainte Anne Marie in Abidjan, where tertiary and specialty care are available. The overarching government body is the Ministry of Health.

GHANA
■ **Demography**
Population: 23,008,000

Religions: Christian (69%), Islam (16%), indigenous beliefs (15%)

Languages: English (official), Asante (14.8%), Ewe (12.7%), Fante (9.9%), Boron (4.6%), Dagomba (4.3%), Dangme (4.3%), Dagarte (3.7%), Akyem (3.4%), Ga (3.4%), Akuapem (2.9%), other (36.1%)

Ethnic Makeup: Akan (45.3%), Mole-Dagbon (15.2%), Ewe (11.7%), Ga-Dangme (7.3%), Guan (4%), Gurma (3.6%), Gursi (2.6%), Mande-Busanga (1%), other (9.2%)

Formerly Colonized: United Kingdom

Politics/Governance: Constitutional democracy

HIV Prevalence: Adult—1.9%

TB: 12,000 deaths annually. Prevalence: 353/100,000 (2007). DOTS coverage: 100%; DOTS rx success: 76%[5]

Malaria: 7,282,377 cases (2006 estimate)[6]

Percent of Population Vaccinated: 95–98% vaccinated with BCG, OPV, MMR, DPT, HBV, and Hib

Infant Mortality Rate: 51.09 deaths/1000 live births (2009)[3]

Under-5 mortality: 120/1000 live births[8]

Leading Causes of Death: HIV/AIDS (15%), malaria (11%), lower respiratory infections (8%), and perinatal conditions (8%) (2006)[9]

Unusual Pathogens: Tetanus, yellow fever, guinea worm (dracunculiasi), onchocerciasis, measles

Unique Environmental Exposures: Droughts in the north are common and affect agricultural activities; poaching; water pollution; supplies of potable water are inadequate.

■ Traditional Medicine

Practitioners use herbs and spiritual guidance as tools for healing. ~70% of the population utilizes traditional medicine exclusively. There is one traditional practitioner for every 400 people in Ghana, as opposed to one allopathic doctor for every 12,000. Ghana Federation of Traditional Medicine Practitioners' Associations interfaces with the government, making most medicines readily available. Considered the "backbone" of health care in Ghana.

■ Healthcare System

Public, private, and informal sectors operate. Ghana Health Service operates at national, regional, district, sub-district, and community levels. 40% of care provided by teaching hospitals and private sector. 60% of the population lives within 1 hour of a healthcare service provider. User fees for certain health services are at time prohibitive for the poor to access care.

There are a total of 286 hospitals and 1487 clinics in Ghana. As the total number of healthcare facilities has increased over time, the distribution of those facilities has become more disparate—most development has taken place in the Greater Accra region. Korle Bu Teaching Hospital in Accra and Komfo Anokye Teaching Hospital in Kumasi are among the key healthcare institutions.[50] The overarching government body is the Ministry of Health.

GUINEA
■ Demography
Population: 9,181,000

Religions: Islam (85%), Christian (10%), traditional indigenous beliefs (5%)

Languages: French (official), each ethnic group has its own language

Ethnic Makeup: Peuhl (40%), Malinke (30%), Soussou (20%), smaller ethnic groups (10%)

Formerly Colonized: France

Politics/Governance: Republic

HIV Prevalence: Adult—1.6%

TB: 6,500 deaths annually. Prevalence: 448/100,000 (2007). DOTS coverage: 60%; DOTS rx success: 75%[5]

Malaria: 3,766,478 cases (2006 estimate)[6]

Percent of Population Vaccinated: 69% vaccinated with DTP, 73% with measles

Infant Mortality Rate: 65.22 deaths/1000 live births (2009)[3]

Under-5 mortality: 161/1000 live births[8]

Leading Causes of Death: Malaria (15%), perinatal conditions (10%), diarrheal diseases (8%), and measles (8%) (2006)[9]

Unusual Pathogens: Schistosomiasis, yaws, leprosy, sleeping sickness

Unique Environmental Exposures: Deforestation; insufficient supplies of potable water, desertification, soil erosion, overfishing, overpopulation in forest region, poor mining practices.

■ Traditional Medicine
Traditional medicine is practiced in the form of traditional therapists, midwives, herbalists, and medico-druggist. Government does not regulate practitioners, but does recognize them and keep a registry. Traditional healers often involved in primary care at the community level.

■ Healthcare System
Decentralized, community-based healthcare system since 1987, following the Bamako Initiative to provide essential medicines and access to healthcare services. Rural penetration is limited. Private and not-for-profit sectors also active in health care, mostly in urban areas.

Among the key healthcare institutions are the Hopital Nationale Donka and the Hopital Nationale Ignace Deen in Conakry, where tertiary and specialty care are available.[51] The overarching government body is the Ministry of Health.

GUINEA-BISSAU
■ Demography
Population: 1,646,000

Religions: Indigenous beliefs (~50%), Islam (~40%), Christian (~10%)

Languages: Portugese (official), Kriol, French, native languages

Ethnic Makeup: Balanta (30%), Fula (20%), Manjaca (14%), Mandinga (13%), Papel (7%), European/mestizo (<1%)

Formerly Colonized: Portugal

Politics/Governance: Republic

HIV Prevalence: Adult—1.8%

TB: 700 deaths annually. Prevalence: 276/100,000 (2007). DOTS coverage: 87%; DOTS rx success: 69%[5]

Malaria: 603,211 cases (2006 estimate)[6]

Percent of Population Vaccinated: 80% vaccinated with DTP and measles

Infant Mortality Rate: 99.82 deaths/1000 live births (2009)[3]

Under-5 mortality: 200/1000 live births[8]

Leading Causes of Death: Lower respiratory infections (11%), malaria (10%), measles (7%), and HIV/AIDS (7%) (2006)[9]

Unusual Pathogens: Schistosomiasis, typhoid fever, yellow fever, rabies

Unique Environmental Exposures: Deforestation; soil erosion, overfishing; overgrazing.

■ Traditional Medicine
Traditional practitioners are neither recognized nor regulated by the Ministry of Health.

■ Healthcare System
Three divisions of healthcare service provision—national, regional, and local, but less than 40% of the population had access in 1995. Decentralized community model that has relied heavily upon aid from the WHO and UNICEF.

Specialty hospitals exist for tuberculosis, leprosy, psychiatry, and physical handicaps. Simão Mendes National Hospital is the main referral hospital in the country. The overarching government body is the Ministry of Health.

LIBERIA
■ Demography
Population: 3,579,000

Religions: Indigenous beliefs (40%), Christian (40%), Islam (20%)

Languages: English (official), ~20 indigenous languages

Ethnic Makeup: Indigenous African, 16 ethnic groups, Kpelle most populous (95%), Americo-Liberians (2.5%), Congo (2.5%)

Formerly Colonized: United States (African-Americans)

Politics/Governance: Republic

HIV Prevalence: Adult—1.7%

TB: 2,300 deaths annually. Prevalence: 398/100,000 (2007). DOTS coverage: 100%; DOTS rx success: 76%[5]

Malaria: 1,459,884 cases (2006 estimate)[6]

Percent of Population Vaccinated: 98–99% vaccinated with BCG, OPV, Hib, HBV, DTP, measles

Infant Mortality Rate: 138.24 deaths/1000 live births (2009)[3]

Under-5 mortality: 235/1000 live births[8]

Leading Causes of Death: Lower respiratory infections (12%), HIV/AIDS (10%), malaria (10%), and diarrheal diseases (7%) (2006)[9]

Unusual Pathogens: Schistosomiasis, lassa fever, onchocerciasis, lymphatic filariasis

Unique Environmental Exposures: Tropical rainforest deforestation; soil erosion, pollution of coastal waters from oil residue and sewage

■ **Traditional Medicine**
Practiced widely, especially in rural areas. Liberian government recognizes, regulates, and offers training for traditional healers

■ **Healthcare System**
Civil conflict and regional instability have led to extremely poor penetrance of the healthcare system. Estimated 90% of health services come from NGOs and disaster relief organizations. ~75% of the population has limited or no access to essential health services.[52]

Partnerships with international aid organizations and NGOs have restored some healthcare services. As of 2006, there were 18 functioning hospitals in the country.[53] JFK Memorial Hospital is the functioning tertiary care referral healthcare institution in Liberia. The overarching government body is the Ministry of Health and Social Welfare.

MALI

■ **Demography**
Population: 11,968,000

Religions: Islam (90%), Christian (5%), indigenous beliefs (5%)

Languages: French (official), Bambara (80%), ~40 other indigenous languages

Ethnic Makeup: Mande (50%), Peul (17%), Voltaic (12%), Songhai (6%), Tuareg and Moor (10%), other (5%)

Formerly Colonized: France

Politics/Governance: Republic

HIV Prevalence: Adult—1.5%

TB: 11,000 deaths annually. Prevalence: 599/100,000 (2007). DOTS coverage: 100%; DOTS rx success: 76%[5]

Malaria: 4,317,487 cases (2006 estimate)[6]

Percent of Population Vaccinated: Measles (75%), DTP (76%), HBV (73%)

Infant Mortality Rate: 102.05 deaths/1000 live births (2009)[3]

Under-5 mortality: 217/1000 live births [8]

Leading Causes of Death: Lower respiratory infections (16%), diarrheal diseases (9%), malaria (9%), and perinatal conditions (8%) (2006)[9]

Unusual Pathogens: Schistosomiasis, meningococcal meningitis, cholera, onchocerciasis, trypanosomiasis

Unique Environmental Exposures: Deforestation; soil erosion, supply of potable water is insufficient

■ **Traditional Medicine**
75% of Malians use traditional medicine—there is roughly one practitioner per 500 people. The government regulates, certifies, and authorizes training of healers. Collaboration is extensive for implementation of primary care.

■ Healthcare System

Most healthcare delivery takes place through a decentralized public health system—national policies are created in Bamako by the Ministry of Health, but each country implements them according to their needs. Limited private services are available, mostly in Bamako. Point G Hospital and Gabriel Toure Hospital in Bamako are key referral institutions in Mali. The overarching government body is the Ministry of Health and Social Welfare.

■ MAURITANIA

■ Demography

Population: 3,044,000

Religions: Islam (religion of state, 99%), Christianity (rare, <1%)

Languages: Arabic (official and national), Pulaar, Soninke, Wolof, French, Hassaniya

Ethnic Makeup: Mixed Moor/black (40%), Moor (30%), black (30%)

Formerly Colonized: France

Politics/Governance: Military junta, Islamic republic

HIV Prevalence: Adult—0.8%

TB: 2,400 deaths annually. Prevalence: 559/100,000 (2007). DOTS coverage: 82%; DOTS rx success: 41%[5]

Malaria: 559,484 cases (2006 estimate)[6]

Percent of Population Vaccinated: 64% vaccinated with measles, 70% with DTP

Infant Mortality Rate: 63.42 deaths/1000 live births (2009)[3]

Under-5 mortality: 125/1000 live births[8]

Leading Causes of Death: Lower respiratory infections (17%), perinatal conditions (11%), diarrheal diseases (9%), and malaria (7%) (2006)[9]

Unusual Pathogens: Schistosomiasis, trachoma, Rift Valley fever, meningococcal meningitis, rabies

Unique Environmental Exposures: Drought, overgrazing, deforestation, locust infestation, limited natural fresh water resources

■ Traditional Medicine

Traditional healing is widely utilized, mostly based on written Arabic medical knowledge. No formal framework exists for regulation or certification of traditional practices.[54]

■ Healthcare System

Most healthcare delivery is through the public sector via a decentralized, community-based model. Over the past decade, increasing private services have become available (mostly in the capital Nouakchott). Medications are provided to community clinics free of charge, but are often in short supply. Access is limited, especially in rural areas.

Key healthcare institutions in Mauritania are the National Hospital in Nouakchott and Kaedi Regional Hospital in the southern part of the country near the Senegal border. The overarching government body is the Ministry of Health.

SENEGAL

■ Demography
Population: 12,072,000

Religions: Islam (95%), Christian (4%), indigenous religions (1%)

Languages: French (official), Wolof, Pulaar, Jola, Mandinka

Ethnic Makeup: Wolof (43.3%), Pular (23.8%), Serer (14.7%), Jola (3.7%), Mandinka (3%), Soninke (1.1%), European and Lebanese (1%), other (9.4%)

Formerly Colonized: France

Politics/Governance: Republic

HIV Prevalence: Adult—1%

TB: 8,000 deaths annually. Prevalence: 468/100,000 (2007). DOTS coverage: 100%; DOTS rx success: 76%[5]

Malaria: 1,456,336 cases (2006 estimate)[6]

Percent of Population Vaccinated: 57% vaccinated against measles, 87% against DTP, and 54% against HBV

Infant Mortality Rate: 58.94 deaths/1000 live births (2009)[3]

Under-5 mortality: 116/1000 live births[8]

Leading Causes of Death: Lower respiratory infections (16%), malaria (13%), perinatal conditions (9%), and diarrheal diseases (7%) (2006)[9]

Unusual Pathogens: Crimean-Congo hemorrhagic fever, dengue, Rift Valley fever, schistosomiasis, meningococcal meningitis

Unique Environmental Exposures: Poaching, deforestation, overgrazing, overfishing, soil erosion

■ Traditional Medicine
Traditional medicine is widely practiced, mostly in the form of herbalism. Center for Experimental Traditional Medicine in Fatick features collaboration between allopathic doctors and traditional healers.

■ Healthcare System
Most of the population is covered by the public sector, with some private services mostly in Dakar. Access to health care in rural areas is ~33% and attributed to distance from points of care.[55]

Key healthcare institutions in Senegal include the Hopital Principale de Dakar and various private clinics. The overarching government body is the Ministry of Health and Preventive Medicine.

SIERRA LEONE

▥ Demography

Population: 5,743,000

Religions: Islam (60%), Christianity (10%), indigenous religions (30%)

Languages: English (official, limited), Mende (most common in the south), Temne (most common in the north), Krio (first language for 10%, understood by 95%)

Ethnic Makeup: 20 African ethnic groups including Temne and Mende (90%), Creole (10%), Liberian refugees, Europeans, Pakistanis, Indians (minimal)

Formerly Colonized: United Kingdom

Politics/Governance: Constitutional democracy

HIV Prevalence: Adult—1.7%

TB: 8,700 deaths annually. Prevalence: 941/100,000 (2007). DOTS coverage: 100%; DOTS rx success: 87%[5]

Malaria: 2,272,651 cases (2006 estimate)[6]

Percent of Population Vaccinated: 64% vaccinated against measles, 61% received DTP

Infant Mortality Rate: 154.43 deaths/1000 live births (2009)[3]

Under-5 mortality: 269/1000 live births[8]

Leading Causes of Death: Lower respiratory infections (13%), diarrheal diseases (10%), perinatal conditions (10%), and malaria (7%) (2006)[9]

Unusual Pathogens: Lassa fever, schistosomiasis, yellow fever, typhoid fever, onchocerciasis

Unique Environmental Exposures: Rapid population growth, deforestation and soil exhaustion, civil war depleted natural resources, overfishing

▥ Traditional Medicine

Traditional medicine widely used, mostly in rural areas, and mostly herbalism. Sierra Leone Traditional Healers Association works with the government to enhance primary care.

▥ Healthcare System

Decentralized community model of public health care since 2005, divided into 13 district councils managing funds for community health. ~70% of health care costs are out-of-pocket, ~20% are public, and ~0.4% are private.[56]

Connaught Hospital in Freetown represents the main referral hospital for Sierra Leone. The overarching government body is the Ministry of Health and Sanitation.

TOGO

▥ Demography

Population: 6,410,000

Religions: Indigenous beliefs (51%), Christianity (29%), Islam (20%)

Languages: French (official), Ewe and Mina (most common in the south), Kabye and Dagomba (most common in the north)

Ethnic Makeup: 37 African tribes including Ewe, Mina, and Kabre (99%), European and Syrian-Lebanese (<1%)

Formerly Colonized: France

Politics/Governance: Republic in transition to multiparty democracy

HIV Prevalence: Adult—3.3%

TB: 9,100 deaths annually. Prevalence: 750/100,000 (2007). DOTS coverage: 100%; DOTS rx success: 67%[5]

Malaria: 2,085,590 cases (2006 estimate)[6]

Percent of Population Vaccinated: 70% are vaccinated against measles, 71% with DTP

Infant Mortality Rate: 56.24 deaths/1000 live births (2009)[3]

Under-5 mortality: 107/1000 live births[8]

Leading Causes of Death: HIV/AIDS (17%), lower respiratory infections (14%), malaria (11%), perinatal conditions (7%) (2006)[9]

Unusual Pathogens: Typhoid fever, yellow fever, schistosomiasis, meningococcal meningitis, H5N1 (avian) influenza, yaws, leprosy, guinea worm

Unique Environmental Exposures: Deforestation, water pollution, air pollution, Iodine deficiency has led to endemic goiter. There is limited access to safe drinking water and sanitation.

■ Traditional Medicine
Female genital mutilation occurs in up to 50% of Togolese women. Traditional herbs often used to treat malaria. The government recognizes and registers traditional healers. Many are involved in primary care at the community level.

■ Healthcare System
Decentralized public health system serves ~2/3 of the population. Limited private services are available, mostly in urban areas.

Tokoin National Hospital in Lome and Hopital Baptiste Biblique in Adeta represent the key healthcare institutions in Togo. The overarching government body is the Ministry of Health and Sanitation.

REFERENCES

1. Africa Development indicators 2008/2009. The World Bank. 50 factoids about Sub Saharan Africa. Available at: http://web.worldbank.org/WBSITE/EXTERNAL/COUNTRIES/AFRICAEXT/EXTPUBREP/EXTSTATINAFR/0,,contentMDK:21106218~menuPK:3094759~pagePK:64168445~piPK:64168309~theSitePK:824043,00.html

2. Smallman-Raynor MR, Cliff AD. Civil war and the spread of AIDS in Central Africa Epidemiology and Infection, 1991. Available at: www.jstor.org/stable/3863924

3. CIA World Factbook

4. UNAIDS, 2008 Report on the global AIDS epidemic. Available at: http://data.unaids.org/pub/GlobalReport/2008/jc1510_2008_global_report_pp211_234_en.pdf

5. WHO, Global Tuberculosis Control: Epidemiology, Strategy, Financing, 2009. Available at: http://www.who.int/tb/publications/global_report/en/index.html

6. WHO, World Malaria Report 2008. Available at: http://www.who.int/malaria/wmr2008/

7. UNICEF. Country Statistics. Available at: http://www.unicef.org/infobycountry/

8. WHO, World Health Statistics 2009. Available at: http://www.who.int/whosis/whostat/2009/en/index.html

9. WHO Mortality Country Fact Sheet. Available at: http://www.who.int/whosis/mort/profiles/en/

10. WHO Global Alert and response. Disease outbreaks by country. Available at: http://www.who.int/csr/don/archive/country/en/

11. Aflatoxin levels in locally grown maize from Makueni District, Kenya. Available at: http://www.find-health-articles.com/rec_pub_19133419-aflatoxin-levels-locally-grown-maize-makueni-district-kenya.htm

12. Barrett J. Liver cancer and aflatoxin: new information from the Kenyan outbreak. Environmental Health Perspectives. Dec 2005.

13. WHO. Legal Status of Traditional Medicine and Complementary/Alternative Medicine: A Worldwide Review. Available at: http://apps.who.int/medicinedocs/en/d/Jh2943e/4.21.html

14. Kenya Government. Health Care and Medical Services. Available at: http://www.kenya.go.ke//index.php?option=com_content&task=view&id=37&Itemid=32

15. Government of Uganda. Annual Health Sector Performance Report. 2007/2008. Available at: http://www.health.go.ug/docs/AHSPR0708.pdf

16. Wikipedia. Hospitals in Uganda. Accessed Aug 11, 2009.

17. Lawyer's Environmental Action Team. Major environmental problems in Tanzania. Available at: http://www.leat.or.tz/publications/decentralization/1.3.env.problems.php

18. Msuya TS, Kideghesho JR. 2009. The Role of Traditional Management Practices in Enhancing Sustainable Use and Conservation of Medicinal Plants in West Usambara Mountains, Tanzania. Tropical Conservation Science. 2;(1): 88–105.

19. Tanzania Ministry of Health and Social Welfare. Available at: www.moh.go.tz

20. Rwanda Ministry of Health. Health facilities. Available at: http://www.moh.gov.rw/index.php?option=com_content&view=category&layout=blog&id=37&Itemid=54

21. Dr Miaka. *Health Reform in DRC. Steering harmonisation and alignment.* Ministry of Health-DRC. 2006. Available at: www.hlfhealthmdgs.org/HLF4Presentations/DRC%20Presentation.ppt

22. Index Mundi. Zambia Environment issues. Available at: http://www.index-mundi.com/zambia/environment_current_issues.html

23. Global Religious Health Assets Mapping. Listing and summary of hospitals. Available at: http://www.ccih.org/grham/country/zambia/Tables_2.htm

24. WHO. Health action in crises—Malawi. 2006. Available at: http://www.who.int/hac/crises/mwi/background/Malawi_June06.pdf

25. Malawi MOH. Malawi Health Care institutions. Available at: http://www.malawi.gov.mw/Health/Listofgovtinstitutions.htm

26. International Insulin Foundation. Mozambique's Health Care System. Available at: http://www.access2insulin.org/html/mozambique_s_health_system.html

27. Mozambique MOH. SAM - Inventário Nacional de Infra- Estruturas de Saúde 2007. Available at: http://www.misau.gov.mz/pt/misau/dpc_direccao_de_planificacao_e_cooperacao/departamento_de_informacao_para_a_saude/documentos_chave_do_sistema_de_informacao_para_a_saude/sam_inventario_nacional_de_infra_estruturas_de_saude_2007

28. South Africa Info. Health care in South Africa. Available at: http://www.southafrica.info/about/health/health.htm

29. Lesotho Ministry of Health and Social Welfare. Available at: http://www.health.gov.ls

30. Staugard F. Traditional medicine in a transitional society: Botswana moving towards the year 2000. Gaborone, Ipelegeng Publishers, 1989.

31. Botswana Ministry of Health. Available at: http://www.moh.gov.bw/

32. Namibia Ministry of Health and Social Services. Available at: http://www.mhss.gov.na/

33. Namibia Health Facilities directory. Available at: http://www.healthnet.org.na/health_facilities/Regional%20Directory.pdf

34. Catherine Connor, Yogesh Rajkotia, Ya-Shin Lin, Paula Figueiredo. 2005. Angola Health system assessment. Partners for Health Reform *plus*. Abt Associates Inc. Available at: http://www.healthsystems2020.org/content/resource/detail/1672/

35. Madagascar Ministry of Health. Available at: http://www.sante.gov.mg/

36. Bishaw M. Promoting traditional medicine in Ethiopia: a brief historical review of government policy. *Social Science and Medicine.* 1991; 33: 193–200.

37. Ethiopia Federal Ministry of Health. Available at: www.moh.gov.et

38. Yusuf et al. Traditional medical practices in some Somali Communities. *Journal of Tropical Pediatrics.* 1984;30(2):87–92.

39. WHO-EMRO. World Health Day 2001. Somalia country profile. Available at: http://www.emro.who.int/mnh/whd/CountryProfile-SOM.htm

40. WHO-EMRO. World Health Day 2001. Sudan country profile Available at: http://www.emro.who.int/mnh/whd/CountryProfile-SUD.htm

41. WHO-EMRO. World Health Day 2001. Djibouti country profile. Available at: http://www.emro.who.int/mnh/whd/CountryProfile-DJI.htm

42. Commonwealth of Australia. Eritrean Community profile. 2006. Available at http://www.immi.gov.au/living-in-australia/delivering-assistance/government-programs/settlement-planning/_pdf/community-profile-eritrea.pdf

43. World Bank. 2004. The Health sector in Eritrea.

44. Gambian Health Policy Framework. Available at: www.statehouse.gm/health.html

45. The Atlas of the Gambia. Health care. Available at: http://www.columbia.edu/~msj42/Education%20and%20Healthcare.htm

46. Equatorial Guinea. Ministry of Health and Social Well-being. Available at: http://www.ceiba-guinea-ecuatorial.org/guineeangl/minsante1.htm

47. Swaziland Ministry of Health and Social Welfare. Available at: http://www.gov.sz/home.asp?pid=142

48. Cameroon Ministry of Health. Available at: http://www.minsante.cm/

49. World Health Organization, *Bamako Initiative revitalizes primary health care in Benin*, Health: a key to prosperity, Success stories in developing countries, http://www.who.int/inf-new/child6.htm

50. Ghana Statistical Service. Health, Nutrition, and Environmental Statistics. http://www.statsghana.gov.gh/Health_Nutrition.html, accessed on December 8th, 2009.

51. Ministere de la Sante Publique. Republic of Guinea. Plan National de Developpement Sanitaire. Conakry: August, 2003.

52. World Health Organization, "Liberia: Health sector needs assessment," World Health Organization: 2006.

53. Ministry of Health and Social Welfare. National Health Policy, National Health Plan 2007–2011. Republic of Liberia: Monrovia, 2007.

54. Graz B. "Assessing traditional healers: an observational clinical study of classical Arabic medicine in Mauritania, with comparison of prognosis and outcome," *Trop Doct*. Vol. 35, No. 4, Oct 2005.

55. Senegal Ministere de la Santé, "Santé pour tous," *Enquete Senegalaise sur les indicateurs de Santé*, 1999.

56. World Health Organization, "Sierra Leone: Country cooperation strategy," WHO: 2008.

XVI ■ MIDDLE EAST AND NORTH AFRICA*

Fadi El-Jardali, MPH, PhD
Diana Jamal, MPH
* Israel country profile prepared by Matthew Dacso, MD, MSc

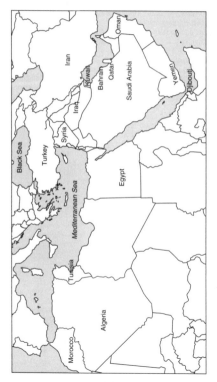

The Middle East and North Africa (MENA) region is characterized by the vast diversity of its political, social, economic, and health indicators.

Despite tremendous improvements in the health of their populations over the last quarter century, MENA countries have experienced epidemiological and demographic transitions, political instability, wars, and natural disasters, against a backdrop of wide variations in social and economic development. Dual disease burden—of communicable and noncommunicable diseases—exists in almost all MENA countries, irrespective of their level of socioeconomic development.

In many countries in the region, especially the low, and low-to-middle income countries, the demographic transition shows a complex picture of a relatively high fertility rate together with a decline in the mortality rate. Population growth in the MENA region is high (almost 2% per year). Over the past half-century, the MENA region has witnessed the highest population growth in the world and, more recently, the annual population growth of the region is second only to sub-Saharan Africa.[1] In several MENA countries, the average fertility rate is 3.6 births per woman.

While the countries of the region continue to maintain a large share of their populations under the age of 18 (and children under age 5 account for as much as 10–40%), in most countries more than 5% of the population are over the age of 65. These characteristics have led to dual challenges of infectious diseases and malnutrition among children and mothers together with a substantial rise in chronic diseases, injuries, and disabilities associated with aging. It is estimated that by 2020 chronic diseases will account for 60% of the disease burden and 70% of all deaths. This is expected to be associated with a decline in the burden of communicable diseases to 20% for the same year.

Urbanization in many countries has been rapid and extensive. On average, almost 60% of MENA populations live in urban areas, ranging from 24% in the Republic of Yemen to 97% in Kuwait.

HEALTH CONCERNS

Chronic diseases will account for almost three-quarters of all deaths in the MENA region by 2020. Risk factors include smoking, poverty and inequality, improper diet, unsafe sex, physical inactivity, alcohol consumption, and pollution. In 1990, the percentage of deaths in the MENA region attributed to tobacco use was 2.4%; a figure which is expected to rise to 9.5% in 2020.[2] Mortality rates by road-traffic injuries are among the highest in the world (26.4 per 100,000 in low- and middle-income countries of the region compared with 19 per 100,000 globally).[3]

Over the past two decades, the MENA countries have achieved notable improvements in the health status of their citizens, as seen by an almost 10-year increase in life expectancy between 1980 and 2003 (to 69 years in 2003) and halving of the infant mortality rate over the same period.[4]

Despite improvements in life expectancy in MENA countries, health disparities between the rich and the poor continue to widen, in terms of both health status and access to care. Most major killers (cancer, coronary heart disease, stroke, etc.) and their associated risk factors are linked to socioeconomic inequality.

The majority of MENA countries lack universal access to healthcare services and have many inequalities. Health spending by most governments in the region ranges between 3% and 8.5%. Some outliers, such as Lebanon and Jordan, are spending 11.5% and 9.3%, respectively. These levels of spending are posing serious challenges to countries in terms of ensuring comprehensive access to high quality preventive, curative, and rehabilitative services. In many countries, access is still based on the ability to pay rather than need. Out-of-pocket household spending on health services accounts for nearly half the total health spending in the MENA region. Many individuals and households have little financial protection (insurance) against illness.[5]

Currently, most health services in the MENA region are based on a curative model, which is becoming ineffective in the face of emerging health challenges.

Research and development funding in the region is the lowest in the world, with expenditure for the Arab world at 0.4% of gross domestic product (GDP) in 1996 compared with 1.26% for Cuba in 1995 and 2.9% for Japan in 1994.[6]

Many health issues affect the entire region: the control of communicable diseases (malaria, pulmonary tuberculosis, and measles are responsible for a substantial proportion of the region's morbidity) and lack of qualified doctors and skilled workforce. Vast geographical inequalities are observed for medical assistance at delivery. The situation can be described as very good in the Gulf States, Jordan, and Palestine (where 96% to 98% of deliveries are attended by skilled health personnel), relatively good (around 90%) in Algeria and Tunisia, and seriously deficient in Iraq, Mauritania, Morocco, and Egypt (between 60 and 70%). Yemen and Somalia lag far behind. The completed vaccination coverage is relatively good (above 75%) in most countries, but some are deficient (below 50%) including Djibouti, Comoros, Mauritania, and notably in Sudan (5%).

According to World Health Organization (WHO) estimates, by 2010, communicable diseases will account for 29% of the disease burden (down from 40% in 2000) and noncommunicable diseases will account for 53% (up from 45% in 2000).[2] By 2020, the respective figures are estimated to be 20% and 60%.[5]

Upper-income and urban areas in middle-income countries of the region are mainly burdened by noncommunicable diseases, having largely eliminated communicable diseases. However, newer communicable diseases such as HIV/AIDS are emerging; in some places, tuberculosis is reemerging.[7] Tuberculosis (TB) incidence and prevalence in several MENA countries is mostly below 200 per 100,000, except for Sudan, Djibouti, Mauritania, and Somalia where considerable higher rates were reported.[8]

Malaria in the region is concentrated in the low-income countries of Sudan, Yemen, Somalia, and Mauritania. These countries also suffer from high rates of childhood death due to malaria.[8]

It is estimated that more than 600,000 people are living with HIV/AIDS, and three countries (Djibouti, Somalia, and Sudan) are experiencing generalized epidemics (defined as HIV prevalence >1% in the general adult population aged 15–45), accounting for the majority of estimated HIV infections in the region (Sudan alone has 512,000 cases). These numbers may be underestimations given the lack of surveillance systems in many countries.

More than 12 million people in the MENA region suffer from sexually transmitted infections (STIs) such as syphilis, gonorrhea, and chlamydia.[9] Although the prevalence of STIs in MENA countries is relatively low, reflecting cultural condemnation of sexual relationships outside of marriage, it is increasing rapidly. In addition, STIs are significantly underreported in the region, as they are elsewhere. For the most part, MENA countries are not equipped with effective systems for detecting and reporting these infections.[9]

Substantial progress has been achieved in several MENA countries toward polio eradication. Sudan and Somalia had some reported cases over the past few years.

Reproductive health care is a major challenge for MENA governments. The rural–urban gap is particularly large in lower-income countries in the region. In Egypt only 42% of pregnant women in rural areas receive any antenatal checkups, compared with 70% of those living in urban areas; in Morocco, the rates are 56% and 88%, respectively.[9]

Maternal mortality is relatively low in many MENA countries. Progress has been made in reducing infant and child mortality and in improving health. But wide disparities between countries, between social groups, and even between sexes remain.[10]

Each year, roughly 13,000 women in the MENA region die of complications related to pregnancy and childbirth, although the mortality ratios vary greatly by country. Yemen and Iraq have some of the highest levels of maternal death, with around 300 maternal deaths per 100,000 live births. Morocco's maternal death ratio remains high, at more than 200 deaths per 100,000, although there have been improvements in maternal health in the country over the past 20 years. The lowest maternal mortality ratios in the MENA region are found in countries with the highest levels of health expenditure per capita and the smallest gender gaps in education.[9]

Only Kuwait and the United Arab Emirates have managed to reduce their maternal mortality ratios to levels considered low by international standards. Maternal mortality is fairly low in Oman, Qatar, and Saudi Arabia, but ratios in all three countries remain higher than those in countries outside the region that have comparable per capita incomes.[11]

COUNTRY PROFILES OF MIDDLE EAST AND NORTH AFRICA

ALGERIA

■ Demography

Population: 33,852,676 in 2007[13]

Religions: The state religion is Sunni Muslim (99% of population), the remaining 1% is mostly Christian (Roman Catholic but also Methodist and Evangelical Christians) while the Jewish population is estimated at around 60 persons.[14]

Languages: Arabic (official), French, Berber[14]

Ethnic Makeup: Arab-Berber

Formerly Colonized: France, independence in 1962

Politics/Governance: Constitutional Republic

■ Healthcare System

Ninety-eight percent of the population has access to health care and the past few decades have witnessed improvement in health indicators. Utilization of primary health care is minimal; the majority of the population seeks tertiary care despite the lack of maintenance and upkeep of facilities. The private sector in Algeria is expanding but quality of care and regulation is not much better than that of the public sector.[15]

Health services in Algeria are partially financed by the state budget, from a social health insurance scheme called the Cassise National des Assurance Sociale (CNAS) in addition to out-of-pocket payments.[16]

The key health institutions are the Clinique Chirurgicale Sidi Yahia, Clinique de Chirurgie Cardio Vasculaire PR Kara, Clinique El Hikma, Clinique Medico Chirurgicale Ediya, Clinique Medico Chirurgicale en Nadjah, Clinique Medico Chirurgicale et Cardio Vasculaire Abou Marwan, and Clinique Saada.[20]

Medicinal herbs are widely used in traditional medicine.

HIV/AIDS Prevalence: Adults ≥ 15 years: 87 per 100,000 (2007)[17]

Prevalence of TB: 56/100,000 (2006)[18]

Malaria: No data reported (2007)[17]

Percent of Population Vaccinated: 90–95%[17,18]

Leading Causes of Death: Cerebrovascular disease, ischemic heart disease, respiratory infections, perinatal conditions.[19]

Infant Mortality Rate: 33/1000 live births[19]

Unusual Pathogens: Plague in Oran district in 2003[19]

BAHRAIN

■ Demography

Population: 752,789 in 2007[13]

Religions: Muslim majority; Christian, Jewish, Hindu, and Zoroastrian minorities[21]

Languages: Arabic, English[21]

Ethnic Makeup: 38% of the population is non-Bahrainis[21]

Formerly Colonized: United Kingdom, independence in 1971[21]

Politics/Governance: Constitutional hereditary monarchy[21]

■ Healthcare System

The Ministry of Health is responsible for planning, policy, provision, and regulation of health services. The private healthcare sector in Bahrain has been limited and largely unregulated.[21]

A wide range of prevention, promotion, curative, and rehabilitative services are available free of charge to Bahrainis and heavily subsidized to non-Bahrainis.[21]

The key health institutions are the Salmaniya Medical Complex, Al Amal Specialist Hospital, American Mission Hospital Society, Bahrain Defence Force Royal Medical Services, Bahrain Specialist Hospital, Dr. Ahmed Eye Clinic, Dr. Ebtisam Eye Care Eye Clinic, Ibn Al Nafees Medical Complex, Noor Specialist Hospital, and International Hospital of Bahrain.[20,21]

HIV/AIDS Prevalence: Adults aged ≥ 15 years: no cases reported[17]

Prevalence of TB: 45/100,000 (2006)[18]

Malaria: No cases reported (2007)[18]

Percent of Population Vaccinated: 97–99%[17,18]

Leading Causes of Death: Heart disease, diabetes, trauma[19]

Infant Mortality Rate: 9/1000 live births[17]

DJIBOUTI

■ Demography

Population: 832,992 in 2007[13]

Religions: Islam

Languages: Afar, Standard Arabic, Spoken Arabic, French, and Somali

Ethnic Makeup: Somali Issa (60%) and the Afar (35%)[19]

Formerly Colonized: Formerly the French Territory of the Afars and Issas, gained independence in 1977

Politics/Governance: Republic

■ Traditional Medicine

Traditional healers represent 12% of the providers. Nomads rely on traditional healers and only go to a dispensary or hospital in cases of severe illness.[22]

■ Healthcare System

Public health services available virtually free of charge.[22]

Officially, medications are provided free of charge by "Pharmacie Nationale d'Approvisionnernent," however. in reality drugs are rarely available.[22]

The main general hospital (Hospital Peltier) in Djibouti City has a capacity of 610 beds. The Paul Faure Center (204 beds), the second largest hospital, specializes in TB and other respiratory diseases. There is also a 60-bed maternity, pediatric, and obstetric hospital (Balbala). Four district hospitals with a total capacity of 300 beds act as referral hospitals for the rural dispensaries.[22]

HIV/AIDS Prevalence: Adults—2870/100,000 (2007)[17]

Prevalence of TB: 1300/100,000 (2006)[18]

Malaria: 4708 reported cases (2007)[17]

Percent of Population Vaccinated: 25–74%[17,18]

Leading Causes of Death: Respiratory infections, waterborne illness, heart disease, perinatal conditions[19]

Infant Mortality Rate: 84/1000 live births[17]

Unusual Pathogens: Remote regions have a very poor access to healthcare facilities and have high rates of infectious diseases such as HIV/AIDS, malaria, and cholera.[19]

Unique Environmental Exposures: Drought, heavy rainfall, and flooding.[19]

EGYPT

■ Demography

Population: 75,466,539 in 2007[13]

Religions: 94% of the population is Muslim (mostly Sunni), 6% is Coptic Christian[23]

Ethnic Makeup: Egyptians and Bedouins make up 99% of the population. Remaining 1% includes Greeks, Nubians, Armenians, and others.[23]

Languages: Arabic (official), English and French are widely used

Formerly Colonized: United Kingdom

Politics/Governance: Republic

■ Traditional Medicine

Laws and regulations regarding traditional medicine (mostly in the form of herbal medicine) were developed in 1955 and a national policy was developed in 2001.[24]

■ Healthcare System

A wide range of public and private providers is available. Public health services are oriented toward poor and underprivileged population groups.[23]

HIV/AIDS Prevalence: Adults—18/100,000 (2007)[17]

Prevalence of TB: 31/100,000 (2006)[18]

Malaria: 30 cases reported (2007)[17]

Percent of Population Vaccinated: 97–98%[17,18]

Leading Causes of Death: Heart disease, cerebrovascular disease, respiratory infections[19]

Infant Mortality Rate: 30/1000 live births[17]

Unusual Pathogens: H5N1 avian influenza virus cases in humans reported.[19]

Unique Environmental Exposures: Visitors should be protected against yellow fever and malaria.[23] There is also the danger of being exposed to the Bilharzias parasite in the Nile River.

IRAQ
■ Demography
Population: 28,993,000 in 2007[17]

Religions: 97% Muslim (60–65% Shiites and 32–37% Sunnis). The Christians that remained in Iraq in the post-Hussein era are estimated at 40,000 and mainly follow the Eastern-rite Chaldean Catholic Church.[25]

Ethnic Makeup: Arab (75–80%), Kurdish[25]

Languages: Arabic and Kurdish (official), Turkmen and Assyrian neo-Aramaic[25]

Formerly Colonized: United Kingdom, obtained its independence in 1932[25]

Politics/Governance: After the overthrow of Saddam Hussein, Iraq has passed through several stages of governance and has transitioned into a Democratic Republic[25]

■ Healthcare System
The Ministry of Health is the main body responsible for the provision of health care to the people throughout the country. Numerous private providers supplement public health services.[26]

Pharmaceutical products are highly subsidized by the government. They are usually distributed by Kimadia, a state company for drugs and medical appliances. All primary healthcare services like immunization, antenatal care, health education, and others are provided free of charge at the PHC centers.[26]

HIV/AIDS Prevalence: Not available

Prevalence of TB: 78/100,000 (2006)[18]

Malaria: 3 reported cases (2007)[17]

Percent of Population Vaccinated: 58–69% (2007)[17,18]

Leading Causes of Death: Respiratory infections, heart disease, perinatal conditions, waterborne illness[19]

Infant Mortality Rate: 36/1000[17]

Unusual Pathogens: Malaria, cholera, and leishmaniasis are endemic in several parts of the country.[26]

Unique Environmental Exposures: There is a wide belief that some of the rural regions in the country have been exposed to hazardous, solid, and radioactive waste that has resulted in birth anomalies among residents of these regions.[26]

ISLAMIC REPUBLIC OF IRAN

■ Demography
Population: 71,021,039 in 2007[13]

Religions: Majority Shiite Muslims. Minority Sunni Muslims composed mainly of Kurds in the northwest and Baluchi tribes in the southeast[27]

Ethnic Makeup: Although Iran is ethnically diverse, it can claim homogeneity based on the shared literary history and traditions[27]

Languages: Persian[27]

Formerly Colonized: Never colonized

Politics/Governance: Islamic republic[27]

■ Traditional Medicine
Traditional medicine (mostly herbal medicine) is practiced in the private sector. Other procedures such as homeopathy, cupping, and leeching are also practiced. The office of the Deputy Minister for Food and Drugs is responsible for overseeing herbal medicine treatments.[27]

■ Healthcare System
At the national level, the government exercises the governance, policy making, planning, financing, and steering of the programs. This changes at the provincial level where the Universities of Medical Sciences and Health Services (UMSHS) are the major government institutions providing health services to the population. The country also has an active and well-developed private sector—private facilities are mainly concentrated in urban areas and provide secondary and tertiary care.[27]

Iran produces its own generic pharmaceuticals and 65% of vaccines over which the government has control over pricing and quality. Prices are kept low and affordable.[27]

Iran's key health institutions are the Alzahra University Hospital, Azadi Psychiatric Hospital, Babol University Hospitals, Center Shariati Hospital In Tehran, Erfan Hospital, Farabi Hospital, Guilan University Hospitals, Hamedan University of Medical Science Hospitals, Imam Khomeini Hospital, Iranian Psychiatric Hospital, Jam Hospital, Kashan University of Medical Sciences and Health Services, Khatam Hospital, Madaen Hospital, Milad Hospital, Mofid Children's Hospital, Nour and Ali Asghar University Hospital, Sadi Hospital, Shariati Hospital, Shiraz University of Medical Sciences Hospitals, Sina Hospital, Tabriz University Hospitals, and Taleghani General Hospital.[20]

HIV/AIDS Prevalence: Adults—163/100,000[17]

Prevalence of TB: 28/100,000 (2006)[18]

Malaria: 15,712 cases reported (2007)[17]

Percent of Population Vaccinated: 97–99%[17,18]

Leading Causes of Death: Heart disease, trauma, cerebrovascular disease, perinatal conditions[19]

Infant Mortality Rate: 29/1000 live births (2007)[17]

Unusual Pathogens: Meningococcal disease, serogroup W135 (disease outbreak reported in 2000)[19]

ISRAEL

Profile prepared by Matthew Dacso, MD, MSc

■ Demography

Population: 6,810,000

Religions: Jewish (75.5%), Muslim (16%), Christian (2%), Druze (1.5%)

Languages: Hebrew, Arabic

Ethnic Makeup: Jewish (76%), Arab (20%)

Formerly Colonized: British Mandate of Palestine, declared independence May 14, 1948

Politics/Governance: Parliamentary democracy

Type of Health Care System: National Health Insurance (NHI) provides universal coverage—4 non-for-profit health plans compete for patients. Enrollment is mandatory. Supplementary voluntary health insurance (VHI) available, 65% of Israelis participate.[57,58]

Life expectancy (years): 79 (male), 82 (female)[59]

Under 5 mortality: 5/1000 live births[59]

Vaccinations: >93% vaccinated with DTP, HBV, MMR, IPV, Hib[60]

HIV adult Prevalence: 0.1%[61]

TB Prevalence: 6/100,000, 5.7% of new cases are MDR[62]

Malaria: Not endemic to Israel

Leading causes of death: Cardiovascular disease, cancer, respiratory diseases, intentional/unintentional injuries[57]

Key health institutions: Ministry of Health, Knesset, Public Health Service, Ichilov Hospital, Tel Hashomer Hospital, Ben Gurion University of the Negev, Tel Aviv University Faculty of Medicine)

Unusual pathogens: West Nile Virus

Unique environmental exposures: Extremes of temperature—desert climate

JORDAN

▥ Demography

Population: 5,718,855 in 2007[13]

Religions: Muslim Sunnis (92–95%), Christians (Greek Orthodox, Roman Catholic, Greek Catholic, Armenian Orthodox, Assyrian, Maronite, assorted Protestant churches, and others; 3–6%)[28]

Ethnic Makeup: Arab

Languages: Arabic, English

Formerly Colonized: United Kingdom, independence in 1949

Politics/Governance: Constitutional monarchy[28]

▥ Traditional Medicine
Medicinal plants play an important role in traditional medicine in Jordan.[30]

▥ Healthcare System
Jordan has a modern healthcare infrastructure and three major sectors: public, private, and donors.[29]

 The Ministry of Health (MOH) and the Royal Medical Services (RMS) are the two major public programs that finance as well as deliver care in Jordan. Other smaller public programs include several university-based programs, such as Jordan University Hospital (JUH) in Amman and King Abdullah Hospital (KAH) in Irbid.[29]

HIV/AIDS Prevalence: No data available

Prevalence of TB: 6/100,000 (2006)[18]

Malaria: No data available[17]

Percent of Population Vaccinated: 95–98%[17,18]

Leading Causes of Death: Heart disease, trauma, cerebrovascular disease[19]

Infant Mortality Rate: 18/1000[17]

KUWAIT

▥ Demography
Population: 2,662,966 in 2007[13]

Religions: Sunni Muslim

Ethnic Makeup: Arab majority, Indians (19.8%), Bangladeshis (10.9%), Pakistanis (7%), and Sri Lankan (6.9%)[31]

Languages: Arabic, English

Formerly Colonized: United Kingdom, independence in 1961[32]

Politics/Governance: Nominal constitutional monarchy[32]

■ Traditional Medicine

Kuwaiti law prohibits the open practice of traditional medicine, though herbal medications can be purchased.[19,31]

■ HealthCare System

The healthcare system is organized into two levels: the central Ministry of Health and regional authorities. Despite the comprehensive services provided by the MOH, private hospitals and clinics thrive in Kuwait.[31] Provision of health services is free of charge to Kuwaiti nationals.[31]

The key health institutions include Al Sabah Nbk Pediatric Hospital, Al Salam International Hospital, British Medical Centre Manqaf, Dar Al Shifa Hospital, Ibn Sina Hospital Department of Pediatric Surgery, New Mowasat Hospital, Royale Hayat Hospital, and Shaab Medical Center.[20]

HIV/AIDS Prevalence: No data available

Prevalence of TB: 25/100,000 (2006)[18]

Malaria: No data available

Percent of Population Vaccinated: 99%[17]

Leading Causes of Death: Heart disease, infectious diseases, trauma[19,33]

Infant Mortality Rate: 9/1000 live births (2007)[17]

Unusual Pathogens: Meningococcus outbreak (2000), SARS (2003)[19]

LEBANON

■ Demography

Population: 4,097,076 in 2007[13]

Religions: An estimated two-thirds of the resident population is Muslim (Shia, Sunni, or Druze), and the rest is Christian (predominantly Maronite, Greek Orthodox, Greek Catholic, and Armenian). Shia Muslims make up the single largest sect.[34]

Languages: Arabic, English, French

Formerly Colonized: France, independence in 1943

Politics/Governance: Republic, secular Arab state, parliamentary democracy[34]

■ Healthcare System

The healthcare system in Lebanon is highly fragmented, with the governmental bodies acting as the official regulators. The private sector provides the bulk of services. The main features in the market are the public, the private, and the public-private mix.[34]

Medications are paid for out of pocket, and immunizations have been provided under the EPI since 1995.[35]

The American University of Beirut Medical Center, Beirut General Hospital, Hammoud Hospital University Medical Center, Hayek Hospital, Khoury General Hospital Doctors Center, Makassed General Hospital, Mount Lebanon Hospital Gharios Medical Center, Rafic Hariri Foundation, Rafik Hariri University

Hospital Beirut Governmental University Hospital, and the Saint George Hospital University Medical Center are the key health institutions in Lebanon.

HIV/AIDS Prevalence: Adults—101/100,000 (2007)[17]

Prevalence of TB: 12/100,000 (2006)[18]

Malaria: No cases reported

Percent of Population Vaccinated: 92–96%[17,18]

Leading Causes of Death: Heart disease, cerebrovascular disease, trauma[19]

Infant Mortality Rate: 26/1000 live births (2007)[17]

LIBYA
■ Demography
Population: 6,156,488 in 2007[13]

Religions: Islam (Sunni majority and Shia minority)

Ethnic Makeup: Mixed Arab and Berber ancestry makes up 90% of the population[36]

Languages: Arabic (offical), English, Berber, Italian, and French

Formerly Colonized: Italy, gained its independence in 1951[36]

Politics/Governance: Libya's political system is based on the philosophy of Colonel Qadhafi's Green Book, which blends socialist and Islamic theories. According to the principles of the Green Book Charter, Libyan Jamahiriya is a grass-roots democracy, with local People's Congresses and Committees constituting the basic instrument of government.[37]

■ Traditional Medicine
Libya has a small, unregulated herbal and traditional medicine market.[37]

■ Healthcare System
Health care is provided by a mixed public and private system. The public sector is the main provider of services including preventive, curative, and rehabilitation services that are provided free of charge to citizens.[37]

Libya's key health institutions are the Al Afia Clinic, Al Hikma Medical Services Al Bassatein Clinic, Alfatah Clinic, Almaraa Clinic, Almokhtar, Brothers Clinic, Fardous Clinic Libya, Nowras Clinic, and Tripoli Clinic Libya.[20]

HIV/AIDS Prevalence: No data reported (2007)[17]

Prevalence of TB: 18/100,000 (2006)[18]

Malaria: No data available

Percent of population vaccinated: 98%[17,18]

Leading Causes of Death: Heart disease, cerebrovascular disease, respiratory infections

Infant Mortality Rate: 17/1000 live births (2007)[17]

MOROCCO

■ Demography

Population: 30,860,595 in 2007[13]

Religions: Sunni Muslim majority, with a small local Jewish minority accounting for 0.02% of population[42]

Ethnic Makeup: Arab and/or Berber

Languages: Arabic (official), Berber, French, Spanish

Formerly Colonized: France, independence in 1956[43]

Politics/Governance: Constitutional monarchy[43]

■ Traditional Medicine

This sector is active mainly in the disadvantaged suburbs and among the low socioeconomic level populations.[42]

■ Healthcare System

Morocco provides free public healthcare services. The private healthcare system is composed of modern for profit, modern not-for-profit, and traditional medicine.[42]

Morocco's key health institutions are the Centre Hospitalier et Universitaire Hassan II Fes, Centre Hospitalier Ibn Sina Rabat, Centre Hospitalier Mohammed VI Marrakech, Centre Hospitalier Universitaire Ibn Rochd Casablanca, and Polyclinique International de Rabat.[20]

HIV/AIDS Prevalence: Adults—95/100,000 (2007)[17]

Prevalence of TB: 79/100,000 (2006)[18]

Malaria: 75 cases reported (2007)[17]

Percent of Population Vaccinated: 90–95% (2007)[17]

Leading Causes of Death: Heart disease, perinatal conditions, perinatal diseases, respiratory infections

Infant Mortality Rate: 32/1000 live births (2007)[17]

Unusual Pathogens: Meningococcal outbreak (2000), human influenza epidemic (2003)[19]

OMAN

■ Demography

Population: 2,599,551 in 2007[13]

Religions: Islam

Ethnic Makeup: Arab

Languages: Arabic

Formerly Colonized: Occupied by Portuguese in the 16th century[44]

Politics/Governance: Islamic Sultanate

■ **Traditional Medicine**

Alternative systems of medicine are practiced by 53 licensed Chinese Medicine and Indian Herbal Medicine clinics.[44]

■ **Healthcare System**

Oman's healthcare system is provided by both public and private institutions. The Muscat Private Hospital and the Royal Hospital are the key health institutions.

HIV/AIDS Prevalence: No reported data

Prevalence of TB: 14/100,000 (2006)[18]

Malaria: 705 cases reported (2007)[17]

Percent of Population Vaccinated: 95–99% (2007)[17,18]

Leading Causes of Death: Heart disease, diabetes, cerebrovascular disease

Infant Mortality Rate: 3/1000 live births (2007)[17]

Unusual Pathogens: Meningococcal disease, serogroup W135 outbreak in 2000

PALESTINE

■ **Demography**

Population: 3,708,069 in 2007[13]

Religions: Muslim[45]

Ethnic Makeup: No official data, predominantly Arab

Languages: Arabic, English

Formerly Colonized: United Kingdom, mandate expired in 1948, currently occupied territory

Politics/Governance: The Palestinian authority political system is the new system for the Palestine following the Oslo Accord in 1993. It is built to be a Parliamentary system where there is an elected legislative council formed of 80 members elected from the northern and southern provinces (West Bank and Gaza Strip).[45]

■ **Healthcare System**

There are four major health service providers in Palestine: the Ministry of Health, the United Nations Relief and Work Agency (UNRWA), NGOs, and private for-profit providers.[45] The key health institutions include Alzari Hospital, European Gaza Hospital, Holy Family Hospital Bethelehem, Saint Joseph Hospital, and Saint John of Jerusalem Hospital.[20]

Prevalence of HIV/TB and Malaria: Data not available

Percent of Population Vaccinated: Data not available

Leading Causes of Death: Data not available

Infant Mortality Rate: Data not available

QATAR
■ Demography
Population: 836,082 in 2007[13]

Religions: Islam

Ethnic Makeup: 30% are Qatari nationals. The remainder is expatriates, mostly from India and Pakistan.[46]

Languages: Arabic, English

Formerly Colonized: United Kingdom, independence in 1971[46]

Politics/Governance: Islamic traditional monarchy[46]

■ Healthcare System
The Ministry of Health is the statutory health authority in the country. Private hospitals play a vital role in health provision. Medical services are provided free of charge to nationals. Al Emadi Hospital, Amercian Hospital Doha, and the Apollo Clinic Qatar are the key healthcare institutions.

HIV/AIDS Prevalence: No data available

Prevalence of TB: 73/100,000 (2006)[18]

Malaria: No data available

Percent of Population Vaccinated: 92–94% (2007)[17,18]

Leading Causes of Death: Heart disease, trauma, diabetes

Infant Mortality Rate: 8/1000 live births[17]

SAUDI ARABIA
■ Demography
Population: 24,157,431 in 2007[13]

Religions: Islam

Ethnic Makeup: Arab (90%), Afro-Asian (10%)[47]

Languages: Arabic (official), English[47]

Formerly Colonized: None

Politics/Governance: Monarchy

■ Traditional Medicine
The Ministry of Health recently established a traditional medicine department to supervise and control traditional medicine in the market.[48]

■ Healthcare System
There is a three-tier health care system: primary, secondary, and tertiary, corresponding respectively to health centers, general hospitals, and specialist hospitals.[48]

Saudi Arabia's key health institutions include the Jeddah Clinic Hospital Al Kandarah, Jeddah National Hospital (New Jeddah Clinic Hospital), King

Abdulaziz University Hospital, King Fahad Armed Forces Hospital, King Fahad Medical City, King Fahad Specialist Hospital Dammam, King Fahd General Hospital, King Fahd Hospital-Jeddah, and the Riyadh Care Hospital.

HIV/AIDS Prevalence: No data available

Prevalence of TB: 62/100,000 (2006)[18]

Malaria: 2864 cases reported (2007)[17]

Percent of Population Vaccinated: 96% (2007)[17,18]

Leading Causes of Death: Heart disease, respiratory infections

Infant Mortality Rate: 20/1000 live births (2007)[17]

Unusual Pathogens: Meningococcal disease, serogroup W135 outbreaks 2000 and 2001, Rift Valley fever in 2000[19]

SYRIA
■ Demography
Population: 19,890,585 in 2007[13]

Religions: Muslim majority, Christian minority

Ethnic Makeup: 90% of the population is Arab (90%), Kurds (9%)[50]

Languages: Arabic, Kurdish, Armenian, English, French

Formerly Colonized: France, independence in 1946

Politics/Governance: Constitutional Republic (single party)

■ Healthcare System
The healthcare system is a mixed public and private system. The key health institutions are the Al Bassel Heart Institute in Damascus, Al Kindi Hospital, Al Razi Hospital, Farah Hospital, Future Hospital, Lattakia National Hospital, Medical Cure Center Soufi Hospital, New Medical Center Dr. Hisham Sinan, Soued Hospital, and the Syrian American Medical Center.

HIV/AIDS Prevalence: No data available

Prevalence of TB: 40/100,000 (2006)[18]

Malaria: 37 cases reported (2007)[17]

Percent of Population Vaccinated: 96–99% (2007)[17,18]

Leading Causes of Death: Heart disease, Cerebrovascular disease, Perinatal diseases

Infant Mortality Rate: 15/1000 live births[17]

TUNISIA
■ Demography
Population: 10,225,400 in 2007[13]

Religions: Islam

Ethnic Makeup: Arab

Languages: Arabic (official), French

Formerly Colonized: France, obtained its independence in 1956

Politics/Governance: Republic

■ Healthcare System
The healthcare providers are mixed public and private sector. Patients pay user fees in public sector facilities. The key health care institutions are the Établissement Public de Santé Charles Nicolle, Institut Salah-Azaïz, Nouvelle Clinique du Parc, Polyclinique Chams, Polyclinique El Farabi, Polyclinique El Yassmine, Polyclinique Errahma, Polyclinique Hammamet, Polyclinique Les Berges du Lac, Polyclinique Les Palmiers, Polyclinique Les Violettes, Polyclinique Meignie, and the Polyclinique Taoufik.

HIV/AIDS Prevalence: 46/100,000 (2007)[17]

Prevalence of TB: 28/100,000 (2006)[18]

Malaria: No data reported

Percent of Population Vaccinated: 98%[17,18]

Leading Causes of Death: Heart disease, cerebrovascular disease, trauma

Infant Mortality Rate: 18/1000 (2007)[17]

TURKEY
■ Demography
Population: 73,885,055 in 2007[13]

Religions: Sunni Muslim majority, Christian and Jewish minorities

Languages: Turkish, Kurdish, Bulgarian, Armenian

Ethnic Makeup: Turkish, Kurdish, Arab, Armenians, Greeks

Formerly Colonized: Republic formed in 1923, formerly part of the Ottoman Empire

Politics/Governance: Secular Democracy

■ Traditional Medicine
Traditional medicine is common in turkey. Folk remedies are generally obtained from local plant species.[41]

■ Healthcare System
Turkey's health care is provided by public, semipublic, private, and philan-thropic institutions. Planning and provision of health services is done by the Provincial Health Directorates found in 81 provinces.[38]

HIV/AIDS Prevalence: Adults—3700 (2007)[38]

Prevalence of TB: 34/100,000 (2007)[17]

Malaria (2007): 358 cases reported (2007)[17,39]

Percentage of Population Vaccinated: 96%[17,18]

Leading Causes of Death: Cerebrovascular disease, heart disease, respiratory infections, perinatal conditions

Infant Mortality Rate: 21/1000 live births (2007)[17]

Unique Environmental Exposures: Asbestos contaminated soil mixtures have been found to cause malignant pleural mesothelioma in Anatolia, mainly in rural areas.[40]

UNITED ARAB EMIRATES
■ Demography
Population: 4,364,746 in 2007[13]

Religions: Sunni Muslim

Ethnic Makeup: UAE Arabs (20%), expatriate workers from South and Southeast Asia (60%), Arabs (Palestinians, Egyptians, Jordanians, Yemenis, and Omanis) as well as Iranians, Pakistanis, Indians, Bangladeshis, Afghanis, Filipinos, and Western Europeans (20%)[52]

Languages: Arabic (official), English

Formerly Colonized: United Kingdom, independence in 1971

Politics/Governance: Federation of seven monarchies

■ Traditional Medicine
Traditional remedies were widely prevalent in the years before the discovery of oil.[53] Although no policy currently exists for the regulation of traditional medicine, a policy is being developed.[54]

■ Healthcare System
Currently the UAE has a comprehensive, government-funded health service and is also developing a private health sector.[53]

HIV/AIDS Prevalence: No data reported (2007)[17]

Prevalence of TB: 24/100,000 (2006)[18]

Malaria: No data available

Percent of Population Vaccinated: 92% (2007)[17,18]

Leading Causes of Death: Heart disease, trauma, cerebrovascular disease

Infant Mortality Rate: 7/1000 live births (2007)[17]

YEMEN
■ Demography
Population: 22,383,108 in 2007[13]

Religions: Muslim majority (70% sunni, 30% Shia), Jewish minority[55]

Ethnic Makeup: Arab

Languages: Arabic (official), English

Formerly Colonized: The Northern part of the country was colonized by the Ottoman Empire and obtained independence in 1918. The southern part of the country was colonized by the United Kingdom and obtained independence in 1967.[55]

Politics/Governance: Republic since its unification in 1990

■ Traditional Medicine
Traditional medicine still plays an important role in Yemen. In many rural areas, it is the only medical assistance available.[56] The country lacks a national policy, laws, regulations, or national program for traditional medicine and there is no current plan to develop such policies. Herbal medicines are widely used and readily available.[54]

■ Healthcare System
The Public Health system provides 95% of the total health care and services.[56] Medications and vaccinations are provided by the public sector.

HIV/AIDS Prevalence: No data available

Prevalence of TB: 132/100,000 (2006)[18]

Malaria: 223,299 cases reported (2007)[17]

Percent of Population Vaccinated: 74–87% (2007)[17,18]

Leading Causes of Death: Respiratory infections, waterborne illness, perinatal conditions, heart disease

Infant Mortality Rate: 55/100 live births[17]

Unusual Pathogens: Acute hemorrhagic fever syndrome outbreak in 2000, poliomyelitis outbreak in 2005,[19] Rift Valley fever outbreak in 2000.

REFERENCES

1. Population Reference Bureau. Population trends and challenges in the Middle East and North Africa. http://www.prb.org/pdf/PoptrendsMiddleEast.pdf
2. Anne Maryse Pierre-Louis, Francisca Ayodeji Akala, and Hadia Samaha Karam. World Bank Institute. Public health in the Middle East and North Africa: meeting the challenges of the twenty-first century. http://www.wds.worldbank.org/servlet/WDSContentServer/WDSP/IB/2004/06/02/000112742_20040602161309/Rendered/PDF/291630Public0Health0in0theOMiddle0East.pdf. Accessed August 19, 2009.
3. Margie Pedenetal. World report on road traffic injury prevention, 2004. http://whqlibdoc.who.int/publications/2004/9241562609.pdf. Accessed August 19, 2009.

4. World Bank Institute. Better governance for development in the Middle East and North Africa Region: enhancing inclusiveness and accountability. 2004. http://www-wds.worldbank.org/servlet/WDSContentServer/WDSP/IB/2003/11/06/000090341_20031106135835/Rendered/PDF/271460PAPER0Be1ance0for0development.pdf. Accessed August 19, 2009.

5. WHO East Mediterranean Regional Office. The Work of the WHO in the East Mediterranean Region: Annual Report of the Regional Director. Cairo: World Health Organization 2005.

6. Anonymous. Public-health challenges in the Middle East and North Africa. *Lancet.* 367(2006):961–964.

7. The Middle East Forum. How the Arabs compare: Arab Human Development Report, 2002. http://www.meforum.org/article/513. Accessed August 19, 2009.

8. Jenkins C, Robalino DA. HIV/AIDS in the Middle East and North Africa: the costs of inaction, 2003. http://lnweb18.worldbank.org/MNA/mena.nsf/Attachments/menaaids-complete/$File/menaaids-complete.pdf. Accessed March 15, 2006.

9. Prüss-Üstün A, and Corvalán C. World Health Organization. Preventing disease through healthy environments: towards an estimate of the environmental burden of disease, 2006. http://www.who.int/quantifying_ehimpacts/publications/preventingdiseasebegin.pdf. Accessed March 15, 2007.

10. Farzaneh Roudi-Fahimi; Population Reference Bureau. Women's Reproductive Health in the Middle East and North Africa. http://www.prb.org/pdf/WomensReproHealth_Eng.pdf.

11. United Nations Children's Fund (UNICEF). Antenatal Care by Region. www.childinfo.org/eddb/antenatal/grpreg.htm.

12. United Nations Development Program (UNDP). Arab Human Development Report 2002: Creating Opportunities for Future Generations. http://www.arab-hdr.org/publications/other/ahdr/ahdr2002e.pdf.

13. The World Bank Group Quick Query. http://ddpext.worldbank.org/ext/DDPQQ/member.do?method=getMembers&userid=1&queryId=135. Accessed July 7, 2009.

14. American Library of Congress Federal Research Division. Country Profile: Algeria, 2008. http://memory.loc.gov/frd/cs/profiles/Algeria.pdf

15. AFDB & OECD. Algeria: African Economic Outlook, 2008. http://www.oecd.org/dataoecd/14/40/40573850.pdf

16. El-Jardali F, Makhoul J, Jamal D, and Tchaghchaghian V. Identification of Priority Research Questions Related to Health Financing, Human Resources for Health, and the Role of the Non-State Sector in Low and Middle Income Countries of the Middle East and North Africa Region. *Final Research Report—Alliance for Health Policy and Systems Research.* 2008.

17. World Health Organization. World Health Statistics. 2009.

18. WHO Statistical Information System (WHOSIS). http://www.who.int/statistics/en/

19. World Health Organization Country Information. http://www.who.int/ countries/en/

20. Ranking Web of World Hospitals. http://hospitals.webometrics.info/ hospital_by_country.asp?country=dz. Accessed July 27, 2009.

21. World Health Organization. Health System Profile: Bahrain, Regional Health Systems Observatory of the Eastern Mediterranean Regional Office. Geneva, Switzerland: World Health Organization; 2007.

22. World Health Organization. Health System Profile: Djobouti, Regional Health Systems Observatory of the Eastern Mediterranean Regional Office. Geneva, Switzerland: World Health Organization; 2006.

23. World Health Organization. Health System Profile: Egypt, Regional Health Systems Observatory of the Eastern Mediterranean Regional Office. Geneva, Switzerland: World Health Organization; 2006.

24. World Health Organization. National policy on traditional medicine and regulation of herbal medicines, Report of a WHO global survey, 2005. http://apps.who.int/medicinedocs/collect/medicinedocs/pdf/s7916e/ s7916e.pdf

25. American Library of Congress Federal Research Division, 2006. Country Profile: Iraq. http://memory.loc.gov/frd/cs/profiles/Iraq.pdf

26. World Health Organization. Health System Profile: Iraq, Regional Health Systems Observatory of the Eastern Mediterranean Regional Office. Geneva, Switzerland: World Health Organization; 2006.

27. World Health Organization. Health System Profile: Islamic Republic of Iran, Regional Health Systems Observatory of the Eastern Mediterranean Regional Office. Geneva, Switzerland: World Health Organization; 2006.

28. American Library of Congress Federal Research Division. Country Profile: Jordan. 2005. http://memory.loc.gov/frd/cs/profiles/Jordan.pdf

29. World Health Organization. Health System Profile: Jordan, Regional Health Systems Observatory of the Eastern Mediterranean Regional Office. Geneva, Switzerland: World Health Organization; 2006.

30. Afifi FU. Abu Irmaileh B. Herbal medicine in Jordan with special emphasis on less commonly used medicinal herbs. *Journal of Ethnopharmacology.* 72(2000):101–110.

31. World Health Organization. Health System Profile: Kuwait, Regional Health Systems Observatory of the Eastern Mediterranean Regional Office. Geneva, Switzerland: World Health Organization; 2006.

32. Division for Public Administration and Development Management (DPADM), Department of Economic and Social Affairs (UNDESA), United Nations, 2004. State of Kuwait Public Administration Country Profile. http://unpan1.un.org/intradoc/groups/public/documents/un/ unpan023178.pdf

33. United Nations 2006 Demographic Yearbook. Department of Economic and Social Affairs, 58th Issue, New York (ST/ESA/STAT/SER.R/37): United Nations; 2008.

34. World Health Organization. Health System Profile: Lebanon, Regional Health Systems Observatory of the Eastern Mediterranean Regional Office. Geneva, Switzerland: World Health Organization; 2006.

35. Ammar W. *Health Beyond Politics*. Beirut, Lebanon: World Health Organization: Eastern Mediterranean Regional Office and Ministry of Public Health in Lebanon; 2009.

36. American Library of Congress Federal Research Division, 2005. Country Profile: Libya. http://memory.loc.gov/frd/cs/profiles/Libya.pdf

37. World Health Organization. Health System Profile: Libya, Regional Health Systems Observatory of the Eastern Mediterranean Regional Office. Geneva, Switzerland: World Health Organization; 2007.

38. http://memory.loc.gov/frd/cs/profiles/Turkey.pdf

39. http://www.who.int/countryfocus/cooperation_strategy/ccsbrief_tur_en.pdf

40. Metintas S, Metintas M, Ucgun I, and Oner U. Malignant Mesothelioma due to Environmental Exposure to Asbestos: Follow-Up of a Turkish Cohort Living in a Rural Area. *Chest*. 122(2002):2224–2229.

41. Sezik, E., Yesilada, E., Honda, G., Takaishi, Y., Takeda, Y., and Tanaka, T. Traditional medicine in Turkey. X. Folk medicine in Central Anatolia. *Journal of Ethnopharmacology*. 75(2001):95–115.

42. World Health Organization. Health System Profile: Morocco, Regional Health Systems Observatory of the Eastern Mediterranean Regional Office. Geneva, Switzerland: World Health Organization; 2006.

43. American Library of Congress Federal Research Division, 2006. Country Profile: Morocco. http://memory.loc.gov/frd/cs/profiles/Morocco.pdf

44. World Health Organization. Health System Profile: Oman, Regional Health Systems Observatory of the Eastern Mediterranean Regional Office. Geneva, Switzerland: World Health Organization; 2006.

45. World Health Organization. Health System Profile: Palestine, Regional Health Systems Observatory of the Eastern Mediterranean Regional Office. Geneva, Switzerland: World Health Organization; 2006.

46. World Health Organization. Health System Profile: Qatar, Regional Health Systems Observatory of the Eastern Mediterranean Regional Office. Geneva, Switzerland: World Health Organization; 2006.

47. American Library of Congress Federal Research Division, 2006. Country Profile: Saudi Arabia. http://memory.loc.gov/frd/cs/profiles/Saudi_Arabia.pdf

48. World Health Organization. Health System Profile: Saudi Arabia, Regional Health Systems Observatory of the Eastern Mediterranean Regional Office. Geneva, Switzerland: World Health Organization; 2006.

49. World Health Organization. Health System Profile: Syria, Regional Health Systems Observatory of the Eastern Mediterranean Regional Office. Geneva, Switzerland: World Health Organization; 2006.

50. American Library of Congress Federal Research Division, 2005. Country Profile: Syria. http://memory.loc.gov/frd/cs/profiles/Syria.pdf

51. World Health Organization. Health System Profile: Tunisia, Regional Health Systems Observatory of the Eastern Mediterranean Regional Office. Geneva, Switzerland: World Health Organization; 2006.

52. American Library of Congress Federal Research Division, 2007. Country Profile: United Arab Emirates. http://memory.loc.gov/frd/cs/profiles/UAE.pdf

53. World Health Organization. Health System Profile: United Arab Emirates, Regional Health Systems Observatory of the Eastern Mediterranean Regional Office. Geneva, Switzerland: World Health Organization; 2006.

54. World Health Organization. World Health Organization National policy on traditional medicine and regulation of herbal medicines, Report of a WHO global survey. Geneva, Switzerland, World Health Organization; 2005. http://apps.who.int/medicinedocs/collect/medicinedocs/pdf/s7916e/s7916e.pdf

55. American Library of Congress Federal Research Division, 2008. Country Profile: Yemen. http://memory.loc.gov/frd/cs/profiles/Yemen.pdf

56. World Health Organization. Health System Profile: Yemen, Regional Health Systems Observatory of the Eastern Mediterranean Regional Office. Geneva, Switzerland: World Health Organization; 2006.

57. World Health Organization, *Highlights on Health in Israel, 2004*, WHO: 2004.

58. B. Rosen, H. Samuel, S. Merkur (ed), Israel, Health System Review, *Health Systems in Transition*, Vol. 11, No.2, 2009.

59. World Health Organization, Country Profile: Israel

60. World Health Organization, Immunization Profile: Israel

61. CIA Factbook, Israel

62. World Health Organzation, TB Country Profile: Israel

XVII ■ CENTRAL ASIA

Catherine Todd, MD, MPH
Samuel Yingst, DVM, PhD
Dmitriy Pereyaslov, MD, MPH

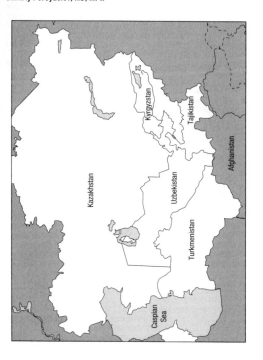

Central Asia is a geographical and cultural area including Kazakhstan, Kyrgyzstan, Tajikistan, Turkmenistan, and Uzbekistan. For the purposes of this chapter, we will be considering these countries with the addition of Afghanistan, which is often considered part of South Asia. Historically, this area has been host to traders, prophets, and armies from various regions, including the ancient Greeks (the empire of Alexander the Great extended through much of Central Asia), the pre-Islamic Sassanid Persians, and Mughal and Turkic tribes from whom the Khanates arose. These tribes included the historic rulers Timur Shah (Tamerlane) and Babur Shah, under whose Mughal Dynasty the arts, science, and education flourished. Islam became the predominant religion as trade routes opened through this region via the Silk Road connecting East and West.

Over the next centuries, the region was divided by a set of Khanates and other small tribal holdings, each with their own dialects and customs. The British Empire never made significant incursions into this region, challenged by Russian pressure from the north, in what is generally referred to as the Great Game.[1] Russian influence in the region became formalized when the Central Asian countries were absorbed into the Soviet Union, with the exception of Afghanistan, whose decade-long occupation is widely credited with having dissolved the Soviet Union.

Following the dissolution of the Soviet Union, these countries, with the exception of Afghanistan, have joined a loose political coalition, the Commonwealth of Independent States. Tajikistan and Afghanistan are emerging from prolonged civil wars with struggling democracies. Kazakhstan and Turkmenistan have a single party political system and relatively vigorous economies based on petroleum and natural gas reserves. Uzbekistan has a depressed economy with a single party political system that is still closely aligned with Russia. Kyrgyzstan had the most robust democracy in the region and is now strengthening ties with Russia.

CLIMATE AND GEOGRAPHY

The climate of Central Asia is one of extremes, with summer months characterized by very high temperatures and low humidity and winters with cold temperatures and snow throughout much of the region. The region itself has great geographic variation. There are desert regions in Turkmenistan (Karakum desert), southwestern Afghanistan (the Registan and Margow deserts), and parts of Uzbekistan (Kyzylkum and Karakum deserts). The Pamir, Altai, Tian Shan, and Hindu Kush mountain ranges run through multiple countries in the region and remain snow-covered most of the year. The Aral Sea, once one of the largest inland seas, has been the site of one of the largest ecological disasters in the former Soviet Union, where river waters feeding the sea were diverted for agriculture—predominantly cotton cultivation. By 2007, the sea had shrunk to 10% of its original size with excessive salinity and pollution resulting in loss of sea-based life, fallow surrounding land due to salt contamination, polluted drinking water and air, and climate change throughout the region. Due to the excessive shrinkage of the waters, there are now three lakes rather than one large body of water.[2] In 2005, a dam was erected to divert fresh water into the Small Aral Sea, the northernmost of the bodies of water in Kazakhstan; this is the sole body of water now able to sustain fish.

HUMAN DIVERSITY AND REGIONAL CULTURAL ISSUES

Central Asia has seen human presence for thousands of years and has been a region of substantial ethnic mixing for centuries, largely through trade routes and invading armies. The Central Asian states take their names from the predominant ethnic group in each country, with the exception of Afghanistan, which is comprised of three distinct ethnic groups. Islam is the predominant religion in the region though there are different sects and significant cultural variations on its practice present in each country.

During Soviet times, Russian served as a unifying language and there was a substantial influx of diverse groups from other parts of the Soviet Union, generally part of Stalin's resettlement campaign to dilute restive populations. Following the collapse of the Soviet Union, each country has returned to some extent to its local language and many ethnic minorities from other areas of the former Soviet Union have left the region, notably the Jewish, Ukrainian, and German populations forcibly resettled in Central Asia. Most local languages spoken in Central Asia (Kazakh, Kyrgyz, and Uzbek) are Turkic, while Tajik and Dari (spoken in Afghanistan) are derived from Persian Farsi. Pashto is spoken through most of Southern and Eastern Afghanistan and is linguistically dissimilar to the other languages in the region.

MAJOR HEALTH ISSUES

The major health issue for most of Central Asia is the challenge of meeting expectations for socialized medicine within impoverished, post-Soviet economies. Physical facilities, while having basic utilities and sturdy construction, are outdated and limited by overcrowding, inadequate technologic resources, and lack of availability of up-to-date diagnostics and medicines. Further, human resources, while sufficient in number in urban areas, are insufficient in supply in rural areas and provider training needs considerable updating. Lack of widespread, high-speed Internet access limits the use of resources available for continuing education; evidence-based practice is a largely unfamiliar concept. Private health care is available and most providers supplement their meager state salaries through private clinics; however, this standard of care is enjoyed by a small fraction of the population.

That said, health indicators for most of the Central Asian countries are generally far superior to the post-conflict settings of Tajikistan and Afghanistan.

Following the 1997 armistice of the civil war, Tajikistan has worked to rebuild its health infrastructure in the Soviet model and grapples with many of the same issues as its neighbor, Uzbekistan. However, Tajikistan has the lowest per capita spending for health at $71/person, as compared to $315 in Kazakhstan, $221 in Turkmenistan, $161 in Kyrgyzstan, and $159 in Uzbekistan.[3] Not surprisingly, this financial limitation translates to worse health indicators.

Afghanistan is still emerging from civil war, as armed conflict and displaced populations continue to present challenges to the nascent health system. The challenges are great: during the relative isolation of thirty years of civil war, there was essentially no remaining infrastructure and the health indicators for the Afghan population are among the worst in the world. A national health system is currently operating in all provinces, with 70% of the population estimated to have healthcare coverage.[4] However, low per capita health spending, reliance on international donors for the bulk of health subsidies, lack of trained health providers, and lack of access due to poor infrastructure and conflict present ongoing obstacles to available health care.

COUNTRY PROFILES OF CENTRAL ASIA

AFGHANISTAN

■ Demography

Population: 33.6 million people[5]

Religions: Islam, comprised of Sunni (80%) and Shia (19%) groups

Languages: Dari and Pashto, several regional languages (e.g., Uzbek, Turkman, Pashai, etc.)

Ethnic Makeup: Pashtun (42%), Tajik (27%), Hazara (9%), Uzbek (9%), Aimak (4%), Turkmen (3%), Baloch (2%), other (4%)[5]

Historical Background: Multiple invading armies, from the Greeks to the Persians, occupied Afghanistan for various periods in the past. More recently, Afghanistan was a barrier to further British incursion during the British Empire, known as the Great Game, and eventually repelled the Soviets following a 10-year occupation in the 1980s.[1]

Politics/Governance: Islamic Republic; Parliamentary Democracy with mixed civil and Sharia-based legal system

■ Traditional Medicine

Hakim-jis serve as informal medical providers in many communities and provide traditional treatments or charms accompanied by prayers. In many rural areas, modern pharmaceuticals are not available and traditional medications, including those made with opium, are used.

■ Healthcare System

Afghanistan's health system is ranked #173 out of 190 countries in overall performance in 2000. More recently, it has one of the lowest human development index values of 0.312.[6]

There are essentially two healthcare systems: a government system, operated by contracted NGOs, and private practitioners. Based on legislation, all services provided in government facilities are free of charge. However, supplies, medications, and laboratory services may not be available within the government facility, necessitating out-of-pocket expenditures.

Medications are provided by the government for inpatient care and for some illnesses (e.g., tuberculosis) as supplies permit. However, many medications are available from pharmacies with few prescription requirements and of widely varying quality. The government quality assurance system for pharmaceuticals is still in development.

There are roughly two physicians and 0.3 midwives or nurses per every 10,000 people. Cultural limitations prevent widespread distribution of female providers and women are often not permitted to receive care from male providers.[7]

Percent of Population Vaccinated: Vaccination rates are slowly improving, but polio cases are still reported in Afghanistan. The most recent national statistics (2005) indicate coverage rates of 73% for BCG (TB), 76% for oral polio vaccine and DTaP series, and 64% for measles vaccination among one-year olds.[9]

HIV: < 1000 cases reported (< 0.01% of population)

TB: 25,440 were treated in 2005[10]

Malaria: Endemic in several provinces, 591,441 cases were reported in 2003, with *P. vivax* and *P. falciparum* the circulating strains.[11]

Leading Causes of Death: Though the health infrastructure and statistical reporting systems are being established and strengthened, it is difficult to know the definitive cause of death in many cases. That said, infectious diseases (principally diarrheal diseases) among children, and maternal causes (principally hemorrhage and obstructed labor) among women, contribute substantially. Furthermore, ongoing conflict and displacement lead to many deaths by violence and malnutrition.

Infant Mortality Rate: Total: 152.0 deaths/1000 live births; male: 156.0 deaths/1000 live births; female: 147.7 deaths/1000 live births[5]

Life expectancy at birth: 44.6 years (44.4 Male; 44.8 Female)[5]

Unusual Pathogens: H5N1 has been identified in Afghanistan, with risk limited to those handling infected birds.[12] Infectious disease surveillance efforts are expanding but limitations in cold chain and laboratory diagnostics prevent greater availability of accurate data.

Unique Environmental Exposures: Much of Afghanistan's terrain is not accessible by road due to mountains, deserts, or other challenging environments. Health facilities often require travel by horseback or on foot to gain access.

Drug Dependence: Afghanistan is not only the largest global opium producer, but also has one of the highest levels of opium use (1.4% of the population) globally.[13]

KAZAKHSTAN

■ Demography

Population: 15.5 million (2007 estimate)

The population density in Kazakhstan is the lowest in WHO's European Region (with the exception of Iceland).[14]

Religions: Muslim (mostly Sunnis; 47%), Christians (Russian Orthodox; 44%), Protestant (2%), other (7%) (1996 estimate)[15]

Language: Kazakh (official; 64.4%), Russian (official; 95%) (2001 estimate)[15]

Ethnic Groups: Kazakh (53.4%), Russian (30%), Ukrainian (3.7%), German (2.4%), Uzbek (2.5%), Tatar (1.7%), Uighur (1.4%), other (4.9%) (1999 estimate)[15]

Historical Background: Kazakhstan was under tsarist rule from Russia from 1850. After the Revolution, the country began an Autonomous Soviet Socialist Republic of the USSR in 1925, and in 1936 was declared a full Soviet Socialist Republic. Kazakhstan was the last Soviet republic to declare independence on December 16, 1991, after the collapse of the USSR.[16]

Politics/Governance: Republic.

■ Healthcare System

Kazakhstan's health system is ranked 64th of 190 countries by WHO in 2000.[17] The government system is based somewhat on the Soviet Semashko model. The state owns most health facilities. At the top of the health system hierarchy is the Ministry of Health, but the 14 oblast (regional) departments have considerable autonomy in administration health services in their area. The main functions of the Ministry of Health are formulating policy, preparing legislation, commissioning research, developing reform strategies, monitoring population health, supervising the implementation of reforms, and ensuring the training of health personnel.

Health care is funded mainly from the national budget, with 2.5% of the gross domestic product (GDP) allotted for health in 2005. This figure underestimates the actual level of healthcare revenue, since out-of-pocket payments accounted for 35.8% of total health expenditure. WHO-produced estimates accounting for substantial out-of-pocket payments by the population suggest that the total health expenditure in 2005 was 3.9% of GDP.[14] The healthcare facility budget consist of 38 line items, which are estimated based on the previous year expenditures with the addition of a per capita formula.

The Ministry of Health, according to Decree 70 (1999), prepares a list of services that are provided to the public for a fee. Socially vulnerable groups and certain diagnostic groups such as cancer patients are free from outpatient drug charges and the cost is covered by the government.

Official policy states that the medications for inpatient care should be supplied by the hospital, but patients have to buy medications even for inpatient care. Pharmaceutical expenditures accounts for 2.5% of total health expenditures (2000 estimate).[14,18]

Percent of Population Vaccinated: 93–99% of one-year olds complete the basic vaccination series (BCG, DTP, Hepatitis B, Polio, Rubella); 99% of one-year-olds have received the measles vaccination (2007 estimate).[14]

HIV: Estimated incidence = 11.4/100,000 with 1745 incident cases in 2006. The estimated number of people living with HIV/AIDS as of July 1, 2008 was 10,601 (population prevalence < 0.1%). A total of 703 AIDS cases were registered.[14,19,20] A major HIV outbreak occurred among children in Shymkent, attributable to nosocomial transmission.[16]

TB: Estimated incidence = 129/100,000 (2007 estimate); Estimated prevalence = 139/100,000 (2007 estimate); multidrug-resistant tuberculosis (MDR-TB) present in 14% of all new TB cases.[21]

Malaria: In 2007, two cases were reported.[14]

Leading Causes of Death: Ischemic heart disease; cerebrovascular disease; poisoning; self-inflicted injuries; hypertensive heart disease; chronic obstructive pulmonary disease; tuberculosis; respiratory system cancers; lower respiratory infections; and cirrhosis of the liver (2002).[22]

Infant Mortality Rates: 28/1000 live births (2007 estimate)[23]

Life expectancy at birth: Total population: 66.4 years; male: 60.8 years; female: 72.3 years (2007 estimate). Life expectancy among women was 11.5 years greater than among men; this is the highest gap in the Central Asian Region.[14]

Unusual Pathogens: Arboviral diseases,[24,25] leishmaniasis,[26–28] echinococcosis,[29,30] and travelers' diarrhea[31] have all been reported.

Unique Environmental Exposures: The Semipalatinsk (Semey) region was the major nuclear testing area for the USSR.[18] Shrinkage of the Aral Sea has great environmental impacts that could affect human health, including salinization of the water table, pesticides in the environment and food chain, dust storms, and air quality.[32] The Pamir, Tien-shan, and Altai mountain ranges in the east and Himalayas to the south of the country have associated harsh conditions and risk of acute mountain sickness for those traveling at high altitudes.

Drug Dependence: The prevalence of drug abuse is growing (incidence rate of 65.3/100,000), leading to increasing HIV infection rates. Injecting drug use is the main route of transmission of HIV in Kazakhstan, accounting for more than 70% of reported cases. In 2007, 55,286 drug abusers were officially registered.[19,33]

KYRGYZSTAN

■ Demography

Population: 5.4 million[34]

Religions: Muslim (75%), Russian Orthodox (20%), other (5%)[34]

Languages: Kyrgyz (official; 64.7%), Uzbek (13.6%), Russian (official; 12.5%), Dungun (1%), other (8.2%)[34]

Ethnic Makeup: Kyrgyz (64.9%), Uzbek (13.8%), Russian (12.5%), Dungan (1.1%), Ukrainian (1%), Uighur (1%), other (5.7%)[34]

Historical Background: Kyrgyzstan was under tsarist rule from Russia from 1876, then annexed into the Soviet Union from 1936–1991.

Politics/Governance: Republic.

■ Healthcare System

Kyrgyzstan's health system is ranked 151st of 190 countries by WHO in 2000.[3] The government system is based somewhat on the Soviet model with multiple directorates for various aspects of the system organized and answerable to the Ministry of Health. However, the Mandatory Health Insurance Fund is the "single payer" and comes under the auspices of the Ministry of Finance. This insurance plan is compulsory and 40% of funds are derived from out-of-pocket payments. Efforts are underway to combine vertical programs, like immunization, into the national system. Since the 1990s, a private provider system has evolved.[35]

   The government provides medication for inpatients. Most pharmacies have been privatized since 1996 and a chief source of out-of-pocket health expenditures is medications.

Percent of Population Vaccinated: 94–99% of one-year-olds complete the basic vaccination series (e.g., polio, DTaP, and hepatitis B); 99% of one-year-olds have received measles vaccination.[36]

HIV/AIDS: The estimated number of people living with HIV/AIDS by the end of 2007 was 4200 (< 0.1%).

TB: Estimated incidence = 138.2/100,000; Multidrug-resistant tuberculosis (MDR-TB) is present, particularly among incarcerated populations.[14]

Malaria: An epidemic (2267 cases) occurred in 2002 attributed to in-migration from Tajikistan and favorable weather conditions. Cases were largely *P. vivax*, though some cases of *P. falciparum* were diagnosed in areas bordering Uzbekistan. By 2007, only 96 cases were reported.[37]

Leading Causes of Death: Heart disease, pneumonia and influenza, lung cancer, stomach cancer, colon cancer, liver cancer, self-inflicted injuries, kidney disease, and pancreatic cancer.

Infant Mortality Rates: 58 deaths/1000 live births[38]

Life Expectancy: Total population: 69.4 years; male: 65.4 years; female: 73.6 years[34]

Unusual Pathogens: Anthrax and brucellosis outbreaks are common, particularly in rural areas where these diseases are transmitted through contact with infected domestic animals. Tick-borne encephalitis is also present in rural areas and vaccination is recommended.[39]

Unique Environmental Exposures: Approximately 90% of Kyrgyzstan is mountainous, with harsh conditions and risk of acute mountain sickness for those traveling at high altitudes. There is mounting regional concern regarding the rising rates of cancer in areas where uranium tailings are stored, some of which are close to groundwater supplies and are in poor repair. These tailings are from mines that operated during the Soviet period.

Drug Dependence: As with other Central Asian countries, there are opium trafficking routes throughout the country and opiate dependence is rising, with 0.8% of the total population estimated to abuse opiates.[13] Trends towards injection in Kyrgyzstan are particularly concerning, with an explosive HIV epidemic among injecting users reported in Osh in 2005.[40]

TAJIKISTAN

■ Demography

Population: 7.5 million[41]

Ethnic Makeup: Tajik, Uzbek, Russian, Kyrgyz

Religions: Sunni Muslim, Shia Muslim

Languages: Tajik (official), Russian (widely used in government and business)

Historical Background: The Tajik people came under Russian rule in the 1860s and 1870s, but Russia's hold on Central Asia weakened following the Revolution of 1917. Bolshevik control of the area was fiercely contested and not fully reestablished until 1925. Much of present-day Soghd province was transferred from the Uzbek SSR to the newly formed Tajik SSR in 1929. Ethnic Uzbeks form a substantial minority in Soghd province. Tajikistan became independent in 1991 following the breakup of the Soviet Union, and experienced a civil war between regional factions from 1992–1997. There have been no major security incidents in recent years, although the country remains the poorest in the former Soviet sphere. Attention by the international community since the beginning of the NATO intervention in Afghanistan has brought increased economic development and security assistance, which could create jobs and strengthen stability in the long term. Tajikistan is in the early stages of seeking World Trade Organization membership and has joined NATO's Partnership for Peace.

Politics/Governance: Republic

■ Healthcare System

Tajikistan's health system is ranked 154th of 190 countries by WHO in 2000.[3] It has inherited the Soviet medical system, rigidly structured around an elaborate network of health facilities, with emphasis on inpatient care (108 beds/10,000 population) and high numbers of doctors (1 doctor/500 population). Expenditure on health is just US $2.50 per capita (1998)—less than 2% of GDP. The service is financed through central and local taxation: the MOH determines the structure and capacities of the Republican health facilities, but the regional and local facilities are provided by the local administration—the *Hukumat*. Although theoretically free of charge, the underfunding means that patients pay for almost all services—they will pay for drugs, dressings, and doctors will expect additional payments. The 3000 health facilities are in poor condition, ill-equipped, and inaccessible to the considerable population living in isolated areas. Doctors working in the community have received no postgraduate training; nurses are also poorly trained, and held in low esteem. At current rates of exchange, doctors and nurses in the community receive a state salary of between US $1.8–$2.8 per month. As a result, there are an increasing number of rural health posts being unfilled, as well as a reduction in student intake to medical universities and colleges.[42]

Percent of Population Vaccinated: Vaccination rates are rising, though there is still room for improvement (81–89% of one-year-olds complete a basic vaccination series, e.g., measles, polio, DTP, and hepatitis B), but Tajikistan is reportedly polio free.[45]

HIV/AIDS = Estimated HIV/AIDS prevalence is 123/100,000

TB = 16,000 cases per year (approx 16% MDR)

Malaria: 5000 cases per year (mix of *P. falciparum* and *P. vivax*—steadily declining from a peak of incidence of 30,000 per year in 1997)[46]

Leading Causes of Death: Ischemic heart disease, hypertensive heart disease, lower respiratory infections, perinatal conditions, cerebrovascular disease, diarrheal disease, cirrhosis of the liver, tuberculosis, meningitis, and chronic obstructive pulmonary disease

Infant Mortality Rate: 57 deaths/1000 live births[45]

Under-5 Mortality Rate: 118 deaths/1000 live births[47]

Maternal Mortality Rate: 100/100,000 deliveries[47]

Life Expectancy: Male: 63 years of age; female: 66 years of age[47]

Unusual Pathogens: Clean water access remains limited and as a result, fecal-oral diarrheal diseases including cholera, hepatitis A, and rotavirus are common.[42] Hepatitis B and C prevalence is not well defined, but in some subpopulations, rates are reportedly high.[43] Regardless, prevalence appears to be frequent enough that transmission through transfusion may occur.[44] CCHF and other arboviral disease occurs occasionally and Brucellosis incidence is among the highest in the world.[48]

Unique Environmental Exposures: Much of Tajikistan is mountainous, with harsh conditions. Acute mountain sickness is a risk for those traveling at high altitudes. As with Kyrgyzstan, concern regarding the health implications of uranium tailing storage is a current issue.[49]

Drug Dependence: As with other Central Asian countries, there are opium trafficking routes through the country, particularly along the vast, porous border with Afghanistan. Opiate use, particularly injecting use, is on the rise and HIV epidemics related to drug injection have been reported in Dushanbe.[50]

TURKMENISTAN

■ Demography

Population: 4.9 million[51]

Ethnic Makeup: Turkmen, Uzbek, Russian

Religions: Muslim, Eastern Orthodox

Languages: Turkmen, Russian, Uzbek

Historical Background: Eastern Turkmenistan for centuries formed part of the Persian province of Khurasan; in medieval times Merv (today known as Mary) was one of the great cities of the Islamic world and an important stop on the Silk Road. Annexed by Russia between 1865 and 1885, Turkmenistan became a Soviet republic in 1924. It achieved independence upon the dissolution of the USSR in 1991. Extensive hydrocarbon/natural gas reserves could prove a boon to this underdeveloped country if extraction and delivery projects were to be expanded. The Turkmenistan Government is actively seeking to develop alternative petroleum transportation routes to break Russia's pipeline monopoly. President Saparmurat Niyazov ("Turkmenbashi") died in December 2006 after 16 years of rule marked by the continuation of communism and development of a personality cult, where days of the week were named for his family members. Turkmenistan held its first multicandidate presidential electoral process in February 2007. Gurbanguly Berdimuhamedov, a vice premier under Niyazov, emerged as the country's new president.

Politics/Governance: Republic; authoritarian presidential rule, with little power outside the executive branch.

Turkmenistan is a closed society and very little health information is openly available.

Health system ranked 153rd of 190 countries by WHO in 2000.[3]

■ Healthcare System

Although WHO ranked Turkmenistan's health system at 153rd of 190 countries in 2000,[3] it is a closed society and very little health information is openly available.

In the post-Soviet era, reduced funding has put the health system in poor condition. In 2002, Turkmenistan had 50 hospital beds per 10,000 population, less than half the number in 1996. Overall policy has targeted specialized inpatient facilities to the detriment of basic outpatient care. Since the late 1990s, many rural facilities have closed, making care available principally in urban areas. President Niyazov's 2005 proposal to close all hospitals outside Ashgabat intensified this trend. Physicians are poorly trained, modern medical techniques are rarely used, and medications are in short supply. In 2004 Niyazov dismissed 15,000 medical professionals, exacerbating the shortage of personnel. In some cases, professionals have been replaced by military conscripts. Private health care is rare, as the state maintains a near monopoly. Free public health care was abolished in 2004.[52]

Percent of Population Vaccinated: An extensive vaccination system has resulted in 98–99% of one-year-olds completing a basic vaccination series, (e.g., measles, polio, DTP, and hepatitis B), and Turkmenistan is polio free.[53]

HIV/AIDS: Estimated HIV/AIDS rate < 100/100,000

TB (Prevalence): 78/100,000 population, (incidence) = 65/100,000 population per year with a low MDR TB rate (4%)

Malaria: Present, but low incidence[54]

Leading Causes of Death: Cardiovascular disease, cancer, and respiratory disease. Major adverse health factors are poor diet, polluted drinking water, and the industrial and agricultural pollutants that are especially concentrated in the northeastern areas near the Amu Darya River and the Aral Sea.[52]

Infant/Under-5 Mortality Rate: 45–50/1000 live births[53]

Life Expectancy: Male: 60; female: 67 years[54]

Unique Environmental Exposures: Much of Turkmenistan is desert, with harsh conditions and risk of severe dehydration for travelers.

Drug Dependence: As with other Central Asian countries, there are opium trafficking routes through the country; however, little is known regarding opiate consumption within Turkmenistan.[50]

UZBEKISTAN

Population: 26.9 million (2007 estimate)[14]

Religions: Muslim (mostly Sunnis), Christians (Russian Orthodox)[55]

Language: Uzbek (official), Russian, Tajik (4.4%)[55]

Ethnic Makeup: Uzbek, Russian, Tajik, Kazakh, Karakalpak, Tatar[55]

Historical Background: Uzbekistan was under tsarist rule from Russia from 1876. In 1918, after the Revolution, the Autonomous Republic of Turkistan was given official status within the new Soviet state. In 1924 the Soviet Socialist Republic of Uzbekistan was declared. The history of modern Uzbekistan started in 31 August 1991 after a declaration of independence following dissolution of the Soviet Union.[56]

Politics/Governance: Republic

Health system ranked 117th of 190 countries by WHO in 2000.[3]

■ Healthcare System

Uzebekistan's health system ranked 117th of 190 countries by WHO in 2000.[3] The government system is based somewhat on the Soviet Semashko model. The responsibility for developing national health policies falls to the Cabinet of Ministers, headed by President. The Ministry of Health is responsible for organization, planning, and management of the healthcare system. Regional (tuman) health administrations are responsible for developing strategies at the regional level and managing their healthcare services. The healthcare system is financed by taxes. In 1991, user fees were officially permitted. Official user charges are collected for outpatient medicines and some healthcare services, with an exemption or reduction in payments for children, disabled people, and other vulnerable groups. In 2005, the share of official user charges in the public sector accounted for 5.8% of total government funding.

    The healthcare budget includes 18 line items, with the Ministry of Finance determining resource distribution.[56,57] In 1994, the private medical practice was legalized. By 1999, about 20% of health care was provided by private hospitals and polyclinics and accounted for 5.8% of the health budget. Total health care expenditure accounted for 2.4% of gross domestic product (GDP) in 2005. This figure underestimates the actual level of healthcare revenue, since substantial out-of-pocket payments by the population are not included. WHO-produced estimates suggest that total health expenditures in 2005 were 5.0% of GDP.[14]

The government provides medications for inpatients for emergency care, care for "socially significant and hazardous" conditions, and specialized care for vulnerable groups. Patients not included in those categories must purchase medicines out-of-pocket. The government controls the medication prices within a 50% top limit of the purchase price of the wholesaler.[57]

Percent of Population Vaccinated: 94–99% of one-year-olds complete the basic vaccination series (BCG, DTP, Hepatitis B, Polio); 98% of one-year-olds have received measles vaccination (2008 estimate)[58]

HIV/AIDS: Estimated incidence = 8.3/100,000 with 2205 of new persons to whom HIV seropositive test was found during 2007. Estimated number of people living with HIV/AIDS as of July 1, 2008 is 14,033 < 0.1%.[14,59,60]

TB: Estimated incidence = 113/100,000 (2007 estimate); estimated prevalence = 140/100,000 (2007 estimate); MDR TB present in 15% of all new TB cases.[21]

Malaria: In 2007, 89 cases and one death due to malaria were reported with majority of registered cases in the Surkhandarya region.[14,61]

Leading Causes of Death: Heart disease, cerebrovascular disease, respiratory infections, liver disease, tuberculosis, COPD[62]

Infant Mortality Rates: Total: 36/1000 live births (2007 estimate)[22]

Life Expectancy: Total population: 70.5 years; male: 68.2 years; female: 73.0 years[14]

Unusual Pathogens: Arboviral diseases,[63–64] leishmaniasis,[26,27] echinococcosis,[65,66] and travelers' diarrhea[67] have all been reported in Uzbekistan.

Unique Environmental Exposures: The shrinking of the Aral Sea has great environmental impacts that could affect human health—the salinization of the water table, pesticides in the environment and food chain, dust storms, and air quality.[32] Water supply sources are polluted; piped water is not available everywhere, especially in rural areas.[68]

Drug Dependence: The level of drug abuse is increasing, with resultant burgeoning HIV infection prevalence. In 2007, 21,465 drug abusers were registered in Uzbekistan. Injecting drug use is the leading route of HIV transmission; 6446 infections among injecting drug users (46% of total) were reported for 2008. Uzbekistan has the highest HIV prevalence of the Central Asian countries.[33,60]

REFERENCES

1. Hopkirk P. *The Great Game: The Struggle for Empire in Central Asia.* New York: Kodansha International; 1992.
2. Micklin P. The Aral Sea Disaster. *Annu. Rev. Earth Planet. Sci.* 2007; 35:47–72. 10.1146/annurev.earth.35.031306.140120
3. World Health Organization. World Health Report 2006. http://www.eolc-observatory.net/global_analysis/tajikistan_health_care.htm. Accessed July 4, 2009.
4. Waldman R, Strong L, Wali A. Afghanistan's Health System Since 2001: Condition improved, prognosis cautiously optimistic. Afghanistan Research and Evaluation Unit: Kabul, Afghanistan; 2006.
5. Central Intelligence Agency. The World Factbook: Afghanistan. https://www.cia.gov/library/publications/the-world-factbook/geos/AF.html. Accessed July 4, 2009.
6. United Nations Development Program. Human Development Report 2007/2008—Afghanistan. http://hdrstats.undp.org/countries/data_sheets/cty_ds_AFG.html. Accessed July 4, 2009.
7. WHO, Eastern Mediterranean Regional Office. Afghanistan country profile. http://www.emro.who.int/emrinfo/index.asp?Ctry=afg. Accessed July 4, 2009.
8. United Nations Childrens Fund. Statistics—Afghanistan. http://www.unicef.org/infobycountry/afghanistan_statistics.html. Accessed July 4, 2009.
9. Afghanistan Online: Number of Afghan patients treated for TB doubled since 2001. March 29, 2007. http://www.afghan-web.com/health/tb_treat.html. Accessed July 4, 2009.
10. Doocy SC, et al. Population-based tuberculin skin testing and prevalence of tuberculosis infection in Afghanistan. *World Health Popul.* 2008; 10:44–53.
11. World Health Organization. World Malaria Report, Afghanistan Country Page. http://rbm.who.int/wmr2005/profiles/afghanistan.pdf. Accessed July 4, 2009.
12. Leslie T, et al. Knowledge, Attitudes, and Practices regarding Avian Influenza (H5N1), Afghanistan. *Emerg Infect Dis.* 2008;14:1459–1461.
13. United Nations Office on Drugs and Crime. World Drug Report 2007. Slovakia: United Nations Publications.
14. European Health for All Database (HFA-DB) [computer program]. Version January 2009. Copenhagen: World Health Organization, Regional Office for Europe, Health Information Unit; 2009.
15. Central Intelligence Agency. World Fact Book: Kazakhstan. https://www.cia.gov/cia/publications/factbook/index.html. Accessed July 3, 2009.
16. Kulzhanov M, Rechel B. European Observatory on Health Systems and Policies. Health care systems in transition: Kazakhstan: health system review. Copenhagen: World Health Organization, Regional Office for Europe; 2007.
17. World Health Organization. The World Health Report 2000: Health systems: improving performance. Geneva, Switzerland: World Health Organization; 2000.

18. World Health Organization, European Observatory on Health Care Systems. Health care systems in transition: Kazakhstan. Copenhagen: World Health Organization Regional Office for Europe; 1999.

19. United Nations Office on Drugs and Crime. Statistics: Kazakhstan. http://www.unodc.org/uzbekistan/en/fact_sheets.html. Accessed July 3, 2009.

20. World Health Organization, Regional Office for Europe. Kazakhstan: HIV/AIDS Data Summary. August 5, 2008. http://www.euro.who.int/aids/ctryinfo/overview/20060118_24. Accessed July 3, 2009.

21. World Health Organization. Global tuberculosis control: epidemiology, planning, financing: WHO report 2009. Geneva, Switzerland: World Health Organization; 2009.

22. World Health Organization. Mortality Country Fact Sheet 2006: Kazakhstan. World Health Organization. http://www.who.int/whosis/mort/profiles/mort_euro_kaz_kazakhstan.pdf. Accessed July 3, 2009.

23. World Health Organization. World health statistics 2009. Geneva, Switzerland: World Health Organization; 2009.

24. Rudakov N, Shpynov S, Fournier PE, Raoult D. Ecology and molecular epidemiology of tick-borne rickettsioses and anaplasmoses with natural foci in Russia and Kazakhstan. *Ann N Y Acad Sci.* 2006;1078:299–304.

25. Onishchenko GG, Tumanova I, Vyshemirskii OI, Kuhn J, Seregin SV, Tiunnikov GI, et al. [Study of virus contamination of Ixodes ticks in the foci of Crimean-Congo hemorrhagic fever in Kazakhstan and Tajikistan]. *Zh Mikrobiol Epidemiol Immunobiol.* 2005;1:27–31.

26. Rapoport LP. [Landscape and geographical distribution of natural reservoirs of human vector-borne diseases in Southern Kazakhstan and Kirghizia]. *Med Parazitol (Mosk).* 1999;4:26–29.

27. Ponirovskii EN, Strelkova MV, Goncharov DB, Zhirenkina EN, Chernikova Iu A. [Visceral leishmaniasis in the Commonwealth of Independent States (CIS): results and basic lines of further study]. *Med Parazitol (Mosk).* 2006;4:25–31.

28. Utepbergenova GA, Medetov JB, Mamikova HU, Aiapbergenova GS. [Spreading of Zoonotic Cutaneous Leishmaniasis in Southern Kazakhstan]. *Siberian Medical Journal, Irkutsk.* 2008;7:112–113.

29. Torgerson PR, Rosenheim K, Tanner I, Ziadinov I, Grimm F, Brunner M, et al. Echinococcosis, toxocarosis and toxoplasmosis screening in a rural community in eastern Kazakhstan. *Trop Med Int Health.* 2009;14:341–348.

30. Torgerson PR, Shaikenov BS, Rysmukhambetova AT, Ussenbayev AE, Abdybekova AM, Burtisurnov KK. Modelling the transmission dynamics of Echinococcus granulosus in dogs in rural Kazakhstan. *Parasitology.* 2003;126 (Pt 5):417–424.

31. Kazakhstan. http://www.travmed.com/guide/country.php?c=Kazakhstan. Accessed July 3, 2009.

32. Small I, van der Meer J, Upshur RE. Acting on an environmental health disaster: the case of the Aral Sea. *Environ Health Perspect.* 2001;109(6):547–549.

33. United Nations Office on Drugs and Crime, Regional Office for Central Asia. Compendium of Drug Related Statistics, 1997–2008. Tashkent: United Nations Office on Drugs and Crime; June 2008.

34. Central Intelligence Agency. The World Factbook: Kyrgyzstan. https://www.cia.gov/library/publications/the-world-factbook/geos/KG.html. Accessed July 4, 2009.

35. Meimanaliev AS, Ibraimova A, Elebesov B, Rechel B. European Observatory on Health Systems and Policies. Health Care Systems in Transition: Kyrgyzstan, Vol. 7, No. 2, 2005.

36. United Nations Childrens Fund. Statistics—Kyrgyzstan. http://www.unicef.org/infobycountry/kyrgyzstan_statistics.html. Accessed July 4, 2009.

37. World Health Organization, Regional Office for Europe—Malaria—Kyrgyzstan. http://www.euro.who.int/malaria/ctryinfo/affected/20020712_17. Accessed July 4, 2009.

38. United Nations Childrens Fund. Statistics—State of the World's Children 2007: Gender Equality. http://www.unicef.org/sowc07/statistics/statistics.php. Accessed July 4, 2009.

39. Travel Medicine. Kyrgyzstan updated travel health information. http://www.travmed.com/guide/country.php?c=Kyrgyzstan. Accessed July 4, 2009.

40. World Health Organization. Country profile: Kyrgyzstan, WHO 3x5. http://www.who.int/3by5/support/june2005_kgz.pdf. Accessed July 4, 2009.

41. Central Intelligence Agency. The World Factbook: Tajikistan. https://www.cia.gov/library/publications/the-world-factbook/geos/TI.html. Accessed July 4, 2009.

42. Department for International Development Resource Centre for Health Sector Reform. Tajikistan: Health Briefing Paper. http://www.dfidhealthrc.org/publications/Country_health/Tajikistan.pdf. Accessed July 4, 2009.

43. Glikberg F, Brawer-Ostrovsky J, Ackerman Z. Very high prevalence of hepatitis B and C in Bukharian Jewish immigrants to Israel. *J Clin Gastroenterol*. 1997;24:30–33.

44. World Bank. Tajikistan—Blood Risks in Central Asia. http://web.worldbank.org/WBSITE/EXTERNAL/COUNTRIES/ECAEXT/TAJIKISTANEXTN/0,,contentMDK:21788209~pagePK:141137~piPK:141127~theSitePK:258744,00.html. Accessed July 4, 2009.

45. United Nations Childrens Fund. Statistics—Tajikistan. http://www.unicef.org/infobycountry/tajikistan_statistics.html. Accessed July 4, 2009.

46. World Health Organization. Tajikistan. http://www.who.int/countries/tjk/en/. Accessed July 4, 2009.

47. World Health Organization. Mortality Country Fact Sheet: Tajikistan. http://www.who.int/whosis/mort/profiles/mort_euro_tjk_tajikistan.pdf. Accessed July 4, 2009.

48. United Nations Food Agriculture Organization (FAO). Brucellosis in Tajikistan Seroprevalence Survey. http://www.untj.org/files/reports/Tajik%20Brucellosis%20Survey.pdf. Accessed July 4, 2009.

49. Ferghana.Ru Information Agency. Central Asia News: Soviet-Era Uranium Waste Sites Now Threaten Central Asia. May 20, 2009. http://enews.ferghana.ru/article.php?id=2536. Accessed July 4, 2009.

50. Corporal LL. Central Asia: Intravenous Drug Use Feeds HIV Pandemic. August 21, 2007. http://www.aegis.com/news/ips/2007/IP070813.html. Accessed July 4, 2009.

51. Central Intelligence Agency. The World Factbook: Turkmenistan. https://www.cia.gov/library/publications/the-world-factbook/geos/TX.html

52. Library of Congress, Federal Research Division. Country Profile: Turkmenistan. http://lcweb2.loc.gov/frd/cs/profiles/Turkmenistan.pdf. Accessed July 4, 2009.

53. United Nations Childrens Fund. Statistics—Turkmenistan. http://www.unicef.org/infobycountry/turkmenistan_statistics.html. Accessed July 4, 2009

54. World Health Organization. Turkmenistan. http://www.who.int/countries/tkm/en/

55. Central Intelligence Agency. World Fact Book: Uzbekistan. https://www.cia.gov/cia/publications/factbook/index.html. Accessed July 3, 2009

56. Iikhamov FA, Jakubowski E, Hajioff S. World Health Organization, Regional Office for Europe. European Observatory on Health Care Systems. Health care systems in transition: Uzbekistan—2001. Copenhagen: WHO Regional Office for Europe; 2001.

57. Ahmedov M, Azimov R, Alimova V, Rechel B. World Health Organization. Regional Office for Europe. European Observatory on Health Systems and Policies. Health systems in transition: Uzbekistan: health system review. Copenhagen: WHO Regional Office for Europe; 2007.

58. United Nations Childrens Fund/World Health Organization. Review of National Immunization Coverage 1980–2008, Uzbekistan. http://www.who.int/immunization_monitoring/data/uzb.pdf, Draft May, 2009.

59. World Health Organization Regional Office for Europe. Uzbekistan: HIV/AIDS Data summary. 19 June 2008. http://www.euro.who.int/aids/ctryinfo/overview/20060118_50. Accessed July 3, 2009.

60. United Nations Office on Drugs and Crime. Statistics: Uzbekistan. http://www.unodc.org/uzbekistan/en/fact_sheets.html. Accessed July 3, 2009.

61. World Health Organization Regional Office for Europe. Uzbekistan: Overview of the malaria situation. 15 January 2009. http://www.euro.who.int/malaria/ctryinfo/affected/20020712_7. Accessed July 3, 2009.

62. World Health Organization. Mortality Country Fact Sheet 2006: Uzbekistan. http://www.who.int/whosis/mort/profiles/mort_euro_uzb_uzbekistan.pdf. Accessed July 3, 2009.

63. Turell MJ, Mores CN, Dohm DJ, Komilov N, Paragas J, Lee JS, et al. Laboratory transmission of Japanese encephalitis and West Nile viruses by molestus form of Culex pipiens (Diptera: Culicidae) collected in Uzbekistan in 2004. J Med Entomol. 2006;43(2):296–300.

64. Iashina LN, Petrov VS, Vyshemirskii OI, Aristova VA, Moskvina TM, L'Vov DK, et al. [Characteristics of Crimean-Congo hemorrhagic fever virus circulating in Russia and Central Asia]. Vopr Virusol. 2002;47(3):11–15.

65. Abdiev TA, Vakhabov TA, Zhuravleva NA, Saidakhmedova DB, Abdiev FT, Alimzhanov ZN, et al. [The prognosis for a change in the situation of echinococcosis among the population in Uzbekistan]. *Med Parazitol (Mosk)*. 2000(3):53–54.

66. Biriukov Iu V, Islambekov ES, Streliaeva AV, Sagieva AT, Sadykov VM, Sakykov RV, et al. [Mediastinal echinococcosis]. *Khirurgiia (Mosk)*. 2002(1): 32–33.

67. Uzbekistan. http://www.travmed.com/guide/country.php?c=Uzbekistan. Accessed July 3, 2009.

68. United Nations Development Program. Human development report: Health for All: a Key Goal for Uzbekistan in the New Millenium. Tashkent: United Nations Development Program; 2006.

XVIII ■ SOUTH ASIA

Umakant Kori, MD
Amit Chandra, MD, MSc

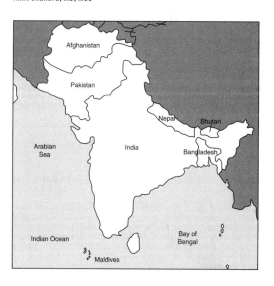

South Asia includes the following seven countries: India, Pakistan, Nepal, Sri Lanka, Bhutan, Bangladesh, and the Maldives. India and Pakistan gained independence from British rule in 1947. Sri Lanka followed a year later. The Maldives was the last British holding in South Asia to gain independence in 1965. Nepal and Bhutan remained independent monarchies throughout the colonial period. The borders of Bangladesh were defined as "East Pakistan" in 1947, but it became an independent country after a civil war in 1971.

The region covers an area of over 4.5 million square kilometers and is home to a population of over 1.5 billion people. Its climate is dominated by the annual monsoon season, and its geography includes deserts, tropical grasslands, mountain tundra, and rain forests.

The modern history of South Asia has been characterized by political upheaval, conflict over border regions, and religious strife. In recent years however, it has also been the source of economic growth and advancements in the fields of science, technology, business process outsourcing, and agriculture.

HEALTH CONCERNS

COMMUNICABLE DISEASE

■ Malaria
687 million people remain at high risk for malaria in South Asia, with an estimated yearly incidence of 90–160 million, and a mortality burden of 120,000.

Two types of malaria predominate in the region: *P. falciparum* and *P. vivax*, with the former, more deadly form, increasing in prevalence. Antimalarial resistance is increasing at a higher rate than any other region of the world.[1] Climate change has increased mosquito-habitable environments, to the extent that previously nonendemic regions have registered new malaria cases in recent years.

■ Tuberculosis
The region carries one-third the world burden of tuberculosis (TB)—India itself carries 20% of the world's burden of TB. DOTS has decreased TB deaths since it was introduced, and is available in all countries of the region.

Although TB is generally considered to be the most deadly opportunistic infection for people living with HIV in the region, it has not altered the epidemiology of the disease overall. Some areas where HIV prevalence is high have reported minimal increases in TB incidence.[2]

■ Polio
Currently only three countries in Asia still report cases of polio: Afghanistan, India, and Pakistan. Surveillance and detection systems have been stepped

up, with a resulting decrease in case numbers. Though easily prevented by oral vaccination, efforts remain hampered due to political instability and cultural myths in some regions that the vaccine leads to impotence and other ailments.

■ HIV/AIDS

The region has the second largest burden in the world of people living with HIV/AIDS (PLHA)—India and Nepal account for the large portion of this burden. As in other areas of the world, incidence and prevalence is highest among commercial sex workers, their clients, men having sex with other men (MSM), and IV drug abusers.

As a region, incident rates have stabilized, if not declined, but intercountry statistics vary greatly. The region continues to lag in adequate treatment of those in need of antiretroviral treatment—in the best of situations, only one-fourth of advanced cases receive antiretroviral therapy.[3]

■ Water Safety

Access to drinking water, as a millennium development goal, has improved over recent years, with 84% coverage in the region. Sanitation, by contrast, is still very much an issue—only 37% of the population has access to adequate sanitation facilities, latrines, and toilets. The variable annual rainfall in the region contributes to an unreliable water supply. Urban population growth is unsustainable given current water delivery infrastructure.

■ Maternal/Child Health

Most countries in South Asia suffer from high maternal and child mortality. Malnutrition, micronutrient deficiency, female illiteracy/poverty, and lack of women's empowerment programs remain hurdles to progress, despite an overall improving economic climate in the region.

A lack of focus on antenatal and neonatal health has contributed to elevated childhood mortality—40% of under-5 mortality is concentrated in the first month of life.[4] In addition to childbirth, infectious disease plays a large role in contributing to childhood mortality—many could be preventable with adequate vaccination. Rates of vaccination in the region range widely, from 67–99%.[5]

ALTERNATIVE MEDICAL PRACTICES: AYURVEDA, HOMEOPATHY, UNANI

As conventional allopathic remedies can be expensive, many people in the region still rely on traditional and alternative forms of medicine. Ayurveda, native to India, defines health as a state of mental, intellectual, and spiritual well being, relying on natural remedies and lifestyle modification. It is particularly useful for chronic disease maintenance and treatment.

Unani, a medicinal system of Greek origin, found its way to the region via the Middle East and has found some favor among South Asians. It is similar to Ayurveda, making use of cheap, locally available herbs. In India, there are over one hundred Unani medical colleges.

Homeopathy, a medical system of European origin, has also found favor in the region, despite its present-day decline in the west. The basis of this system of medicine, "like cures like," integrates the idea that substances that cause certain symptoms can be used to cure diseases producing a similar constellation of symptoms. With 186 colleges and more than a quarter-million licensed practitioners, it is the third most commonly accessed system of medicine in South Asia.

REGIONAL ORGANIZATIONS

All seven nations of South Asia plus Afghanistan are members of the South Asian Association for Regional Cooperation (SAARC). In 2006, they agreed to work toward a regional free trade zone by ratifying the South Asia Free Trade Agreement, which begins by lowering tariffs on goods traded in the region.

The World Health Organization operates in these countries via their regional office for South-East Asia, in New Delhi, India (www.searo.who.int). Another good resource is the South Asia Public Health Forum (www.saphf.org).

COUNTRY PROFILES OF SOUTH ASIA

BANGLADESH
■ Demography
Population: 156,050,883

Religions: Islam (83%), Hindu (16%), other (1%)

Languages: Bangla (previously known as Bengali), English

Ethnic Makeup: Bengali (98%), other (2%; tribal, non-Bengali Muslims)

Formerly Colonized: British

Politics/Governance: Parliamentary democracy, recent elections 2008, following two years of a military-backed caretaker government

■ Traditional Medicine
Traditional medicine includes Unani, Ayurveda, and traditional faith healers such as pirs and fakirs.

■ Healthcare System
Public primary care is organized at subdistrict centers that employ government-trained health assistants, family welfare assistants, and more recently, skilled birth attendants. Private sector care includes traditional healers, homeopathic practitioners, and easily accessible pharmacies dispensing on-demand allopathic remedies often without any formally trained personnel to properly diagnose disease. Vaccinations are provided with government, donor, and NGO support.

The key health institutions are the Dhaka Medical College and Hospital, Bangladesh Medical College Hospital, and Apollo Hospitals Dhaka.

HIV/AIDS Prevalence: < 0.1%, highest among IV drug users

TB: Ranks 6th among countries of highest TB burden with 70,000 deaths annually

Malaria: *P. falciparum* most common; 1,000,000 cases treated annually

Percent of Population Vaccinated: Children in rural areas (59%) are less likely to be immunized than their urban counterparts (70%), but children in urban slums are even less likely to be immunized.[6]

Leading Causes of Death: Ischemic heart disease (12%), lower respiratory infection (11%), perinatal conditions (8%), TB (7%), waterborne diarrheal disease (6%)[7]

Infant Mortality Rate: 59.02 deaths/1000 live births[8]

Under-5 Mortality: 61/1000 (2007 estimate)[9]

Unusual Pathogens: Dengue, malaria, filariasis

Unique Environmental Exposures: Much of the country experiences floods during the monsoon, high incidence of water-borne diarrheal illness

BHUTAN
■ Demography
Population: 691,141 (2005 census)

Religions: Buddhism (75%), Hindu (25%)

Languages: Dzonka (official), various Tibetan and Nepali dialects

Ethnic Makeup: Bhote (50%), ethnic Nepalese (35%), indigenous tribes (15%)

Formerly Colonized: None

Politics/Governance: Monarchy

■ Traditional Medicine
The Institute of Traditional Medicine Services maintains indigenous units in all districts for the purpose of developing traditional medical services in the country. The traditional medicine system was established around the 16th century and passed on through oral tradition until formalized in 1967.[10]

■ Healthcare System
The primary healthcare approach focuses on maternal and child health and makes extensive use of village health workers. There is a four-tiered system; the National Referral Hospital in Thimphu is the key healthcare institute. Then there are regional referral hospitals, district hospitals, and basic health units. There are 29 hospitals, 3 training institutes, and no formal medical schools. An extended program for immunization launched in 1979.

Percent of Population Vaccinated: Universal child Immunization was achieved in 1991 (maintained above 85%).

HIV/AIDS Prevalence: 0.1% (< 500 PLHA 2007 estimate)[11]

TB: < 0.1% incidence, 90% DOTS coverage, 91% DOTS rx success[12]

Malaria: 1.69/1000. Endemic to the country[13]

Leading Causes of Death: Perinatal conditions (14%), ischemic heart disease (13%), lower respiratory infection (8%), CVA (7%), diarrheal disease (6%)[14]

Under-5 Mortality: 80/1000

Unusual Pathogens: Malaria

Unique Environmental Exposures: High altitude illness

INDIA

■ Demography

Population: 1,166,079,217 (2009 estimate)

Religions: Hindu (80.5%), Muslim (13.4%), Christian (2.3%), Sikh (1.9%), other: Jain, Parsi, Buddhist (1.8%)

Languages: Hindi (41%), Bengali (8.1%), Telugu (7.2%), Marathi (7%), Tamil (5.9%), Urdu (5%), Gujarati (4.5%), Kannada (3.7%), Malayalam (3.2%), Oriya (3.2%), Punjabi (2.8%), Assamese (1.3%), Maithili (1.2%), other (5.9%). English is important for national and commercial communication.

Ethnic Makeup: Indo-Aryan (72%), Dravidian (25%), other (3%)

Formerly Colonized: British

Politics/Governance: Federal republic

■ Traditional Medicine

Traditional medicine in India includes Ayurveda, Siddha Medicine, Unani, Homeopathy, and spiritual healers.

■ Healthcare System

India maintains a public healthcare system. The rural areas employ a three-tier system consisting of a subcenter for every 5000 people, a primary health center for every 30,000 people, and a community health center for every 100,000 people with inpatient/basic specialist availability. The urban two-tiered system consists of an urban health center/urban family welfare center for every 100,000 people and a general hospital facility. Sixty-eight percent of all hospitals exist in the private system. The government provision of medications is divided between the Ministry of Chemicals and Fertilizers, and the Ministry of Health and Family Welfare.

The key health institutions include the All India Institute of Medical Sciences, New Delhi (AIIMS); Christian Medical College, Vellore; Armed Forces Medical College, Pune; and Jawaharlal Nehru Institute of Postgraduate Medical Education and Research, Puducherry.

Vaccinations: Provided under the Universal Immunization Program in partnership with the WHO

Percent of Population Vaccinated: 70% of children[15]

HIV/AIDS Prevalence: 0.3% (38% female)

TB: 299/100,000 prevalence. 2.4% MDR TB. 100% DOTS coverage; 86% DOTS treatment success.

Malaria: Endemic; 1.67/1000 cases, 990 deaths (2003)

Leading Causes of Death: Ischemic heart disease, lower respiratory infection, CVA, perinatal conditions, COPD[16]

Infant Mortality Rate: 34.61/1000 live births (2007 estimate)

Under-5 Mortality: 85/1000

Unusual Pathogens: Dengue, malaria, chikungunya, leprosy

MALDIVES
■ Demography
Population: 396,300

Religions: Predominantly Islam (Sunni)

Languages: Maldivian Dhivehi, English

Ethnic Makeup: South Indian, Sinhalese, Arab

Formerly Colonized: First Dutch then British

Politics/Governance: Republic

■ Healthcare System
The publicly funded, five-tiered system includes the Indira Gandhi Memorial Hospital, six regional hospitals, atoll hospitals, atoll health centers, and island health posts. There is near universal vaccination of the population provided by the central government.

The Indira Gandhi Memorial Hospital, located in the capital Male, is the sole tertiary care, referral hospital for the country.

HIV/AIDS Prevalence: 0.1% (2001 estimate)[17]

Tuberculosis Prevalence: 0.1/1000 (2003 estimate)[18]

Leading Causes of Death: Circulatory system (41%), respiratory disease (10%), infectious/parasitic diseases (2.25%)[19]

Life Expectancy: 72 (male), 73 (female) (2006 estimate)[20]

Infant Mortality Rate: 16/1000 live births (2006 estimate)[21]

Unusual Pathogens/Diseases: Dengue fever, dengue hemorrhagic fever, high incidence of thalassemia, no significant incidence of malaria

NEPAL

■ Demography
Population: 28,500,000

Religions: Hinduism, Buddhism

Languages: Nepali

Formerly Colonized: Not applicable

Politics/Governance: Democratic Republic (monarchy dissolved in 2008)

■ Traditional Medicine
Ayurveda and Nepali Folk Medicine are traditionally practiced. Traditional medicine is recognized through the Department of Ayurvedic Medicine.

■ Healthcare System
Primary Health Centers and Hospitals, administered by the Department of Health Services and the Department of Ayurvedic Medicine, are located in cities and regional capitals. There are health posts and sub-health posts at the village level. The key health institutions include the Institute of Medicine of Nepal, Tribhuvan University Teaching Hospital, Department of Health Services, and the Department of Ayurvedic Medicine.

HIV/AIDS Prevalence: 0.5% (2007 estimate)[22]

Tuberculosis Prevalence: 0.28% (2005 estimate)[23]

Percent of Population Vaccinated: 74–87% (2006 estimate)[24]

Leading Causes of Death: Perinatal conditions, respiratory infections, ischemic heart disease, waterborne illness

Life Expectancy: 64.3 (male), 66.6 (female)[25]

Infant Mortality Rate: 48/1000 live births[26]

Unusual Pathogens: Malaria, kala azar, Japanese encephalitis, filariasis

Unique Environmental Exposures: High altitude and cold related illness

PAKISTAN

■ Demography
Population: 166,273,000

Religions: Islam (Sunni Muslim majority)

Languages: Urdu, Punjabi, Pashto, Sindhi, Seraiki, English

Ethnic Makeup: Punjabi, Pashtun, Sindhi

Formerly Colonized: British

Politics/Governance: Islamic Republic

■ Traditional Medicine
Traditional medicine in Pakistan includes Unani healers, herbalists, hakeems, and spiritual healers.

■ Healthcare System

Pakistan's healthcare system consists of separate public and private hospitals. The government-trained community health workers are provided at the village level. Key health institutions include the National Institute of Health (Islamabad), The Children's Hospital (Lahore), and the Pakistan Institute of Medical Sciences (Islamabad).

HIV Prevalence: 0.1% (2008 estimate)[27]

Tuberculosis Prevalence: 423,011 (all forms)[28]

Malaria: 125,152 reported annual cases (2003)[29]

Percent of Population Vaccinated: 83–89% of one-year-olds[30]

Leading Causes of Death: Lower respiratory diseases, heart disease, waterborne illness, perinatal conditions

Life Expectancy: 62[31]

Infant Mortality Rate: 78/1000 live births[32]

Unusual Pathogens: Malaria, dengue fever, tuberculosis

REFERENCES

1. Narain JP. Malaria in the South-East Asia Region: Myth & the reality [editorial]. *Indian J Med Res*. 2008;128:1–3. http://www.searo.who.int/LinkFiles/Malaria_editorial_Myth&reality.pdf. Accessed May 12, 2009.
2. Tuberculosis:TBinSouth-EastAsia.http://www.searo.who.int/en/Section10/Section2097/Section2100_10639.htm. Updated March 4, 2009. Accessed May 12, 2009.
3. World Health Organization. TB/HIV in the South-East Asia Region: Status Report. http://www.searo.who.int/LinkFiles/Tuberculosis_Status_paper_TB-HIV-SEAR.pdf. Updated December 2008. Accessed May 12, 2009.
4. World Health Organization. Child Health and Development: Child Survival in the South-East Asia Region. http://www.searo.who.int/en/Section13/Section37/Section135.htm. Updated August 30, 2005. Accessed May 12, 2009.
5. Bhutta ZA, Gupta I, de'Silva H, et al. Maternal and child health: is South Asia ready for change? *BMJ*. 2004;328:816–819. doi:10.1136/bmj.328.7443.816.
6. Chowdhury AMR, Bhuiya A, Mahmud S, et al. Immunization Divide: Who Do Get Vaccinated in Bangladesh? *J Health Popul Nutr*. 2003;21(3):193–204.
7. World Health Organization. Mortality Country Fact Sheet: Bangladesh 2006. http://www.who.int/whosis/mort/profiles/mort_searo_bgd_bangladesh.pdf. Accessed May 12, 2009.
8. Central Intelligence Agency. World Factbook: Bangladesh. https://www.cia.gov/library/publications/the-world-factbook/geos/bg.html. Accessed May 12, 2009.

9. UNICEF. Bangladesh Statistics of Basic Indicators. http://www.unicef.org/infobycountry/bangladesh_bangladesh_statistics.html. Updated February 26, 2004. Accessed May 12, 2009.

10. World Health Organization. Bhutan Health Information. http://www.whobhutan.org/EN/Section4.htm. Updated July 31, 2006. Accessed May 12, 2009.

11. Kaiser Global Health. Bhutan: Statistics on HIV, TB, and Malaria. http://www.globalhealthfacts.org/country.jsp?c=41. Accessed May 12, 2009.

12. Kaiser Global Health. Bhutan: Statistics on HIV, TB, and Malaria. http://www.globalhealthfacts.org/country.jsp?c=41. Accessed May 12, 2009.

13. Kaiser Global Health. Bhutan: Statistics on HIV, TB, and Malaria. http://www.globalhealthfacts.org/country.jsp?c=41. Accessed May 12, 2009.

14. World Health Organization. Mortality Country Fact Sheet: Bhutan 2006. http://www.who.int/whosis/mort/profiles/mort_searo_btn_bhutan.pdf. Accessed May 12, 2009.

15. World Health Organization: India. Universal Immunization Programme Review. http://www.whoindia.org/LinkFiles/Routine_Immunization_Acknowledgements_contents.pdf. Accessed May 12, 2009.

16. World Health Organization. Mortality Country Fact Sheet: India 2006. http://www.who.int/whosis/mort/profiles/mort_searo_ind_india.pdf. Accessed May 12, 2009.

17. Central Intelligence Agency. World Factbook: India. https://www.cia.gov/library/publications/the-world-factbook/geos/in.html. Accessed May 12, 2009.

18. Ministry of Health, Republic of Maldives. The Maldives Health Report 2004. http://www.unicef.org/maldives/Maldives_Health_Report_2004.pdf. Accessed May 12, 2009.

19. Ministry of Health, Republic of Maldives. The Maldives Health Report 2004. http://www.unicef.org/maldives/Maldives_Health_Report_2004.pdf. Accessed May 12, 2009.

20. Ministry of Health, Republic of Maldives. The Maldives Health Report 2004. http://www.unicef.org/maldives/Maldives_Health_Report_2004.pdf. Accessed May 12, 2009.

21. Ministry of Health, Republic of Maldives. The Maldives Health Report 2004. http://www.unicef.org/maldives/Maldives_Health_Report_2004.pdf. Accessed May 12, 2009.

22. Central Intelligence Agency. World Factbook: Nepal. https://www.cia.gov/library/publications/the-world-factbook/geos/np.html. Accessed May 12, 2009.

23. World Health Organization Regional Office for South-East Asia. Nepal Mini-profile—2007. http://www.searo.who.int/LinkFiles/Country_Health_System_Profile_8-Nepal.pdf. Accessed May 12, 2009.

24. World Health Organization Regional Office for South-East Asia. Nepal National Health System Profile. http://www.searo.who.int/LinkFiles/Nepal_Profile-Nepal.pdf. Accessed May 12, 2009.

25. Central Intelligence Agency. World Factbook: Nepal. https://www.cia.gov/library/publications/the-world-factbook/geos/np.html. Accessed May 12, 2009.

26. World Health Organization Regional Office for South-East Asia. Nepal: National Health System Profile. http://www.searo.who.int/LinkFiles/Nepal_Profile-Nepal.pdf. Accessed May 12, 2009.

27. World Health Organization. Epidemiological Fact Sheet on HIV and AIDS: Pakistan. http://apps.who.int/globalatlas/predefinedReports/EFS2008/full/EFS2008_PK.pdf. Update 2008. Accessed May 12, 2009.

28. The Global Fund. Overview of HIV/AIDS, TB and Malaria in Pakistan. http://www.theglobalfund.org/programs/countrystats/?CountryId=PKS&lang=. Accessed May 12, 2009.

29. World Health Organization. World Malaria Report 2005. http://whqlibdoc.who.int/publications/2005/9241593199_section2_eng.pdf. Accessed May 12, 2009.

30. The World Health Organization. Pakistan Country Profile. http://www.who.int/countries/pak/en/. Accessed May 12, 2009.

31. World Health Organization. Mortality Country Fact Sheet: Pakistan 2006. http://www.who.int/whosis/mort/profiles/mort_emro_pak_pakistan.pdf. Accessed May 12, 2009.

32. The World Health Organization. Pakistan Country Profile. http://www.who.int/countries/pak/en/. Accessed May 12, 2009.

XIX ■ SOUTHEAST ASIA

Jonathan Bertram, MD

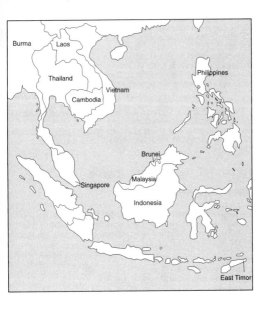

Southeast Asia is a subregion of Asia, consisting of the countries that are geographically south of China, east of India, and north of Australia. The region lies on an intersection of geological plates, with heavy seismic and volcanic activity.

Southeast Asia consists of two geographic regions: the Asian mainland and the island arcs and archipelagos to the east and southeast. The mainland section consists of Burma (Myanmar), Cambodia, Laos, Thailand, Vietnam, and Malaysia. The maritime section consists of Brunei, East Timor, Indonesia, Malaysia, the Philippines, and Singapore.

The region covers an area of approximately 4,523,000 square kilometers and has a population of 568,300,000 with a population density of 126 people per square kilometer. The climate in Southeast Asia is mainly tropical—hot and humid all year round with significant rainfall. Exceptions can be found in the mountain areas in the northern region, where high altitudes lead to milder temperatures and a drier landscape.

The modern history of Southeast Asia has been characterized by colonization, boundary conflicts, political strife, and third party warfare. In recent years however, some areas have proved to be a continued and renewed source of global economic growth and advancements in the fields of science, technology, and business.

MAIN HEALTH CONCERNS

COMMUNICABLE DISEASES

■ Tuberculosis
The prevalence of tuberculosis (TB) is widely variable in the region. With aggressive smear-positive testing and surveillance of multidrug resistant (MDR) TB, declining rates are being achieved in previously high-incident regions of Cambodia, Thailand, and Vietnam.

Although TB is generally considered to be the most deadly opportunistic infection for people infected with HIV in the region, it has not altered the epidemiology of the disease overall. Some areas where HIV prevalence is high have reported minimal increases in TB incidence.[1]

■ HIV/AIDS
Though, by numbers, this region does not rank among the areas with the highest burden of HIV/AIDS, Southeast Asia accounts for the largest proportion of new infections in Asia. As in other areas of the world, incidence and prevalence is highest among commercial sex workers, their clients, men having sex with other men, and IV drug abusers.

The epidemics in Cambodia, Myanmar, and Thailand all show declines in HIV prevalence, with national HIV prevalence in Cambodia falling from 2% in 1998 to an estimated 0.9% in 2006. However, epidemics in Indonesia (especially in its Papua province) and Vietnam are growing rapidly. In Vietnam, the estimated number of people living with HIV more than doubled between 2000 and 2005.[2]

■ **Rural Access**

The distribution of most countries in the region reflects a stark urban/rural divide with resources concentrated in urban areas. In restructuring the organization of healthcare providers, government spending, and health policy, many of these countries have, in recent years, concentrated on primary care.[3]

TRADITIONAL MEDICINE

Traditional medicine has existed throughout the region for thousands of years. Its integration into modern health care has driven the work of the World Health Organization (WHO) Regional Committee for the Western Pacific. This has extended to a concerted program that now includes such areas as standardization of traditional medicine, control of heavy metal and pesticide residues in herbal medicines, monitoring adverse reactions to herbal medicines, conservation of plants with medicinal value, and intellectual property rights.

REGIONAL ORGANIZATIONS

Established in 1986, The Association of Southeast Asian Nations' (ASEAN; http://www.aseansec.org) declaration states that its aims and purposes are: (1) to accelerate economic growth, social progress and cultural development in the region; and (2) to promote regional peace and stability through abiding respect for justice and the rule of law in the relationship among countries in the region and adherence to the principles of the United Nations Charter.

For the WHO, both the Regional Office for Southeast Asia (SEARO; http://www.searo.who.int) and the Regional Office for Western Pacific (WPRO; http://www.wpro.who.int) deal with the issues of countries within the region.[4]

COUNTRY PROFILES OF SOUTHEAST ASIA

BRUNEI

■ **Demography**

Population: 388,190 (2009 estimate)

Religions: Muslim (official; 67%), Buddhist (13%), Christian (10%), other (includes indigenous beliefs; 10%)

Languages: Malay (official), English, Chinese

Ethnic Makeup: Malay, Chinese, indigenous

Formerly Colonized: In 1888, Brunei became a British protectorate; independence was achieved in 1984. The same family has ruled Brunei for over six centuries.

Politics/Governance: Constitutional sultanate[5]

■ **Healthcare System**

Brunei maintains a free universal health system, with health centers and health clinics throughout the whole country. Flying Medical Services provide care in remote areas. Each administrative district has four government hospitals, and the military has its own system for their members and their dependents. The Ministry of Health's Public Health Services branch (the key health institution in Brunei) is responsible for the immunization program.[6]

HIV/AIDS: No data available

TB: 59/100,000[7]

Malaria: Not endemic

Percent of Population Vaccinated: 96–99%[8]

Infant Mortality Rate: 12.27/1000 live births[9]

BURMA
■ **Demography**

Population: 48,137,741

Religions: Buddhist, Christian, Muslim, animist, other

Languages: Burmese

Ethnic Makeup: Burman, Shan, Karen, Rakhine, Chinese, Indian

Formerly Colonized: British (1824–1886), self-administered colony under India (1937–1948)

Politics/Governance: Military junta (in power since 1990), newly instituted parliamentary elections planned for 2010[10]

■ **Healthcare System**

Most of Burma's health care is funded by international sources, with the government spending only about 3% on health annually, compared with 40% on the military. Burma's population, high in internally displaced persons (IDP), notably relies in part on refugee clinic care from its neighboring countries; Thailand, for instance, provides local NGO support from nearby Chiang Mai.[11]

Vaccinations are distributed via the Expanded Programme on Immunization (EPI)—via a collaboration between UNICEF and Myanmar health officials.

HIV/AIDS Prevalence: 7%

Tuberculosis Prevalence: 78,846 reported cases

Malaria: 4,208,818 reported cases[12]

Percent of Population Vaccinated: 81–89%[13]

Leading Causes of Death: Heart disease, respiratory illness, COPD, water-borne illness, prematurity, birth complications, trauma, neonatal infections, malaria[14]

Infant Mortality Rate: 47.61/1000 live births[14]

Unusual Pathogens: Hepatitis A, typhoid fever, dengue fever, leptospirosis, highly pathogenic H5N1 avian influenza

CAMBODIA

■ Demography

Population: 14,494,293

Religions: Buddhist, Muslim, Christian

Languages: Khmer, French, English

Ethnic Makeup: Khmer, Vietnamese, Chinese

Formerly Colonized: French protectorate 1863–1953, followed by Khmer Rouge regime, Vietnamese occupation 1979–1993

Politics/Governance: Multiparty democracy under a constitutional monarchy[15]

■ Healthcare System

Separate public and private health care is available in Cambodia, but access is directed by the individual's ability to pay.[16] Vaccinations are provided under the EPI, in conjuction with Cambodian health officials.[17]

HIV/AIDS Prevalence: 0.8%

Tuberculosis Prevalence: 71,504 reported cases

Malaria: 261,956 reported cases[18]

Percent of Population Vaccinated: 82–90%[1]

Leading Causes of Death: Respiratory infection, TB, HIV/AIDS, diarrheal disease, neonatal infections, heart disease

Infant Mortality Rate: 54.79/1000 live births[20]

EAST TIMOR

■ Demography

Population: 1,131,612

Religions: Roman Catholic (majority), Muslim, Protestant

Languages: Tetum, Portuguese, Indonesian, English,

Ethnic Makeup: Austronesian (Malayo-Polynesian), Papuan, small Chinese minority

Formerly Colonized: Portugal (16th century–19th century), Japan (1942–1945), Indonesia (late 20th century)

Politics/Governance: Republic

■ Healthcare System

East Timor's healthcare system is entirely dependent on NGO support.[21,22]

HIV/AIDS: No data available

TB: 4371 reported cases

Malaria: Not endemic[23]

Percent of Population Vaccinated: 63–76%[24]

Infant Mortality Rate: 40.65/1000 live births[25]

Unusual Pathogens: Malaria, filariasis

INDONESIA
■ Demography

Population: 240,271,522

Religions: Muslim (majority); Christian and Hindu (minorities)

Languages Spoken: Bahasa Indonesia (official, modified form of Malay), English, Dutch, Javanese

Ethnic Makeup: Javanese, Sundanese, Madurese, Minangkabau, Betawi, Bugis, Banten

Formerly Colonized: Portuguese, 16th century; Dutch, 19th century; Japanese, during WWII

Politics/Governance: Republic, legal system based on Roman-Dutch Law[26]

■ Traditional Medicine
It is documented that over 40,000 traditional medicines originate from Indonesia and are widely used across the region. Many of these plants are threatened by deforestation and commercial logging.[27]

■ Healthcare System
Indonesia offers both public and private coverage. Government insurance is available for the very poor.[28] Vaccinations are provided under the EPI in conjunction with Indonesian health officials.[29] The Ministry of Health and the National Health Information Systems are the key health institutions in Indonesia.

HIV Prevalence: 0.2%

TB: 565,614 cases reported

Malaria: 2,518,046 cases reported[30]

Percent of Population Vaccinated: 83–91%[31]

Leading Causes of Death in Adults: Heart disease, respiratory infections, trauma, diabetes

Leading Causes of Death in Children: Diarrheal diseases, other childhood infectious diseases, perinatal morbidity

Infant Mortality Rate: 31.04/1000[32]

LAOS

■ Demography

Population: 6,834,942

Religions: Buddhist (majority), Christian (small minority)

Languages: Lao, French, English

Ethnic Makeup: Lao, KhmouHmong

Formerly Colonized: Thailand, French Indochina (indirectly)

Politics/Governance: Communist state headed by president and prime minister[33]

■ Traditional Medicine

Alternative therapies are emphasized by the Ministry of Public Health and are marketed by the Institute of Traditional Medicine.

■ Healthcare System

The public health system of hospitals, district clinics, and subdistrict clinics suffers from chronic underfunding and understaffing. Slow improvements have been noted in recent years as a market-oriented economy has emerged.[34,35] Vaccinations are supplied via the EPI in conjunction with Laotian health officials.[36] The key health institutions are the Ministry of Public Health and the Institute of Traditional Medicine.

HIV/AIDS: 0.2%

TB: 16,906 cases reported

Malaria: 21,809 cases reported[37]

Percent of Population Vaccinated: 46–59%[38]

Leading Causes of Death: Respiratory infections, heart disease, waterborne illness

Infant Mortality Rate: 77.82/1000 live births[39]

Unusual Pathogens: Hepatitis A, typhoid, dengue fever, malaria

MALAYSIA

■ Demography

Population: 25,715,819

Religions: Muslim, Buddhist, Christian, Hindu

Languages: Bahasa Malaysia (official), English, Chinese dialects

Ethnic Makeup: Malay, Chinese, indigenous, Indian

Formerly Colonized: Under British control until 1963

Politics/Governance: Constitutional monarchy[40]

■ **Traditional Medicine**
Malaysia has a large herbal medication industry, and the government sponsors the Malaysian Herbal Corporation under the Ministry of Science.[41]

■ **Healthcare System**
Malaysia provides universal public health care with a parallel private system.[42] Vaccinations are provided via the EPI in conjunction with Malaysian health officials.[43]

HIV/AIDS: 0.5%

TB: 32,251 cases reported

Malaria: 14,600 cases reported[44]

Percent of Population Vaccinated: 90–99%[45]

Infant Mortality Rate: 15.87/1000 live births[46]

PHILIPPINES
■ **Demography**
Population: 97,976,603

Religions: Roman Catholic (majority), Muslim (minority)

Languages: Filipino (based on Tagalog) and English

Ethnic Makeup: Tagalog, Cebuano, Ilocano, Bisaya/Binisaya, Hiligaynon Ilonggo

Formerly Colonized: By Spain in 1565. Under British control in the 18th century and American control over the 20th century.

Politics/Governance: Presidential democracy with a bicameral congress[47]

■ **Healthcare System**
The Philippines has a mixed public and private healthcare system. There are provincial run hospitals and rural health units, along with a large private health system.[48] Vaccinations are provided by the EPI in conjunction with Filipino health officials.[49] The Philippines Health Promotion Programme is the key healthcare institute.

HIV/AIDS: 0.1%

TB: 440,035 cases reported

Malaria: 124,152 cases reported[50]

Percent of Population Vaccinated: 88–92%[51]

Leading Causes of Death: Respiratory infections, heart disease, waterborne illness

Infant Mortality Rate: 20.56/1000 live births[52]

SINGAPORE
■ Demography

Population: 4,657,542

Religions: Buddhist, Muslim, Taoist, Hindu, Christian

Languages: Mandarin, English, Malay, Hokkien, Cantonese, Teochew, Tamil

Ethnic Makeup: Chinese, Malay, Indian

Formerly Colonized: Founded as a British trading colony in 1819, later a part of the Malaysian Federation, became independent in 1965.

Politics/Governance: Parliamentary republic[53]

■ Healthcare System

Public healthcare services concentrate on infectious disease prevention and health promotion. The government provides an optional low-cost, catastrophic health insurance plan. An advanced private healthcare sector offers a full range of health services.[54]

Under the National Immunization Program, failure to vaccinate children is punishable by law under the Infectious Diseases Act of Singapore.[55]

HIV/AIDS: 0.8%

TB: 93,974 cases reported

Malaria: 261,956 cases reported[56]

Percentage of Population Vaccinated: 95–98%[57]

Leading Causes of Death: Heart disease, lung cancer, respiratory infections

Infant Mortality Rate: 2.31/1,000[58]

THAILAND
■ Demography

Population: 65,905,410

Religions: Buddhist (majority), Muslim, and Christian (minorities)

Languages: Thai, English

Ethnic Makeup: Thai, Chinese

Formerly Colonized: Never colonized

Politics/Governance: Constitutional monarchy[59]

■ Healthcare System

Thailand's healthcare system includes government health centers, district hospitals, provincial hospitals, and tertiary care centers. Hospitals are mainly concentrated in urban areas.[60] Vaccinations are provided under the EPI in conjunction with Thai health officials.[61]

HIV/AIDS: 1.4%

TB: 122,826 cases reported (MDR TB in southern Thailand, especially post-tsunami)

Malaria: 257,020 cases reported[62]

Percent of Population Vaccinated: 96–99%[63]

Leading Causes of Death: HIV/AIDS, heart disease, diabetes, COPD, liver and lung cancer, waterborne illness

Infant Mortality Rate: 17.63/1000[64]

VIETNAM
■ Demography

Population: 86,967,524

Religions: Buddhist and Catholic minorities, majority state no religion

Languages: Vietnamese, English, French

Ethnic Makeup: Kinh (Viet), Tay, Thai, Muong, Khome, Hoa, Nun, Hmong

Formerly Colonized: France 19th century, American occupation in mid-20th century

Politics/Governance: Communist state with elected national assembly[65]

■ Healthcare System
Vietnam has parallel public and private healthcare systems. The public system is administered by the Ministry of Health through the National Health Programs. Over the past decade, the public system has expanded from an urban, tertiary care focus to promote rural health and disease prevention.[66] Vietnam Health Insurance (VHI) is provided particularly for the nations poorest—approximately one-third of the population.
   Vaccinations are provided under the EPI in conjunction with Vietnamese health officials.[67]

HIV/AIDS: 0.5%

TB: 192,092 cases reported

Malaria: 70,324 cases reported[68]

Percent of Population Vaccinated: 86–94%[69]

Leading Causes of Death: Heart disease, respiratory infections, HIV/AIDS, TB, stomach and lung cancer

Infant Mortality Rate: 22.88/1000[70]

Unusual Pathogens: *Diantemeba fragilis* (intestinal pathogen endemic to Vietnam linked to poultry), *Chromobacterium vialaceum* (soil and water pathogen causing a fatal bacteremia)

REFERENCES

1. World Health Organization.Tuberculosis Control in the Western Pacific Region, 2009 Report. http://www.wpro.who.int. Accessed Aug 14, 2009
2. UNAIDS. Region profile, Asia 2009. http://www.unaids.org/en/CountryResponses/Regions/Asia.asp. Accessed Aug 7, 2009.
3. World Health Organization. Department of Health and Measurement Information, February 2009 Report. Geneva, Switzerland: World Health Organization.
4. World Health Organization. Regional Committee for the Western Pacific. http://www.wpro.who.int. Accessed Aug 14, 2009.
5. Central Intelligence Agency. World Fact Book: Brunei. https://www.cia.gov/library/publications/the-world-factbook/geos/bx.html. Accessed Aug 13, 2009.
6. Brunei National Development Plan. http://www.brunei.gov.bn/government/plan.htm. Accessed Aug 3, 2009.
7. Kaiser Family Foundation. US Global Health Policy. http://globalhealthfacts.org/country.jsp?c=47. Accessed Aug 3, 2009.
8. Child Info. Updated Jan 2009. http://www.childinfo.org/immunization_countrydata.php. Accessed Aug 3, 2009.
9. World Health Organization. Department of Health and Measurement Information, February 2009 Report. Geneva, Switzerland: World Health Organization.
10. Central Intelligence Agency. World Fact Book: Myanmar. https://www.cia.gov/library/publications/the-world-factbook/geos/bm.html. Accessed Aug 10, 2009.
11. World Health Organization. SEARO. (Update Dec. 9th, 2009). http://www.searo.who.int. Accessed Dec 15, 2009.
12. Kaiser Family Foundation. US Global Health Policy. http://globalhealthfacts.org/country.jsp?c=152. Accessed Aug 10, 2009.
13. Child Info. Update Jan 2009. http://www.childinfo.org/immunization_countrydata.php. Accessed Aug 3, 2009.
14. World Health Organization. Department of Health and Measurement Information, February 2009 Report. Geneva, Switzerland: World Health Organization.
15. Central Intelligence Agency. World Fact Book: Cambodia. https://www.cia.gov/library/publications/the-world-factbook/geos/cb.html. Accessed Aug 1, 2009.
16. Asian Development Bank. http://www.adb.org/Documents/Periodicals/ADB_Review/2004/vol36_3/healing.asp. Accessed Aug 1, 2009.
17. World Health Organization. Regional Committee for the Western Pacific. http://www.wpro.who.int. Accessed Aug 1, 2009.
18. Kaiser Family Foundation. US Global Health Policy. http://globalhealthfacts.org/country.jsp?c=51. Accessed Aug 1, 2009.
19. Child Info. update Jan 2009. http://www.childinfo.org/immunization_countrydata.php. Accessed Aug 1, 2009.

20. World Health Organization. Department of Health and Measurement Information, February 2009 Report. Geneva, Switzerland: World Health Organization.
21. Central Intelligence Agency. World Fact Book: East Timor. https://www.cia.gov/library/publications/the-world-factbook/geos/tt.html. Accessed July 30.
22. World Health Organization. SEARO. Update Dec 9th, 2009. http://www.searo.who.int Accessed Jan 2, 2010.
23. Kaiser Family Foundation. US Global Health Policy. http://www.globalhealthfacts.org. Accessed July 30, 2009.
24. Child Info. Update Jan 2009. http://www.childinfo.org/immunization_countrydata.php. Accessed July 30, 2009.
25. World Health Organization. Department of Health and Measurement Information, February 2009 Report. Geneva, Switzerland: World Health Organization.
26. Central Intelligence Agency. World Fact Book: Indonesia. https://www.cia.gov/library/publications/the-world-factbook/geos/id.html. Accessed July 30, 2009.
27. Traditional Medicine in Indonesia. http://www.thejakartapost.com. Accessed July 30, 2009.
28. Integrated Regional Information Networks. http://www.unhcr.org/country/idn.html. Accessed July 30, 2009.
29. World Health Organization. SEARO. Updated Dec. 9th, 2009. http://www.searo.who.int. Accessed Jan 2, 2010.
30. Kaiser Family Foundation. US Global Health Policy. http://http://globalhealthfacts.org/country.jsp?c=107. Accessed July 30, 2009.
31. Child Info. Update Jan. 2009. http://www.childinfo.org/immunization_countrydata.php. Accessed July 30, 2009.
32. World Health Organization. Department of Health and Measurement Information, February 2009 Report. Geneva, Switzerland: World Health Organization.
33. Central Intelligence Agency. World Fact Book: Laos. https://www.cia.gov/library/publications/the-world-factbook/geos/la.html. Accessed Aug 4, 2009.
34. Ireson WR. Health Infrastructure. In: Savada AM. *A country study: Laos.* Washington, DC: Library of Congress Federal Research Division; 1994.
35. Primary Health Care Review in LaoPDR (2001). http://www.wpro.who.int/NR/rdonlyres/D24349FC-7D82–4D2B-9A6E-B3F721E33229/0/lao.pdf
36. World Health Organization. WPRO. http://www.wpro.who.int/internet/resources.ashx/EPI/docs/Meetings/MTGRPT_HepBWrkGrpTokyo02.pdf
37. Kaiser Family Foundation. US Global Health Policy. http://globalhealthfacts.org/country.jsp?c=123. Accessed Aug 4, 2009.
38. Child Info. Update Jan. 2009. http://www.childinfo.org/immunization_countrydata.php. Accessed Aug 4, 2009.
39. World Health Organization. Department of Health and Measurement Information, February 2009 Report. Geneva, Switzerland: World Health Organization.

40. Central Intelligence Agency. World Fact Book: Malaysia. https://www.cia.gov/library/publications/the-world-factbook/geos/my.html. Accessed Aug 4, 2009.

41. Traditional Medicine: Malaysia. http://www.wpro.who.int/NR/rdonlyres/ADDFE18E-58EB-4F5C-9DDE-DC6B331D0ACB/0/RC5207.pdf

42. End of Life-Care Observatory: Health Care Systems Analysis. http://www.eolc-observatory.net. Accessed Aug 4, 2009.

43. World Health Organization. WPRO. http://www.wpro.who.int/NR/rdonlyres/ADDFE18E-58EB-4F5C-9DDE-DC6B331D0ACB/0/RC5207.pdf

44. Kaiser Family Foundation. US Global Health Policy. http://globalhealthfacts.org/country.jsp?c=136. Accessed Aug 4, 2009.

45. Child Info. Update Jan. 2009. http://www.childinfo.org/immunization_countrydata.php. Accessed Aug 4, 2009.

46. World Health Organization. Department of Health and Measurement Information, February 2009 Report. Geneva, Switzerland: World Health Organization.

47. Central Intelligence Agency. World Fact Book: Philippines. https://www.cia.gov/library/publications/the-world-factbook/geos/rp.html. Accessed July 21, 2009.

48. End of Life-Care Observatory: Health Care Systems Analysis. http://www.eolc-observatory.net. Accessed July 21, 2009.

49. World Health Organization. WPRO. http://www.wpro.who.int/NR/rdonlyres/3E195EDF-0585-4540-BF71-F3E4D1978553/0/RC5511.pdf

50. Kaiser Family Foundation. US Global Health Policy. http://globalhealthfacts.org/country.jsp?c=173. Accessed July 21, 2009.

51. Child Info. Update Jan. 2009. http://www.childinfo.org/immunization_countrydata.php. Accessed Aug 4, 2009.

52. World Health Organization. Department of Health and Measurement Information, February 2009 Report. Geneva, Switzerland: World Health Organization.

53. Central Intelligence Agency. World Fact Book: Singapore. https://www.cia.gov/library/publications/the-world-factbook/geos/sn.html. Accessed July 21, 2009.

54. Singapore's Health Care System. http://www.economist.com

55. World Health Organization. WPRO. http://www.wpro.who.int/internet/resources.ashx/EPI/docs/HepB/POA_HepB.pdf

56. Kaiser Family Foundation. US Global Health Policy. http://globalhealthfacts.org/country.jsp?c=192. Accessed July 21, 2009.

57. Child Info. Update Jan. 2009. http://www.childinfo.org/immunization_countrydata.php. Accessed Aug 4, 2009.

58. World Health Organization. Department of Health and Measurement Information, February 2009 Report. Geneva, Switzerland: World Health Organization.

59. Central Intelligence Agency. World Fact Book: Thailand. https://www.cia.gov/library/publications/the-world-factbook/geos/th.html. Accessed Aug 14, 2009.

60. End of Life-Care Observatory: Health Care Systems Analysis. http://www.eolc-observatory.net. Accessed Aug 14, 2009.

61. World Health Organization. SEARO. http://www.searo.who.int/vaccine/LinkFiles/EPI2005/Thailand05.pdf. Accessed Aug 14, 2009.

62. Kaiser Family Foundation. US Global Health Policy. http://globalhealthfacts.org/country.jsp?c=208. Accessed Aug 14, 2009.

63. Child Info. Update Jan. 2009. http://www.childinfo.org/immunization_countrydata.php. Accessed Aug 14, 2009.

64. World Health Organization. Department of Health and Measurement Information, February 2009 Report. Geneva, Switzerland: World Health Organization.

65. Central Intelligence Agency. World Fact Book: Vietnam. https://www.cia.gov/library/publications/the-world-factbook/geos/vm.html. Accessed Aug 14, 2009.

66. Vietnam's Health Care System: A Macroenomic Perspective. http://www.imf.org/external/country/VNM/rr/sp/012105.pdf. Accessed Aug 14, 2009.

67. World Health Organization. WPRO. Updated 2009. http://www.wpro.who.int/vietnam/sites/dhp/epi/. Accessed Aug 14, 2009.

68. Kaiser Family Foundation. US Global Health Policy. http://globalhealthfacts.org/country.jsp?c=228. Accessed Aug 14, 2009.

69. Child Info. Update Jan. 2009. http://www.childinfo.org/immunization_countrydata.php. Accessed Aug 14, 2009

70. World Health Organization. Department of Health and Measurement Information, February 2009 Report. Geneva, Switzerland: World Health Organization.

XX ■ EAST ASIA

Joseph Walline, MD

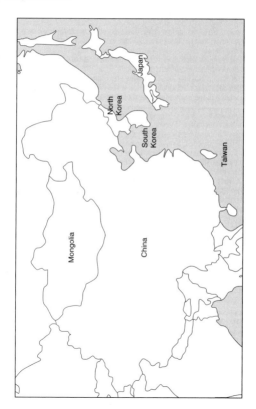

Eastern Asia is a geographical and cultural area defined by the United Nations to include China, Korea, Japan, Mongolia, and Taiwan. Although historically and geographically dominated by China, the late 19th century and the 20th century saw the rapid industrialization and economic expansion of Japan, which competed with European colonial powers for political supremacy in the region. Whole subregions of Eastern Asia (Taiwan, Korea, Mongolia, as well as parts of China) were exploited and fought over amongst the imperial powers during the 19th and early 20th centuries, culminating in World War II.

As a major theatre of war, Eastern Asia saw land battles between Japan and the Allied nations of Australia, China, Great Britain, the United States, and Russia, focusing on South-Western China, while extensive naval battles took place between Japan and the Allies in the Pacific. The war culminated in the world's first use of nuclear weapons by the United States on Japan, an action that continues to impact the health of the peoples of Eastern Asia.

In the aftermath of the war, significant political struggles still remained unresolved. Japan became a constitutional monarchy with a new democratic, and officially pacifist, form of government. China saw a deepening of political crisis as the Nationalist and Communist forces resumed a civil war, resulting in the Nationalist forces retreating to the island of Taiwan. Taiwan has since remained a distinct political entity, developing a democratic form of government while remaining culturally Chinese.

Two other parts of the Chinese political sphere include Tibet and Hong Kong. Tibet used to be an independent nation, although historically it had significant ties to the Chinese government. In 1949, Chinese forces began entering Tibet, which has since been part of the Chinese nation. Hong Kong was a British colony for a hundred years, before returning peacefully to Chinese control in 1997. Hong Kong and Tibet maintain unique local health and political characteristics (although they are quite divergent economically).

Korea remains an active area of political tension. In the aftermath of WWII, and heightened communist/capitalist tensions, Korea became a theater of war between UN forces led by the United States supporting South Korea and Chinese/Soviet Union support for North Korea. This war eventually ended in a stalemate, which continues to this day. Politically and economically, South Korea has moved ahead of North Korea, yet the unease between these two nations and its' implications on neighboring China, Japan, Mongolia, Russia, and even the United States is a major source of global political tension.

Finally, Mongolia has seen significant change since the collapse of the Soviet Union in 1989. Prior to declaring a new parliamentary republic in 1990, Mongolia was aligned very closely with the Soviet Union. Particularly after China and the Soviet Union had a political falling-out in the late 1950s–1960s, Mongolia was the staging ground for Soviet armed forces stationed near China. With the new republic, Mongolia is pursuing a capitalist road with new diplomatic relations with neighboring China, Korea, and Japan.

CLIMATE

The climate of Eastern Asia is dominated by warm, humid air from the south, leading to high temperatures, high humidity, and significant rainfall during the summer months. In the winter, cold, dry air from the north causes occasional snow showers and below-freezing temperatures in the northern parts of Eastern Asia, while cool, moist air dominates the southern regions. Overall, the great majority of Eastern Asia is dominated by relatively high humidity, which is only broken by the great Gobi desert in the northwest and the Himalayan plateau in the southwest.

HUMAN DIVERSITY AND REGIONAL CULTURAL ISSUES

Eastern Asia has seen human presence for over 5000 years. Although Eastern Asia has been populated by a rich diversity of peoples, cultures, and languages, the current ethnic make-up of most of the countries in this overview is remarkably homogeneous. Even China, the most diverse in terms of the percentage of minorities within its borders is over 90% of the Han ethnicity. Whether through war, disease, or migration, the countries discussed here have, until recently, been dominated by single ethnic groups.

As Eastern Asia modernizes and trade and travel accelerate throughout the region, the numbers of minorities living in each of these countries will likely increase, leading to new opportunities and tensions in this most populous of the world's regions.

MAJOR HEALTH ISSUES

The major health issues for Eastern Asia can be divided into two broad categories: health insurance challenges and infectious disease issues.

In terms of public health, the region has seen dramatic improvement commensurate with the world's most rapidly growing economic region. Although somewhat slowed by the "Asian Economic Flu" of 1997, the economic tigers of Japan, South Korea, and Taiwan have been joined by China in making rapid progress in lifting millions of people out of poverty. All of the countries discussed in this overview have some form of nationalized health insurance. Although the degree of public financing of these systems vary greatly, all except North Korea are based on private physicians and a mix of private and public hospitals. All of the countries are struggling to find the most appropriate balance between public funding/control and free-market enterprise. For example, Taiwan has a very successful public health insurance system that is very popular locally. Taiwan is constantly struggling, however, to rein in healthcare costs, and although both physicians and patients are pleased with the quality of their system, the financial stability of the Taiwanese system is in doubt.

On the opposite extreme of the scale is China, which has a few legacy public insurance schemes left from the pre-1980s that generously fund government officials. The bulk of China's middle class, however, depends on employer-provided discount cards that pay a percentage of care at a preferred hospital. Finally, Chinese rural dwellers, who recently suffered the loss of their communal insurance program in the 1990s, have new hope with a new government-sponsored health insurance plan devised for rural farmers.

North Korea, meanwhile, is dealing with significant health disparities compared with its neighboring Eastern Asian countries. After suffering through a severe drought in the mid 1990s, North Korea has become dependent on international aid to maintain its failing healthcare sector—a dependence that is increasingly problematic given North Korea's rollercoaster-like relations with its neighbors in recent years.

Besides the trials of maintaining nationalized healthcare initiatives, the other major threat to regional (and global) health is the emergence of contagious infectious disease. The best example of this is the outbreak in the spring of 2003 of the worldwide SARS (Severe Acute Respiratory Syndrome) corona virus. The rapid escalation of the pandemic sent shockwaves through the worldwide public health community and people from Hong Kong to Toronto quickly donned masks to ward away the impending calamity. Fortunately, the SARS epidemic was short-lived, but the region continues to threaten with the next potential influenza: avian flu.

COUNTRY PROFILES OF EAST ASIA

CHINA

■ **Demography**

Population: 1.3 billion

Religions: Ancestor worship and five state-sanctioned religions: Buddhism, Taoism, Islam, Catholicism, and Protestantism.

Languages: Mandarin Chinese (official state language), many regional dialects (e.g., Cantonese, Shanghainese, etc.)

Ethnic Makeup: Han Chinese (91.5%), Zhuang, Manchu, Hui, Miao, Uyghur, Tujia, Yi, Mongol, Tibetan, Buyi, Dong, Yao, Korean, and other nationalities (8.5%).[

Colonization: Multiple old treaty ports (most famously Shanghai, Tianjin, Dalian, Xiamen, among many others) were controlled by foreign colonial powers until World War II.

Politics/Governance: Communist (single-party)

■ **Healthcare System**

China's health system ranked 132 out of 191 countries in overall performance, but only 188 out of 191 for economic fairness by WHO.[2] There are three competing healthcare systems: fully government operated, operated by state owned enterprises, and government operated based on traditional Chinese medicine (TCM).

Health care is paid for through privately-funded, workplace insurance, with additional niche national insurance plans (retired party officials, rural farmers). China's publicly-funded healthcare system was converted to a privately-funded model in the late 1980s. This conversion has been criticized for worsening rural healthcare coverage and for accelerating the inequality of healthcare coverage based on income. For example, hypertension treatment rates remain low nationally, but only 7% receive treatment in rural areas compared with 12% in urban centers.[3]

Many basic services remain accessible through price controls, although this has discouraged doctors from performing basic health control measures (e.g., vaccinations, first-line antibiotics), and has led to an over-prescription of expensive tests and medications. Medications are not provided by the government, with the exception of a few special programs (e.g., some HIV/TB treatments).

In China there are approximately 162 physicians/100,000 people (c/w India at 48), but most rural "doctors" have no college education.[4]

Percent of Population Vaccinated: Vaccination rates vary widely by location. For example, some rural provinces in China had measles vaccination rates around 50%, while urban centers enjoy rates closer to 100%.[4]

HIV/AIDS: 700,000 (0.1% of population)[1]

TB: 400,000,000 (approximately one-third of population); 5,000,000 with active TB; more Chinese die from TB than from any other infectious disease.[4]

Malaria: Endemic, 42 deaths reported (2002), 25,520 cases reported (0.02/1000 people).[5]

Leading Causes of Death:[6] Cerebrovascular disease, COPD, heart disease, stomach cancer, liver cancer, lung cancer, perinatal conditions, self-inflicted injuries, tuberculosis, pneumonia, and influenza.

Infant Mortality Rate:[1] 20.25/1000 live births (total), 18.87/1000 live births (male), 21.77/1000 live births (female)

Life Expectancy:[1] 73.47 years (total; 71.61 male; 75.52 female)

Unusual Pathogens: China is believed to have been the starting point for the worldwide SARS (Severe Acute Respiratory Syndrome) corona virus outbreak in the spring of 2003. This outbreak led to over 3000 infections and over 100 deaths in 20 countries.[7] There was a second, smaller outbreak of SARS virus from a virology research lab in Beijing in 2004 that was more rapidly contained. Additionally, H5N1 avian influenza "Bird Flu" has been found in China, although it has been limited to people with close contact with birds. Of the 38 cases confirmed to date in China, 25 have been fatal.[8]

Unique Environmental Exposures: China's food supply has come under increasing criticism in recent years for high levels of organic and inorganic contamination. Most recently the finding of high levels of the look-a-like protein melamine in infant formula caused significant loss of faith in the effectiveness of government food safety procedures.

Traditional Medicine: Traditional Chinese medicine (TCM) is one of the world's most developed healing disciplines, with practitioners around the world. TCM exists in China as a competing model of healthcare practice with separate medical schools and hospitals. Modern Chinese TCM as it is practiced in China, however, does rely on some "Western" medications such as antibiotics, steroids, etc. The major difference between TCM and Western medical practice lies in a difference in the basic philosophy of care. TCM sees disease as an imbalance of essential forces in the body and the use of medicinal herbs, drugs, and acupuncture is geared toward correcting this imbalance. One significant difference in Chinese TCM as compared to versions practiced abroad is that herbal remedies represent the majority of TCM treatments prescribed in China while acupuncture is a relatively minor discipline.

JAPAN
■ Demography
Population: 127 million

Religions: Shintoism, Buddhism, Christianity

Language: Japanese

Ethnic Makeup: Japanese, Koreans, Chinese

Colonial History: Never colonized, active colonizer in late 19th and early 20th centuries

Politics/ Governance: Constitutional monarchy, parliamentary democracy

■ Healthcare System
Japan's health system is ranked #1 out of 191 countries overall by WHO.[2] Japan has a universal health insurance mandate (i.e., everyone is required to have health insurance). If someone is too poor to afford insurance, the government provides a basic insurance plan. Employers cover a portion of insurance premiums. Eighty percent of Japan's hospitals are privately owned.[9]

Japan's healthcare system does have some issues, however—there is marked over-crowding in major university-affiliated hospitals, while smaller centers are left out. Financially, many hospitals and physicians are dissatisfied with their income (or deficits, in the case of hospitals), due to a fee schedule kept low by the government.[10] Luckily, for the general populace, medications are covered through mandated insurance programs.

Percent of Population Vaccinated: 94–99%, depending on vaccine type. Eighty-three percent have had the Japanese encephalitis vaccination.[11]

HIV/AIDS[1]: 9600 or 0.1% (estimated number of people living with HIV/AIDS by the end of 2007)

TB: 28,330 (estimated incidence), 29/100,000 (estimated prevalence)

TB Mortality: 3/100,000[12]

Malaria: Not endemic to Japan[5]

Leading Causes of Death:[6] Cerebrovascular disease, heart disease, pneumonia and influenza, lung cancer, stomach cancer, colon cancer, liver cancer, self-inflicted injuries, kidney disease, pancreatic cancer

Infant Mortality Rates:[1] 2.79/1000 live births (total), 2.99/1000 live births (male), 2.58/1000 live births (female)

Life Expectancy:[1] 82.12 years (total), 78.8 years (male), 85.62 years (female)

Unique Environmental Exposures: Air pollution from power plant emissions results in acid rain; acidification of lakes and reservoirs degrades water quality and threatens aquatic life.[1]

Japan was the site of two nuclear weapon detonations in August of 1945 which led to the end of World War II. As a result of the bombings of Hiroshima and Nagasaki, thousands of people were killed and exposed to significant doses of radiation. One of the byproducts of these events has been the following of this population as a cohort study on the effects of radiation.[13] The data collected from these studies is the principal source of information regarding the toxic effects of radiation exposure today.

Traditional Medicine: Herbal therapy with roots in traditional Chinese medicine has seen a resurgence in Japan in recent years. This form of traditional healing, named Kampo, has accelerated in use since government health insurance regulations made it a covered healthcare expense in the mid-1980s.[14]

MONGOLIA
■ Demography
Population: 3 million

Religions: Buddhist Lamaist, Shamanist and Christian, Muslim

Languages: Mongol, Turkic and Russian

Ethnic Makeup: Mongol, Turkic

Colonial History: Mongolia was part of China until 1921 when, with Soviet support, it won independence from China. Mongolia then remained firmly under the influence of the Soviet Union until 1990, when, with the collapse of the Soviet Union, Mongolia became a fully independent republic.

Politics/Governance: Parliamentary Democratic (two major parties: ex-Communist Mongolian People's Revolutionary Party [MPRP] and the Democratic Union Coalition [DUC])

■ Healthcare System
Mongolia's health system is ranked #136 out of 191 countries overall by WHO.[2] On average, there are 4 physicians per 1000 people (80% of physicians are women). The health system is in the process of switching from a centralized system of large hospitals to a greater emphasis on local health centers.[15] The government provides vaccinations and food rations for women and children.

Percent of Population Vaccinated: 88–98%, depending on type of vaccine.[12]

HIV/AIDS: Less than 500 cases (< 0.1%) reported[16]

TB: 4893 (estimated incidence), 191/100,000 (estimated prevalence)

TB Mortality: 15/100,000[13]

Malaria: Not endemic to Mongolia[5]

Leading Causes of Death: Stroke, liver cancer, heart disease, road traffic accidents, perinatal conditions, tuberculosis, diarrheal diseases, pneumonia and influenza, stomach cancer, hypertension-related disease[6]

Infant Mortality Rate:[16] 39.88 /1,000 live births (total), 42.99/1000 live births (male), 36.61/1000 live births (female)

Life Expectancy:[16] 67.65 years (total), 65.23 years (male), 70.19 years (female)

Unique Environmental Exposures: Over 90% of the country is desert, and temperatures in the summer and winter can be extreme.

Traditional Medicine: Traditional herbal remedies and healing Buddhist rituals are increasingly popular in Mongolia. Potentially harmful practices include giving ill children their mother's early morning urine.[17]

NORTH KOREA
■ Demography
Population: 22.6 million

Religions: Buddhist and Confucianist, some Christian and syncretic Chondogyo (Religion of the Heavenly Way)

Languages: Korean

Ethnic Makeup: Korean, as well as small communities of Chinese and Japanese people

Colonial History: Japan annexed Korea as a colony in 1910, following the Russo-Japanese war. Korea became an independent nation once more in 1945 after the defeat of Japan by the Allied powers in World War II. Korea was divided into the North and South sections at the end of the Korean War in 1953.

Politics/Governance: Communist, single-party

■ Healthcare System
North Korea's healthcare system is ranked #149 out of 191 countries in overall performance by WHO.[2] It all but collapsed in the mid-1990s during serious droughts that collapsed the country's food supply. Since then, North Korea has relied on foreign assistance for much of its basic necessities, and such items as vaccines and antibiotics are chronically in short supply—although many are made available through international aid organizations. International assistance has been successful in easing some of this burden, however. Chronic malnutrition was decreased between 1998 (62%) and 2004 (37%).[16] Unfortunately, the country's public health

system is thereby very sensitive to changes in the international political environment.

Percent of Population Vaccinated: 92–99%, depending on vaccine type. Ninety-seven percent have had the BCG antituberculosis vaccination.[12]

HIV: No reported cases[18]

TB: 105,000 (prevalence); 82,000 (annual incidence)[13]

Malaria: Was eradicated in the 1970s, but reemerged in 1997–1998 to peak at nearly 300,000 reported cases in 2001. Since then, medications and education have brought the case burden down to less than 50,000 annually.[5]

Leading Causes of Death:[6] Heart disease, pneumonia and influenza, stroke, hypertensive heart disease, perinatal conditions, COPD, diabetes mellitus, stomach cancer, violence, kidney disease

Infant Mortality Rate:[18] 51.34/1000 live births (total), 58.64/1000 live births (male), 43.6 deaths/1000 live births (female)

Life Expectancy:[18] 63.81 years (total), 61.23 years (male), 66.53 years (female)

Unusual Pathogens: North Korea was probably affected by the worldwide SARS (Severe Acute Respiratory Syndrome) corona virus outbreak in the spring of 2003. However, exact numbers of cases have not been reported. [7] H5N1 avian influenza "Bird Flu" has been found in North Korean poultry, most recently in 2005. No cases of human transmission have yet been reported in North Korea.[8]

Unique Environmental Exposures: In April of 2004, 54 people were confirmed dead and thousands of casualties were reported in a train station explosion when a large supply of ammonium nitrate was accidentally ignited in the northern city of Ryongchon.[17]

Traditional Medicine: With the instability of conventional medical facilities in North Korea, traditional remedies relying on herbs, acupuncture, and massage are likely used.

SOUTH KOREA

■ Demography

Population: 48.5 million

Religions: Christian (26.3%: Protestant 19.7%, Roman Catholic 6.6%), Buddhist (23.2%), other or unknown (1.3%), none (49.3%)[18]

Languages: Korean

Ethnic Makeup: 99% Korean, and approximately 20,000 Chinese[21]

Colonial History: Japan annexed Korea as a colony in 1910, following the Russo-Japanese war. Korea became an independent nation once more in 1945 after the defeat of Japan by the Allied powers in World War II. Korea was divided into the North and South sections at the end of the Korean War in 1953.

Politics/Governance: Democratic republic

■ Healthcare System

South Korea's health system is ranked #35 out of 191 countries overall by WHO.[2]

It used to be based on voluntary employer-funded health insurance up to the late 1970s. Between 1976 and 1988, this system was gradually changed to a mandated health insurance system (medications are provided through this program) overlaid onto an existing private physician and clinic supply. This system is doing fairly well compared with other similar nations, although there are several problems. The percentages that some plans' participants out pay are as high as 50% in some cases.[19] Also, the 1997 economic depression disproportionally affected Korea, and since then, the government-run insurance system has been running ever-higher deficits.[20]

Percent of Population Vaccinated: 94–99%, depending on type of vaccine. Eighty-four percent have had the Japanese encephalitis vaccination.[12]

HIV/AIDS: 13,000 (< 0.1% of population)[21]

TB: 61,000 (prevalence); 43,000 (annual incidence)[13]

Malaria: Eradicated in the 1960s, but reemerged in 1993 to peak at over 4000 cases reported in 2001. Since then, intensive education and public health programs have reduced the case burden to less than 2000 annually.[5]

Leading Causes of Death:[6] Cerebrovascular disease, lung cancer, heart disease, diabetes mellitus, stomach cancer, liver cancer, liver cirrhosis, road traffic accidents, self-inflicted injuries, alzheimer's and other dementias.

Infant Mortality Rate:[21] 4.26/1000 live births (total), 4.49/1000 live births (male), 4.02/1000 live births (female)

Life Expectancy:[21] 78.72 years (total), 75.45 years (male), 82.22 years (female) (2009)

Unusual Pathogens: South Korea was affected by the worldwide SARS (Severe Acute Respiratory Syndrome) corona virus outbreak in the spring of 2003. There were three confirmed cases, but no deaths reported.[7]

Unique Environmental Exposures: Due to South Korea's rapid industrialization and development, the country (like its neighbors) has experienced increasing levels of acid rain and environmental deterioration. As a counterreaction to this (and similarly to other industrialized countries), South Korea has seen in the past decade a dramatic popular embrace of foods, clothing, and personal products that espouse an organic or natural theme.

Traditional Medicine: Herbal therapy, acupuncture, and therapeutic massage are increasingly popular in South Korea.

TAIWAN

■ Demography

Population: 23 million

Religions: Mixture of Buddhist and Taoist (93%), Christian (4.5%), other (2.5%)[21]

Languages: Mandarin Chinese (official state language), Taiwanese (Min-nan), Hakka dialects

Ethnic Makeup: Taiwanese (including Hakka: 84%), mainland Chinese (14%), indigenous (2%)[24]

Colonial History: Taiwan became a Japanese colony after China's 1895 military defeat. It remained part of Japan until the end of WWII, after which it became the primary base for Nationalist forces from 1949 to the present.

Politics/Governance: Parliamentary Democratic (three major parties)

Note: Taiwan is not recognized as an independent country by many of the world's nations, especially China. Taiwan's status as a country or province of China is an active area of political debate both within and outside of Taiwan.

■ Healthcare System

Taiwan has a nationalized health insurance system with a mix of private and public healthcare providers. This national system includes traditional Chinese medicine practitioners. Taiwan implemented the national health insurance (NHI) plan in 1995. Prior to the introduction of NHI, Taiwan had widening disparities in care based on economic class. These disparities decreased in size while maintaining the same percentage of gross domestic product spent on health care (5–6%).[22] Medications, physician visits, and tests and procedures are all covered under the NHI.

Percent of Population Vaccinated: Vaccination rates are greater than 90%. Taiwan implemented a vaccination program directed at hepatitis B in the mid-1980s achieving 80–90% protective effect and decreased hepatic disease in infants by 68%.[12,23]

HIV/AIDS: 17,000 cases reported[24,27]

TB: No data available[24]

Malaria: Eradicated in 1965, no new cases reported[5,27]

Leading Causes of Death:[25] Cancer, stroke, heart disease, diabetes, accidents, chronic liver disease, pneumonia, kidney disease, suicide, hypertension-related disease; also, liver cancer is the most prevalent form of cancer in Taiwan.

Infant Mortality Rate:[24] 5.35/1000 live births (total), 5.64/1000 live births (male), 5.04/1000 live births (female)

Life Expectancy:[24] 77.96 years (total), 75.12 years (male), 81.05 years (female)

Unusual Pathogens: Taiwan was heavily affected by the SARS (Severe Acute Respiratory Syndrome) corona virus outbreak in the spring of 2003. This outbreak led to over 3000 infections and over 100 deaths in 20 countries worldwide.[7] To date, no cases of H5N1 avian influenza "Bird Flu" have been found in Taiwan.[8]

Unique Environmental Exposures: Taiwan's high population density and rapid pace of industrialization have led to significant environmental deterioration on the island. In addition, Taiwan regularly experiences serious earthquakes (most recently in 2003 when a 6.5 Richter-scale quake shook central Taiwan).

Traditional Medicine: Traditional Chinese medicine (TCM) is one of the world's most developed healing disciplines, with practitioners around the world. TCM exists in China as a competing model of healthcare practice with separate medical schools and hospitals. Modern Chinese TCM as it is practiced in China, however, does rely on some Western medications such as antibiotics, steroids, etc. The major difference between TCM and Western medical practice lies in the difference in the basic philosophy of care. TCM views disease as an imbalance of essential forces in the body and the use of medicinal herbs, drugs, and acupuncture is geared toward correcting this imbalance. One significant difference in Chinese TCM as compared to versions practiced abroad is that herbal remedy represents the majority of TCM treatments prescribed in China while acupuncture is a relatively minor discipline.

REFERENCES

1. Central Intelligence Agency. The World Fact Book: China. https://www.cia.gov/library/publications/the-world-factbook/geos/ch.html. Accessed May 12, 2009.
2. World Health Organization. World Health Report 2000. Geneva, Switzerland: World Health Organization: 2000.
3. Liu Y, et al. China's health system performance. *Lancet.* 2008;372(9653): 1914–1923.
4. Ooi EW. The World Bank's Assistance to China's Health Sector. Washington, DC: World Bank; 2005.
5. World Health Organization. World Malaria Report, 2005. http://rbm.who.int/wmr2005/index.html. Accessed May 12, 2009.
6. World Health Organization. Death and DALY estimates by cause, 2002. http://www.who.int/entity/healthinfo/statistics/bodgbddeathdalyestimates.xls. Accessed May 12, 2009.
7. World Health Organization. SARS—One hundred days into the outbreak—Update 83. June 2003. http://www.who.int/csr/don/2003_06_18/en/index.html. Accessed May 12, 2009.
8. World Health Organization. Avian influenza—Situation in China—Update 4. February 2009. http://www.who.int/csr/don/2009_02_02/en/index.html. Accessed May 12, 2009.

9. Ikegami N, Campbell JC. Japan's Health Care System: Containing Costs and Attempting Reform. *Health Affairs*. 2004;23(3):26–36.

10. Reid TR. Japanese pay less for more health care [transcript]. *All Things Considered*. National Public Radio. April 14, 2008. http://www.npr.org/templates/story/story.php?storyId=89626309. Accessed April 13, 2009.

11. World Health Organization. Immunization surveillance, assessment, and monitoring. http://www.who.int/vaccines/globalsummary/immunization/countryprofileresult.cfm?C=%27mng%27. Accessed May 12, 2009.

12. World Health Organization. Global TB database. http://www.who.int/tb/country/global_tb_database/en/index2.html. Accessed May 12, 2009.

13. Schull WJ. The somatic effects of exposure to atomic radiation: The Japanese experience, 1947–1997. *Proc Natl Acad Sci USA*. 1998;95(10):5437–5441.

14. Audet B. Traditional medicine finds a place in technology-oriented Japan. *CMAJ*. 1994;150(9):1473–1474.

15. Manaseki S. Mongolia: a health system in transition. *BMJ*. 1993;25(307)(6919):1609–1611.

16. World Health Organization. Country Profile: Democratic People's Republic of Korea. 2007. http://www.dprk.searo.who.int/EN/Section11.htm. Accessed May 13, 2009.

17. New theory on N Korea rail blast. *BBC News*. April 2004. http://news.bbc.co.uk/2/hi/asia-pacific/3651705.stm. Accessed May 13, 2009.

18. Central Intelligence Agency. World Fact Book: South Korea. 2009. https://www.cia.gov/library/publications/the-world-factbook/geos/ks.html. Accessed May 12, 2009.

19. Mathews B, Jung YS. The Future of Health Care in South Korea and the UK. *Social Policy and Society*. 2006;5(3):375–385.

20. Lee JC. Health Care Reform in South Korea: Success or Failure? *Am J Public Health*. 2003;93(1):48–51.

21. Central Intelligence Agency. World Fact Book: Taiwan. 2009. https://www.cia.gov/library/publications/the-world-factbook/geos/tw.html. Accessed May 12, 2009.

22. Wen CP, et al. A 10-Year Experience with Universal Health Insurance in Taiwan: Measuring Changes in Health and Health Disparity. *Ann Int Med*. 2008;148(4):258–267.

23. Chien YC, et al. Nationwide hepatitis B vaccination program in Taiwan: effectiveness in the 20 years after it was launched. *Epidemiol Rev*. 2006;28:126–135.

24. Centers for Disease Control, R.O.C. HIV/AIDS data. http://www.cdc.gov.tw/content.asp?mp=5&Cultem=6563. Accessed May 12, 2009.

25. Chiu YT. Cancer still top killer. *Taipei Times*. June 15, 2004. http://www.taipeitimes.com/News/taiwan/archives/2004/06/15/2003175103. Accessed May 12, 2009.

APPENDIX 1 ■ WHO DISEASE STAGING SYSTEM FOR ADULTS AND ADOLESCENTS

CLINICAL STAGE 1
- Asymptomatic
- Persistent generalized lymphadenopathy

CLINICAL STAGE 2
- Moderate and unexplained weight loss (< 10% of presumed or measured body weight)
- Recurrent respiratory tract infections (such as sinusitis, bronchitis, otitis media, or pharyngitis)
- Herpes zoster
- Recurrent oral ulcerations
- Papular pruritic eruptions
- Angular cheilitis
- Seborrhoeic dermatitis
- Fungal fingernail infections

CLINICAL STAGE 3
Conditions where a presumptive diagnosis can be made on the basis of clinical signs or simple investigations:
- Unexplained chronic diarrhea for longer than one month
- Unexplained persistent fever (intermittent or constant for longer than one month)
- Severe weight loss (> 10% of presumed or measured body weight)
- Oral candidiasis
- Oral hairy leukoplakia
- Pulmonary tuberculosis (TB) diagnosed in last two years
- Severe presumed bacterial infections (e.g., pneumonia, empyema, meningitis, bacteraemia, pyomyositis, bone or joint infection)
- Acute necrotizing ulcerative stomatitis, gingivitis, or periodontitis
Conditions where confirmatory diagnostic testing is necessary:
- Unexplained anaemia (< 80 g/l), and/or neutropenia (< 500 μl), and/or thrombocytopenia (< 50 000 μl) for more than one month

CLINICAL STAGE 4
Conditions where a presumptive diagnosis can be made on the basis of clinical signs or simple investigations:
- HIV wasting syndrome
- Pneumocystis pneumonia
- Recurrent severe or radiological bacterial pneumonia

- Chronic herpes simplex infection (orolabial, genital, or anorectal of more than one month's duration)
- Oesophageal candidiasis
- Extrapulmonary tuberculosis
- Kaposi's sarcoma
- Central nervous system toxoplasmosis
- HIV encephalopathy

Conditions where confirmatory diagnostic testing is necessary:

- Extrapulmonary cryptococcosis including meningitis
- Disseminated nontuberculous mycobacteria infection
- Progressive multifocal leukoencephalopathy
- Candida of trachea, bronchi, or lungs
- Cryptosporidiosis
- Isopsoriasis
- Visceral herpes simplex infection
- Cytomegalovirus (CMV) infection (retinitis of an organ other than liver, spleen, or lymph nodes)
- Any disseminated mycosis (e.g., histoplasmosis, coccidiomycosis, penicilliosis)
- Recurrent nontyphoidal salmonella septicemia
- Lymphoma (cerebral or B cell non-Hodgkins)
- Invasive cervical carcinoma
- Visceral leishmaniasis

WHO DISEASE STAGING SYSTEM FOR CHILDREN

CLINICAL STAGE 1

- Asymptomatic
- Persistent generalized lymphadenopathy

CLINICAL STAGE 2

- Hepatosplenomegaly
- Papular pruritic eruptions
- Seborrhoeic dermatitis
- Extensive human papilloma virus infection
- Extensive molluscum contagiosum
- Fungal nail infections
- Recurrent oral ulcerations
- Lineal gingival erythema (LGE)
- Angular cheilitis
- Parotid enlargement
- Herpes zoster
- Recurrent or chronic RTIs (otitis media, otorrhoea, or sinusitis)

CLINICAL STAGE 3

Conditions where a presumptive diagnosis can be made on the basis of clinical signs or simple investigations:

- Moderate unexplained malnutrition not adequately responding to standard therapy
- Unexplained persistent diarrhea (14 days or more)
- Unexplained persistent fever (intermittent or constant, for longer than one month)
- Oral candidiasis (outside neonatal period)
- Oral hairy leukoplakia
- Acute necrotizing ulcerative gingivitis/periodontitis
- Pulmonary TB
- Severe recurrent presumed bacterial pneumonia

Conditions where confirmatory diagnostic testing is necessary:

- Chronic HIV-associated lung disease including brochiectasis
- Lymphoid interstitial pneumonitis (LIP)
- Unexplained anaemia (< 80 g/l), and/or neutropenia (< 1000 µl), and/or thrombocytopenia (< 50 000 µl) for more than one month

CLINICAL STAGE 4

Conditions where a presumptive diagnosis can be made on the basis of clinical signs or simple investigations:

- Unexplained severe wasting or severe malnutrition not adequately responding to standard therapy
- Pneumocystis pneumonia
- Recurrent severe presumed bacterial infections (e.g., empyema, pyomyositis, bone or joint infection, meningitis, but excluding pneumonia)
- Chronic herpes simplex infection (orolabial or cutaneous of more than one month's duration)
- Extrapulmonary tuberculosis
- Kaposi's sarcoma
- Oesophageal candidiasis
- Central nervous system toxoplasmosis (outside the neonatal period)
- HIV encephalopathy

Conditions where confirmatory diagnostic testing is necessary:

- CMV infection (CMV retinitis or infection of organs other than liver, spleen, or lymph nodes; onset at age one month or more)
- Extrapulmonary cryptococcosis including meningitis
- Any disseminated endemic mycosis (e.g., extrapulmonary histoplasmosis, coccidiomycosis, penicilliosis)
- Cryptosporidiosis
- Isosporiasis
- Disseminated nontuberculous mycobacteria infection
- Candida of trachea, bronchi, or lungs

- Visceral herpes simplex infection
- Acquired HIV-associated rectal fistula
- Cerebral or B cell non-Hodgkins lymphoma
- Progressive multifocal leukoencephalopathy (PML)
- HIV-associated cardiomyopathy or HIV-associated nephropathy

APPENDIX 2 ■ ANTIRETROVIRAL AGENTS USED FOR HIV INFECTION

(FROM SAX, ESSENTIALS OF HIV, TABLE 3.1)*

Drug (abbreviation; trade name, manufacturer)	Formulations	Usual Adult Dosing⁴
NUCLEOSIDE (AND NUCLEOTIDE) REVERSE TRANSCRIPTASE INHIBITORS (NRTIs)		
Abacavir sulfate (ABC; Ziagen, GlaxoSmithKline)	300-mg tablets; 20-mg/mL oral solution	300-mg BID or 600-mg QD
Abacavir sulfate/lamivudine (Epzicom, GlaxoSmithKline)	600/300-mg tablet	One 600/300-mg tablet QD
Abacavir sulfate/ lamivudine/ zidovudine (Trizivir, GlaxoSmithKline)	300/150/300-mg tablet	One 300/150/300-mg tablet BID
Didanosine (ddI; Videx/ Videx EC, Bristol-Myers Squibb; Oncology/ Immunology; also available generically)	125-, 200-, 250-, 400-mg delayed-release enteric-coated capsules; 100-, 167-, 250-mg powder	Capsule: < 60 kg: 250-mg QD ≥ 60 kg: 400-mg QD 250-mg QD with tenofovir (best avoided) Powder: < 60 kg: 167-mg BID ≥ 60 kg: 250-mg BID probably Administration: Take on empty stomach at least 30 minutes before or 2 hours after meal
Emtricitabine (FTC; Emtriva, Gilead Sciences)	200-mg capsule	200-mg QD
Lamivudine (3TC; Epivir, GlaxoSmithKline)	150-, 300-mg tablets; 10-mg/mL oral solution	150-mg BID or 300-mg QD

Continues

*Sax, P. HIV Essentials. Sudbury, MA:Jones and Bartlett Publishers; 2009:17–21.

NUCLEOSIDE (AND NUCLEOTIDE) REVERSE TRANSCRIPTASE INHIBITORS (NRTIs) Continued		
Drug (abbreviation; trade name, manufacturer)	**Formulations**	**Usual Adult Dosing§**
Lamivudine/ zidovudine (Combivir, GlaxoSmithKline)	150/300-mg tablet	One 150/300-mg tablet BID
Stavudine (d4T; Zerit, Bristol-Myers Squibb Virology)	15-, 20-, 30-, 40-mg capsules; 1-mg/mL oral solution	< 60 kg: 30-mg BID ≥ 60 kg: 40-mg BID
Tenofovir disoproxil fumarate (TDF; Viread, Gilead Sciences)	300-mg tablet	One 300-mg tablet QD
Tenofovir disoproxil fumarate/emtricitabine (Truvada, Gilead Sciences)	300/200-mg tablet	One 300/200-mg tablet QD
Zidovudine (ZDV; Retrovir, GlaxoSmithKline; also available generically)	100-mg capsule; 300-mg tablet; 10-mg/5 mL oral solution; 10-mg/mL IV solution	200-mg TID or 300-mg BID (or with 3TC as Combivir or with abacavir and 3TC as Trizivir) 5–6 mg/kg daily
NON-NUCLEOSIDE REVERSE TRANSCRIPTASE INHIBITORS (NNRTIs)*		
Delavirdine mesylate (DLV; Rescriptor, Agouron)‡	100-, 200-mg tablets	400-mg TID (100-mg tablets can be dispersed in water; 200-mg tablet should be taken intact). Separate dosing from ddI or antacids by 1 hour, with or without food

Continues

NON-NUCLEOSIDE REVERSE TRANSCRIPTASE INHIBITORS (NNRTIs)* Continued		
Drug (abbreviation; trade name, manufacturer)	Formulations	Usual Adult Dosing§
Efavirenz (EFV; Sustiva, Bristol-Myers Squibb Oncology/Immunology; outside USA known as Stocrin)‡	50-, 100-, 200-mg capsules; 600-mg tablet	600-mg QD; best taken prior to bed to reduce incidence of CNS side effects
Etravirine (ETR; Intelence, Tibotec Therapeutics)	100-mg tablets	Two 100-mg tablets after a meal
Nevirapine (NVP; Viramune, Boehringer Ingelheim)‡	200-mg tablet; 50-mg/5 mL oral suspension (pediatric)	200-mg QD × 2 weeks, then 200-mg BID
COMBINATION NRTI/NNRTI		
Efavirenz/emtricitabine/ tenofovir (Atripla, Bristol-Myers Squibb & Gilead)	600/200/300-mg tablet	One 600/200/300-mg tablet daily
PROTEASE INHIBITORS (PIs)†		
Atazanavir sulfate (ATV; Reyataz, Bristol-Myers Squibb Virology)‡	100-, 150-, 200-, 300-mg capsules	400-mg QD, or 300-mg QD in combination with ritonavir 100-mg QD. For treatment-experienced patients, or when used with tenofovir or efavirenz or nevirapine use: 300-mg in combination with 100-mg of ritonavir. Take with food
Darunavir (DRV; Prezista, Tibotec Therapeutics)	400-, 600-mg tablets	600-mg BID with ritonavir 100-mg BID (treatment experienced); 800-mg QD with ritonavir 100-mg QD (treatment naïve)

Continues

PROTEASE INHIBITORS (PIs)[†] Continued		
Drug (abbreviation; trade name, manufacturer)	Formulations	Usual Adult Dosing[§]
Fosamprenavir (FPV; Lexiva, GlaxoSmithKline)[‡]	700-mg tablet	PI-naïve patients: 1400-mg BID, or 700-mg BID in combination with ritonavir 100-mg BID, or 1400-mg QD in combination with ritonavir 200-mg QD or 100-mg QD PI-experienced patients: 700-mg BID in combination with ritonavir 100-mg BID
Indinavir sulfate (IDV; Crixivan, Merck)[‡]	200-, 333-, 400-mg capsules	800-mg TID, or 800-mg BID in combination with ritonavir 100-mg or 200-mg BID Administration: Unboosted: Take 1 hour before or 2 hours after meals; may take with skim milk/low-fat meal. Boosted: Take with or without food. Separate dosing from ddI by 1 hour
Lopinavir/ritonavir (LPV/r; Kaletra, Abbott)[‡]	200/50-mg tablet; 80/20-mg/mL oral solution	Two tablets (400/100-mg) BID; 5 mL oral solution BID. Four tablets (800/200-mg) QD an option for treatment-naïve patients. With EFV or NVP: 3 tablets (600/150-mg) BID or 6.7 mL BID
Nelfinavir mesylate (NFV; Viracept, Agouron/ Pfizer)	250-, 625-mg tablets; 50-mg/ gm oral powder	750-mg TID or 1250-mg BID. Take with food

Continues

PROTEASE INHIBITORS (PIs)[†] Continued		
Drug (abbreviation; trade name, manufacturer)	Formulations	Usual Adult Dosing[§]
Ritonavir (RTV; Norvir, Abbott)[‡]	100-mg capsule; 600-mg/7.5 mL solution; 80-mg/mL oral solution	600-mg BID as sole PI; 100–400-mg daily in 1–2 divided doses as pharmacokinetic booster for other PIs Administration: Take with food or up to 2 hours after a meal to improve tolerability
Saquinavir (SQV; Invirase, Roche)[‡]	200-, 500-mg hard-gel capsules	1000-mg BID in combination with ritonavir 100-mg BID. Take with food
Tipranavir (TPV; Aptivus, Boehringer Ingelheim)[‡]	250-mg soft-gel capsule	500-mg BID in combination with ritonavir 200-mg BID. Take with food
FUSION INHIBITOR		
Enfuvirtide (T-20; Fuzeon, Roche)[‡]	Injectable (lyophilized powder). Each single-use vial contains 108-mg of enfuvirtide to be reconstituted with 1.1 mL of sterile water for injection for delivery of approximately 90-mg/mL	90-mg BID IV. Administered subcutaneously into upper arm, anterior thigh, or abdomen
CCR5 ANTAGONIST		
Maraviroc (MVC; Selzentry, Pfizer)	150-, 300-mg tablets	150-mg, 300-mg or 600 BID depending on concomitant drugs (see p. 224 for details); may be taken with or without food

Continues

INTEGRASE INHIBITOR		
Drug (abbreviation; trade name, manufacturer)	Formulations	Usual Adult Dosing
Raltegravir (RAL; Isentress, Merck)	400-mg tablet	One 400-mg tablet BID with or without food

*Nevirapine and efavirenz are cytochrome p450 CYP3A4 inducers; delavirdine is an inhibitor; etravirine has mixed effects. Consult package insert for full drug interaction profile.

†All protease inhibitors are hepatically metabolized by the cytochrome p450 system; they also are specific inhibitors of CYP3A4 and have induction effects on other enzymes. Consult package insert for full drug-drug interaction profile.

‡Consult package insert for full drug interaction profile.

APPENDIX 3 ■ GLOBAL HEALTH MEDICAL BAG

Consult the following list in creating your personal medical kit. What you will need in the field will depend on where you are going, what your role will be, and what access you will have to pharmacies, stores, etc.

1. Tarascon Global Health Pocketbook
2. Stethoscope
3. Otoscope and ophthalmoscope (with extra batteries)
4. Trauma shears
5. Power converter (if needed)
6. Flashlight (with extra batteries)
7. Map
8. Forceps
9. Suture set and suture materials
10. Steri-strips
11. Skin adhesive glue
12. Syringes/needles
13. Antiseptic (chlorhexidine and/or betadine)
14. Gloves
15. CPR mouth barrier
16. Gauze bandages
17. Tape
18. Dental kit
    a. Dental mirror
    b. Calcium hydroxide paste
19. Eye kit
    a. Morgan lens
    b. Fluorescein strips
    c. Eye shield
20. Paper and pen
21. Water purification tablets
22. Thermometer
23. Silver nitrate sticks
24. Blood pressure cuff
25. Scalpel handle and multiple blades
26. Suggested medicines:
    a. Aspirin
    b. Diphenydramine
    c. Prednisone
    d. Acetaminaphen
    e. Ciprofloxacin and a selection of other ABX
    f. NSAID of choice

g. Famotidine tablets
h. Hydrocortisone cream
i. Anti-fungal cream
j. Erythromycin ophthalmic ointment
k. Loperamide
l. Epi-pen
m. 2% Lidocaine
n. Beta-agonist inhaler (e.g., albuterol)
o. Oral rehydration salts
p. Topical antibiotic ointment

APPENDIX 4 ■ EVALUATION OF MALNUTRITION WITH WEIGHT FOR HEIGHT CHARTS

Weight-for-height BOYS
2 to 5 years (percentiles)

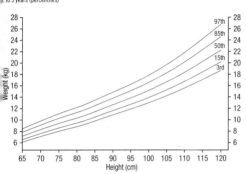

Weight-for-height GIRLS
2 to 5 years (percentiles)

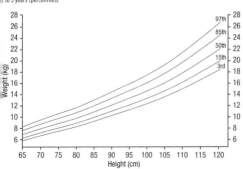

INDEX

Note: Page numbers followed by "*f*" and "*t*" denote figures and tables, respectively.